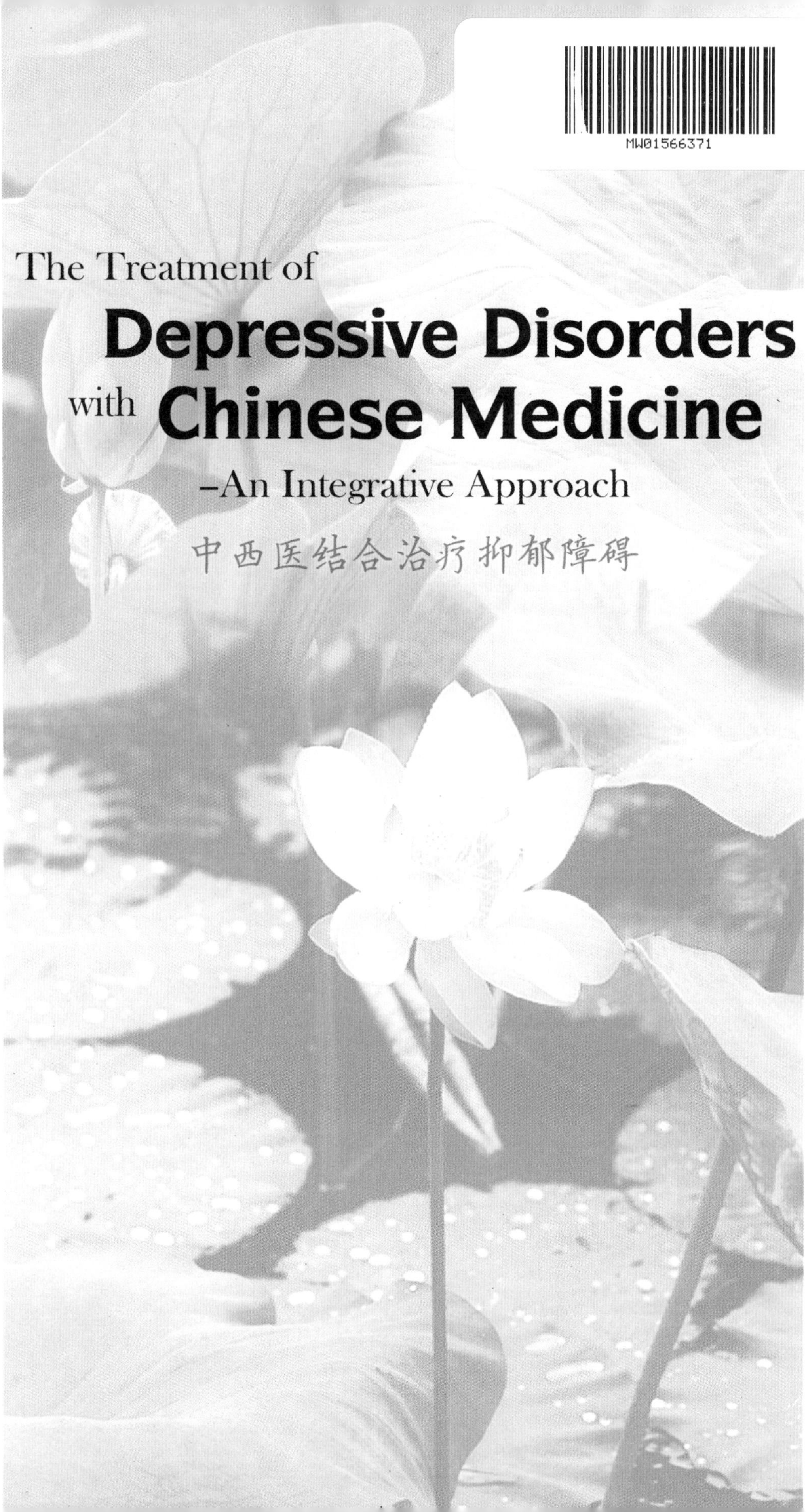

The Treatment of Depressive Disorders with Chinese Medicine
–An Integrative Approach

中西医结合治疗抑郁障碍

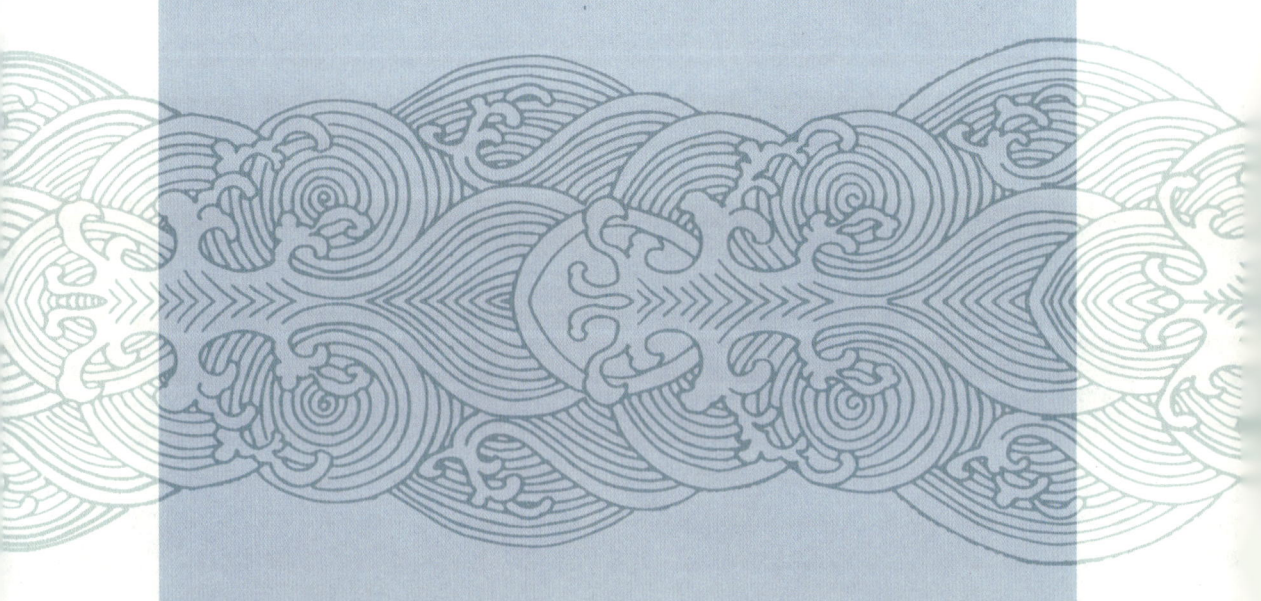

Project Editor: Zeng Chun, Harry F. Lardner & Liu Shui
Copy Editor: Chen Xiao-lei
Book Designer: Dai Shan-shan
Cover Designer: Dai Shan-shan
Typesetter: He Mei-Ling

The Treatment of
Depressive Disorders
with Chinese Medicine
–An Integrative Approach

中西医结合治疗抑郁障碍

Wang Yan-heng

Chief Physican, TCM Psychiatric Department
Beijing An Ding Hospital, Capital Medical University

Kang Yu-chun, M.S. TCM

Attending Physican, TCM Psychiatric Department
The Third Hospital of Chaoyang District, Beijing

Translated by

Li Wan-ling & Zheng Qi

Edited by

Pär Rufus Scott, MOAM Lic Ac.
Douglas Eisenstark, L.Ac.

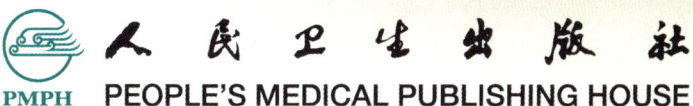

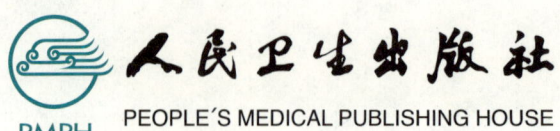

PEOPLE'S MEDICAL PUBLISHING HOUSE

BEIJING · LONDON · NEW YORK

Website: http://www.pmph.com/en

Book Title: The Treatment of Depressive Disorders with Chinese Medicine
　　　　　　—An Integrative Approach
　　　　　　中西医结合治疗抑郁障碍

Copyright © 2010 by People's Medical Publishing House. All rights reserved. No part of this publication may be reproduced, stored in a database or retrieval system, or transmitted in any form or by any electronic, mechanical, photocopy, or other recording means, without the prior written permission of the publisher.

Contact address: No. 19, Pan Jia Yuan Nan Li, Chaoyang District, Beijing 100021, P.R. China, phone/fax: 8610 5978 7338, E-mail: pmph@pmph.com

For text and trade sales, as well as review copy enquiries, please contact PMPH at pmphsales@gmail.com

---

Disclaimer

This book is for educational and reference purposes only. In view of the possibility of human error or changes in medical science, the author, editor, publisher and any other party involved in the publication of this work do not guarantee that the information contained herein is in any respect accurate or complete. The medicinal therapies and treatment techniques presented in this book are provided for the purpose of reference only. If readers wish to attempt any of the techniques or utilize any of the medicinal therapies contained in this book, the publisher assumes no responsibility for any such actions. It is the responsibility of the readers to understand and adhere to local laws and regulations concerning the practice of these techniques and methods. The authors, editors and publishers disclaim all responsibility for any liability, loss, injury, or damage incurred as a consequence, directly or indirectly, of the use and application of any of the contents of this book.

First published: 2010

ISBN: 978-7-117-12729-5/R-12730

Cataloguing in Publication Data:
A catalogue record for this book is available from the CIP-Database China.

ISBN 978-7-117-12729-5

9 787117 127295

Printed in The People's Republic of China

About the Author

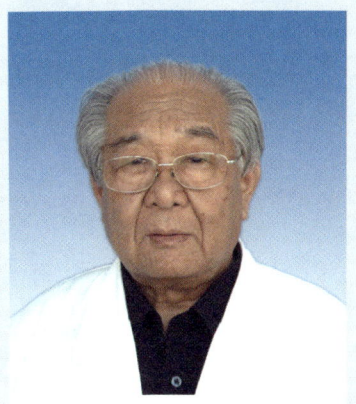

王彦恒

Dr. Wang Yan-heng serves as Chief Physician at Beijing An Ding Hospital in the TCM Psychiatric Department. He began his apprenticeship with Chen Shen-wu in 1956, a renowned physician of the Shanghan School, later graduating in 1961 from Beijing Chinese Medical College. Having remained in clinical practice for nearly 50 years, Dr. Wang is also one of China's leading professors of Chinese medical psychiatry.

Preface

In recent years, the understanding and treatment of depressive disorders in Western medicine has certainly achieved remarkable development. However, a number of key questions and difficulties still remain regarding effective treatment, preventing recurrence, and adverse drug reactions. In fact, the results of standard treatment approaches in many cases are neither satisfactory nor permanent.

In Chinese medicine, the first objective is to assess the underlying patterns of disharmony as related to the etiology, and to follow with modalities of treatment that address both root and branch manifestations. Such methods can benefit both the physical body and the spirit. Due to an accumulation of clinical experiences that span hundreds of years, the flexible and individualized treatment strategies of Chinese medicine can sometimes deliver outstanding results. Of course, there are always cases where the main symptom of mental depression cannot be significantly improved. Clinically speaking, the therapeutic effects are usually less gratifying when Western or Chinese modalities are used alone; treatment with integrative medicine is undoubtedly the best approach.

This book summarizes many years of collected clinical experience and theoretical development, over which time it has become clear that the cause of depression is much more complex than simple liver qi stagnation; depressive disorder is a complex systemic condition. Therefore, only soothing the liver and rectifying qi is not very effective in most cases, nor is the typical application of the representative formula *Chái Hú Tāng* (Bupleurum Decoction). Better results can be obtained by applying individualized pattern differentiation while observing the traditional guideline, "the brain governs spirit-brightness".

However, for best results, integrative medical treatment and psychotherapy are also required. In this book, other alternative treatment methods such as warming yang and opening constraint are provided; we also introduce here our empirical experiences with paired medicinals and also our methods for administering relatively large dosages of raw gypsum.

This book is based on "Treatise on Treatment of Depressive Disorder with Integrative Medicine", published in 2006 by People's Medical Publishing House. Both books have received great support from Liang Yining, Dean of Medicine of Chaoyang Third Hospital in Beijing, along with many others. We are always open to comments from our colleagues.

Wang Yan-heng

June 26, 2010

Editors' Preface

It was my great pleasure to work on the English edition of Dr. Wang's PMPH book on depressive disorders. We are privileged to have such a comprehensive work on a common ailment that afflicts so many around the world, seemingly in many if not most cultures and, if we are to believe art and literature, through the ages as well. Depression and related depressive disorders are forms of mental disease, sometimes minor and fleeting and yet sometimes lifelong and devastating. Its influence is so widespread; one could say that both depression and elation are two opposite yet inevitable components of the human condition.

Depressive disorders are the beginning of a deep well of conflicting questions in the West. We may or may not measure success in treating depression by how well the person is brought back into the workplace and into family life. When an individual measures their own worth by this standard, then social life can reinforce it. However, when the society changes that reinforcement system, then the individual becomes even more "individual" and isolated.

In the West, depression is viewed as a "victimless crime", or one where the criminal and victim are one. The Western perspective may be that the individuals are many elements of an amorphous and changing society. Yet, society remains a background to one's happiness. The Westerner may object to the loss of "self" in the politics of the community, while the Asian model often intertwines the community within the conception of the individual. In the West, depression is often described as "anger turned inward." So we may ask, "To whom is this anger really directed?" Ideas abound.

These concepts in TCM seemed rather abstract until I read the chapter that Par had edited and contributed to. In *Yu*: Constraint and Depression, this is made explicit in the very word that dominates and titles the book. *Yu* is alternatively translated as both constraint and depression only because the English mind and language does not allow for one word to encompass both ideas. How to read *yu* informs this major and contentious translation issue. Yanhua Zhang, in Transforming Emotions with Chinese Medicine: An Ethnographic Account from Contemporary China (Albany, 2007), talks about the way that the Chinese view themselves in the very language of the concept of the self. She writes that the word *shenti*, what we in English most often translate as "body", actually encompasses both body and self. The person is at all times both mind and self, or an integrated body/self/mind.

More than one in our profession has complained erroneously that modern TCM (especially in the PRC) has taken the spirituality out of Chinese Medicine. Western students and practitioners may find much of modern Chinese medical theory on depression decidedly "materialistic", if not simply conservative. However, Yanhua Zhang's research replies that the "spirit" in TCM has never left the body. Bob Flaws also states that the emotional component of CM is located nowhere else but within the qi itself. We here in the West may be obsessed with finding the spiritual aspects of CM only because we ourselves have split this off within our own minds. In distress, from this viewpoint, one is always *yu*: constrained and depressed. This perspective of *yu* and *shenti* is not as one of my students said, "The self is that which is behind the eyes, the body is everything attached to the nose".

Like a depressed patient, estranged from society, in the West, acupuncture and Chinese Medicine patients are most often on the fringes of standard medical care. What impresses me about this book is both the comprehensive scope of what Dr. Wang has written, as well the responsibility that he has imparted to all those who treat patients with depression. No matter how serious the case in my own clinic in Los Angeles, I know that there is always the possibility of referral to a Western physician. Should treatment be unsuccessful, there is the mainstream to supply medications (even if I may not agree with it). Then there are those patients for whom Western medications "don't work". I have a feeling that when I face patients with emotional issues to whom I am the "last resort," this book will be of special value.

I'd like to acknowledge Harry F. Lardner and all those at PMPH Beijing for going the extra mile on this book, Par Scott and both Dr. (Phoenix) Li in Beijing and Lionel Lee (Ph.D in Psychology) in Los Angeles for indulging many lengthy conversations and generous explanations beyond the call of duty.

Douglas Eisenstark, L.Ac.

June 2010

This text represents a fusion of Western medical and traditional Chinese medicinal treatment for depressive disorders. While the format is fairly standard in that it presents a review of pertinent Chinese medical concepts and a series of disease categories and treatments, the author also displays a comprehensive understanding of the topic that is both impressive and helpful. He explores many issues in some depth, and has coined a number of novel ideas that are worth exploring here before reading the main text.

1. The author uses the term brain-spirit (*nao-shen*, 脑神) to indicate an aspect of the spirit function. He associates the curious organ of the brain with the thought function typically ascribed to the heart in classical sources for Chinese medicine. Other classical authors like Li Shi-zhen have attributed the brain with more consciousness-related functions, and this author's displacement of the spirit (which is not complete, as the author often refers to the heart-spirit as well) is following a Western theoretical model for the locus of thought being in the brain. Since he maintains the nature of the brain as the "sea of marrow" as well, in many cases the focus of the treatment of the "brain-spirit" shifts to a deeper strategy of nourishing the essence and maintaining physical brain with medicinals that have a focus in the head. This aspect of Chinese medicine is sometimes overlooked in the management of psychiatric conditions using more typical TCM approaches unless the symptoms are mental deficits clearly related to aging or prenatal conditions associated with essence deficiency. This approach is also relevant in the context of strong psychiatric pharmaceuticals which can damage kidney essence in relatively short periods of time. Regardless of one's final stance on the relevance of the brain-spirit as a concept, the relative depth of his analysis of pattern diagnosis makes this text valuable to anyone seeking a better understanding of the possible mechanisms for mental disorders in patients, beyond the typical knee-jerk diagnosis of a liver pattern or even non-interaction of heart and kidney.

2. The author has created and utilizes many variations of a formula to treat what I would loosely call "brain-spirit stagnation" or "brain-spirit dysregulation". Since most of the other substances of the body

are prone to stagnation, it seems reasonable that even the rarified spirit-material could also become stagnant and thus require treatment to restore proper function. The author attributes the persistent quality of emotional disorders to this tendency for the spirit's environment to become uninhabitable through accumulation and stagnation, whether due to excess or deficiency conditions. This model is linked to the author's discussion of various historical models for "depression" as a disorder and an illness.

The author's modular formula *Jú Shēn Tāng* (Chrysanthemum and Salvia Decoction, 菊参汤) is composed of *jú huā* (Flos Chrysanthemi) 15 - 20g, *chuān xiōng* (Rhizoma Chuanxiong) 10g, and *dān shēn* (Radix et Rhizoma Salviae Miltiorrhizae) 30g. It is added to address concurrent spirit issues in other pathologies or as a modified base formula when the depression is the primary issue.

Jú huā (Flos Chrysanthemi) functions to lightly open, and its light nature, like many flowers, naturally going to the aid of the spirit while also expelling wind and heat evils, moistening, and moderately nourishing metal and water. The effect of this can resolve stagnation related to excess and deficiency heat in the head to allow for clear expression of the spirit.

Chuān xiōng (Rhizoma Chuanxiong) is an herb that functions within the blood, but is primarily related to wind and qi, much like the spirit. When evils and stagnation block the expression of yang, it can facilitate movement and enliven the blood. As with *jú huā* (Flos Chrysanthemi), its functions are also focused in the head.

Dān shēn (Radix et Rhizoma Salviae Miltiorrhizae) has a multitude of functions all focused on the blood, particularly heart blood, which is the traditional "residence" of the heart-spirit. It nourishes and enlivens blood to rehabilitate the "residence" of the spirit.

Since *jú huā* (Flos Chrysanthemi) and *chuān xiōng* (Rhizoma Chuanxiong) are also traditionally associated with pathologies of the head, the correspondence of the formula with the treatment of the relocated "brain spirit" becomes clearer. By clearing and nourishing the upper residence of the spirit, the effect of more substantial treatments involving the physical aspects of depressive patterns can thus be enhanced while the psycho-emotional elements of the pattern can be eliminated, also allowing for a more enduring effect. Whereas more standard treatment of spirit disorders related to depression focus on supporting the free flow of liver qi, this treatment strategy is at once lighter and more profound. Ultimately the nature of spirit in TCM is incorruptible, being the internal emptiness and calm that allows us a space to accommodate ideas and accurately perceive; this method opens and frees the spirit-residence and opens and frees the sensory orifices allowing for clear perception of the world, thus assisting in dispelling the lingering tendency of emotional problems.

3. The author proposes that Western psychiatric medications can have powerful actions that will facilitate and speed up the treatment of psychiatric disorders when combined with TCM medicinal therapies. In the West, however, the acupuncture community tends to generally avoid and even disparage psychiatric medicines. Here we see an integrated collaborative medical model that utilizes the rapid and vigorous actions of pharmacological medicines to stabilize and benefit the patient, while concurrently applying Chinese medicinals to treat the root and reduce side effects. While coordinating such a treatment plan may prove more challenging because we are not as yet well-integrated into the Western medical establishment, the author's model represents an optimistic and pragmatic utilization of powerful psychiatric medications in conjunction with herbal therapies. As we in the West become more integrated into the medical community, it is important that we learn to respect the power and actual limitations of the drugs our patients are taking. In the same vein, the author includes a very helpful analysis of the common side effects of psychiatric medications, including effective treatments for drug-related sexual disorders, weight gain, and more challenging issues like tardive dyskinesia.

While the text recapitulates much information about basic TCM theory, it also parses the origins and development of "depression" patterns in TCM from the *Nei Jing* period through the Qing Dynasty, which, while not surprising, is not a treatment approach that we often see in English language works on Chinese medicine. The "standard" treatment patterns are covered here, but they looked at from a relatively personal perspective. Spending time with this text has clarified and deepened my way of thinking about the nature of emotional disorders in TCM and their management, as I hope it will for you.

Pär Rufus Scott, MOAM Lic Ac.

June 2010

Contents

Chapter 1 Overview — 1
The Concept of Depressive Disorders 2

Chapter 2 The History of Depressive Disorder Theory in Chinese Medicine — 7

Chapter 3 Five Spirits and the Brain — 21
Heart – *Shen* 24
Lung – *Po* 30
Spleen – *Yi* 33
Liver – *Hun* 35
Kidney – *Zhi* 38
The Brain-Spirit 41

Chapter 4 Etiology and Pathomechanism — 47
Etiology 48
Pathomechanisms 52

Chapter 5 *Zang-fu* Patterns and Treatment — 57
Etiology 58
Pathomechanism 58
Clinical Guidelines 58
Pattern Differentiation and Treatment 60
Commentary 76

Chapter 6 Acupuncture and Moxibustion — 79
Main Objectives 80

XV

Pattern Differentiation and Symptomatic Treatment 90
Psychological Guidance.. 95
Compliance and Course of Treatment 96

Chapter 7 Associated Disease Categories — 97

Schizophrenia (Withdrawal) 98
Insomnia 105
Somnolence 116
Poor Memory 123
Sorrow 129
Fear 133
Bulimia 137
Geriatric Depressive Disorder 147
Pediatric Depressive Disorder 155

Chapter 8 Treating Side Effects — 161

Side-effects and Toxicity—the Chinese Medical Perspective 162
Drug-induced Digestive Dysfunction 165
Drug-induced Weight Gain 170
Drug-induced Chest Impediment 177
Drug-induced Urinary Block 184
Tardive Dyskinesia 188
Drug-induced Sexual Disorders 194
Drug-induced Amenorrhea 199

Chapter 9 Recovery and Recurrence — 205

Factors in the Recurrence of Depressive Disorders 206
Preventing Recurrence 207
Dietary Guidelines for Recovery and Rehabilitation 209

Chapter 10 Case Studies   213

1. Liver Constraint with Phlegm Binding 214
2. Spleen and Kidney Dual Deficiency 216
3. Depression due to Dual Depletion of Qi and Blood 218
4. Liver and Stomach Disharmony 221
5. Liver Constraint Transforming into Fire,
   Static Blood Obstruction 223
6. Liver Constraint and Blood Stasis 225
7. Qi Stagnation and Blood Stasis 228
8. Bulimic Depressive Disorder 232

Chapter 11 Applications of Chinese Medicine in Psychiatry   235

Qi 236
Blood 236
Blood Stasis 237
Phlegm 237
Fire 238
Applications and Modifications of *Jú Shēn Tāng*
(Chrysanthemum and Salvia Decoction) 239

Chapter 12 Depression Patterns in Selected Ancient Works   247

Appendix 1 Classifications of Depressive Disorder   275
Appendix 2 Recent Studies   287
Appendix 3 Classical Sources   296

References   **305**

Index by Disease Names and Symptoms 313
Index by Chinese Medicinals and Formulas 317
General Index 325

Chapter 1
Overview

The Concept of Depressive Disorders

In China before the 1980's, there was a relatively narrow concept for the diagnosis of mood disorders in the psychiatric field, and for this reason the diagnosis rate remained low. Later establishment of the ICD-9 and DSM-III modified the diagnostic criteria for mood disorders, thus creating a more complete understanding of these disorders within China. As a result, subsequent studies have reported an increasing prevalence of depressive disorders.

A global cooperative research study from the World Health Organization (WHO) showed that the prevalence of depression in the wards of general hospitals was 4%, and 0.6% for dysthymia. In a comprehensive analysis of 23 cross-sectional epidemiology surveys of elder depressive disorder patients in Taiwan, the prevalence rate for depression was 3.86%, and the risk rate of incidence in rural areas was 5.07%, higher than the 2.61% in cities, but still at a much lower rate than in Western countries (Chen, 1999).

There are a great number of both somatic and psychological symptoms associated with depressive disorders. Somatic symptoms include sleep disorders, appetite changes, fatigue, psychomotor retardation and agitation. According to the DSM-IV, psychological symptoms include low mood, loss of self-esteem or a feeling of self-reproach, difficulties with concentration and indecision, and suicidal thoughts or attempts. All of these symptoms are interrelated, also being based on a biological foundation.

Depressive disorder is a common mood disorder caused by a variety of factors, with the most common clinical manifestation being a significantly persistent depressed mood. Clinical manifestations may also include extreme grief, significant anxiety, and motor agitation, where severe cases can display other psychiatric symptoms such as hallucinations and paranoia. Most cases have a tendency for recurrent episodes, and while the episodic symptoms can often be relieved, some patients may also suffer residual or chronic symptoms.

Chapter 1
Overview

Depressive disorders include depression, dysthymia, psychogenic depression, concurrent depression from brain diseases, post-psychosis depression, somatization, and accompanying depression of a mental disorder caused by psychoactive or non-addictive substances.

Clinically, depression is viewed as a depressive episode of an affective (mood) disorder. At least 10% of these patients have manic episodes, and in these cases, the patient will likely be diagnosed with a bipolar disorder.

There are numerous varying reports on the epidemiology of depressive disorder because of the many different views regarding the concept and criteria of diagnosis. Also, because unipolar depression and bipolar disorders were frequently mixed together in early studies, the prevalence rates and incidences in these reports do vary widely.

In 1984, the National Institute of Health (NIH–USA) found that the lifetime prevalence rate of depression was 4.9%, and 3.3% for dysthymia (Regier, 1988). Another study in 1994 showed that the lifetime prevalence rate of depression was 17.1% (male 12.7%, female 21.3%) and 6% for dysthymia (Kessler, 1998). In 1993, the World Health Organization (WHO) performed a global cooperative study in 15 cities around the world. Their survey on the rates of psychological disorder of patients in general hospitals found that 12.5% suffered from depression and dysthymia. In a community survey of 38,000 independent communities from 10 countries and regions (including the United States, Canada, Lebanon, South Korea, and Taiwan) found a great difference among the lifetime prevalence rates in different countries, with only 1.5% in Taiwan, and up to 19.9% in Lebanon. The annual (non-lifetime) incidence rate was 0.8% in Taiwan, and 5.8% in New Jersey, USA (Myra, 1996).

The World Health Organization's definition of health is: "a state of complete physical, mental, and social well-being; not merely the absence of disease or infirmity". In other words, physical, mental, and social functioning should all be at optimum levels in order for an individual to be considered as healthy, and this is obviously the treatment goal for all depressive disorders. Furthermore, the current trend in medical science development shows a shifting away from a purely biomedical model to a broader biological-psychosocial model. There is no doubt that this emerging medical model will provide a superior theoretical basis for the treatment of depressive disorder.

In recent years, the term "depressive disorder" has been often used by the worldwide psychiatric community. According to the clinical manifestations, these disorders also fall under the category of "depression disease" in traditional Chinese medicine. However, Chinese medicine treatment is based on pattern differentiation with an emphasis on both body and mind, as well as both the manifestation and the root of the disease. For this reason, Chinese medicine also remains relatively flexible in its principles and methods of treatment.

Secondly, an integrated approach gives us more choices by providing new ways to enhance treatment effects while at the same time reducing the side effects of Western drugs. Treating depressive disorders with Western pharmaceutical drugs can have dramatic positive effects, but antipsychotic and antidepressant medicines also display a plethora of side effects; the adverse reactions often prove to be just as challenging as the original condition.

Drug-induced symptoms may include extrapyramidal reactions, urinary retention, dry mouth, constipation, seizures, paralysis agitans, cardiovascular responses, weight gain, sexual dysfunction, amenorrhea and drug-induced mania. Traditional Chinese medicine can be very advantageous in many cases. Chinese medicine also emphasizes the physician-patient relationship and the role of open communication, so in this way therapy and medication can be continually adjusted according to feedback from the patient, thus giving both the patient and the physician an improved sense of control.

Clinical practice also shows that an integrative treatment approach is more effective in many refractory cases. For example, we can look at the case of a severe geriatric depressive disorder patient who on the second day after taking an antidepressant displayed urinary retention and distention of the lower abdomen. The discomfort and pain caused urethral catheterization was unbearable for the patient, and he refused to continue taking the medication. However, all of these symptoms disappeared when a modification of *Zhū Líng Tāng* (Polyporus Decoction) was prescribed together with the antidepressant.

In another example, *Shēng Mài Yǐn* (Pulse-Engendering Beverage) is commonly used for those patients who show adverse cardiovascular reactions following medication. The common side effect of thirst and muscle stiffness can also be relieved effectively by employing this kind of integrative therapy. Furthermore, when patients take Western drugs and Chinese medicinals concurrently, in many cases the dosage of Western drugs can be reduced, but with equal efficacy.

Thirdly, the course of treatment is shorter and results are more rapid. Clinically, those taking Chinese and Western medicine therapies at the same time usually display significant improvement after one or two treatment courses. Therapy takes effect more quickly than when solely using Western drugs, and the effects last longer. This somewhat bold statement reflects the experience of the author as gained by 45 years in clinical practice.

Because of the characteristics of depressive disorders, patients may need to take medications for a long time, potentially for the rest of their lives. This can be a heavy burden for patients, both mentally and financially. However, integrative therapies can enhance efficacy, lessen dosages, shorten the course of disease, and prevent or reduce recurrence.

In the also author's experience that depressive disorder patients should not terminate or reduce medications hastily, they should follow the principle of "slow reduction" and "cautious termination" i.e., dosages of medication must be reduced slowly. For Western drugs, it usually takes 3 months to reduce the dosage by half, another 1 to 3 months to reach 1/3rd of the original, and another six months to a year to reduce to 1/4th of the original dosage. It must be emphasized that any sudden termination of medication is always inadvisable.

For Chinese medicinals, the same principle applies. After elimination of the basic symptoms, patients may take one portion each day for 2 days and then take a day off. Continue this for one course of treatment and then reduce the prescription to one portion every other day. If the condition is stable, medicinals can be reduced to one portion each week and then terminated gradually. If the symptoms return in the course of this reduction, the prescription can be adjusted with increased dosages to prevent relapse.

In modern Chinese medicine, a two-pronged approach is generally applied, but the theoretical basis is different for each system. Therefore, it should be understood that the integration of Chinese and Western medicines is not just simply the combining of Chinese medicinals with Western drugs.

One difference is that Western medicine emphasizes disease diagnosis, whereas Chinese medicine emphasizes syndrome differentiation. Western drugs are rapid in their effect, while Chinese medicinals act to address the root condition. Also, Western drugs target specific symptoms and biological mechanisms, whereas Chinese medicinals are patient-oriented with an emphasis on the overall improvement of both psychosomatic status and changing somatic symptoms. In fact, the strengths of such an integrative approach have already been proven successfully in clinical practice.

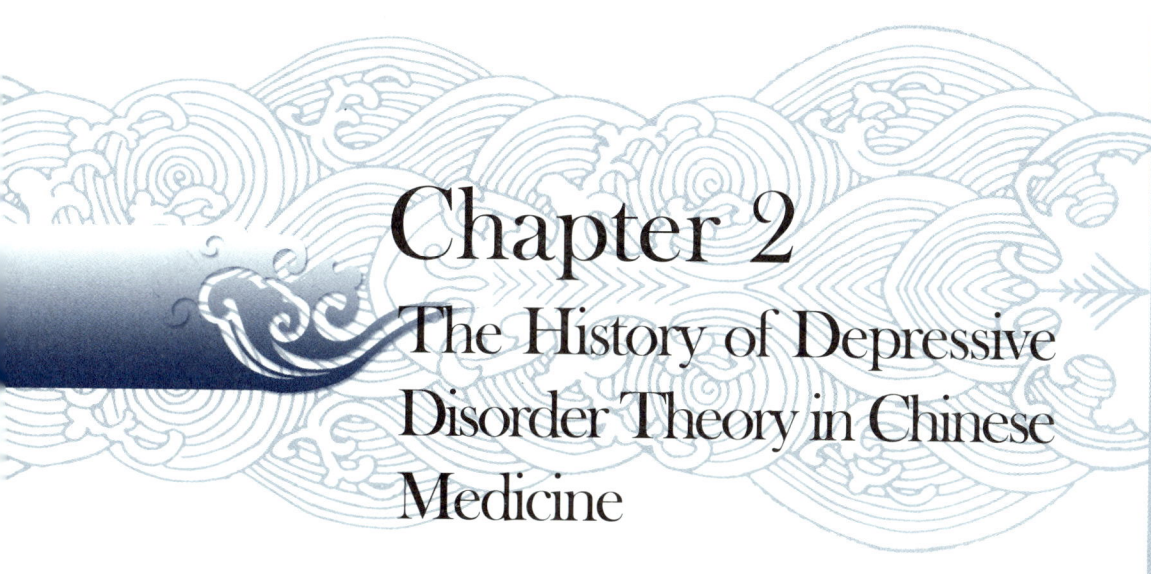

Chapter 2
The History of Depressive Disorder Theory in Chinese Medicine

In both contemporary and ancient times, the word "constraint" has always had multiple meanings. Traditionally, a constraint pattern would include constraint, blockage and stoppage manifesting with accumulations or binding; emotional depression is merely one aspect. In contemporary documents, "depression pattern", "depression disease" and "withdrawal disease" are used to cover what we call "emotional depression" and the depressive status that manifests in different diseases. In fact, depressive disorder may include not only depression, but also other emotional conditions such as a tendency to sorrow, anxiety and preoccupation, vexation and agitation, timidity and fear, or even fuller versions of withdrawal disease more typically associated with a Western diagnosis of schizophrenia. Therefore, to study constraint/depression in Chinese medicine, we have to examine the source and development of both the theories of constraint patterns and emotional diseases, which are related but not identical. In this chapter we will predominantly examine the development of the theory of the constraint pattern as it relates to movement of the qi dynamic.

The character for *yù*, (constraint/depression) is 郁, which itself is a relatively old shorthand version of the character 鬱. Colloquially this means "dense", "pent-up", "anxious" or "grieving", but it also conveys the sense of something "lush", "verdant" or "fragrant". The character for *yù* is composed largely phonetically. The older character contains two 木 (*mù*) wood radicals and 冖 (*mì*) 'cover' and a 缶 (*fǒu*) 'jar', which are, perhaps coincidentally, indicative of the general nature of the disorder, the pent-up energy of the wood phase. The meanings "fragrant" and "lush" come out of the idea of very dense vegetation which has a pungent odor prone to be rich and cloying. Like the nature of the color of the wood phase, 青 (*qīng*), which is described as blue-green-black, this character shows some of the shadow of the wood phase with its roots in the chaos and darkness of yin.

In Chinese medicine, "constraint" means the inability to extend, also referring to a stagnation and stoppage of qi and blood. The *Source of Hundreds of Diseases Names in TCM* (*Zhōng Yī Bǎi Bìng Míng Yuán Kǎo*) states, "Constraint refers to blockage and stoppage. There are five phases

Chapter 2
The History of Depressive Disorder Theory in Chinese Medicine

of the heavens, and seven emotions in mankind. When the five phases are constrained, then heaven and earth are blocked. The 'anger eruption' that results when qi is blocked can cause diseases as well as constraint of the seven emotions. The 'anxiety' of qi stagnation can also cause diseases. All these diseases originate in blockage and stoppage; therefore, the ancient people combined the two categories and named it 'constraint/depression'." As a disease name, constraint/depression can refer to a condition caused by retaliation of the five qi, as well as to a condition caused by internal damage from the seven emotions.

The Inner Classic (*Nèi Jīng*) did not list constraint as a disease category; however, the discussion on the five qi constraints is quite clear. *The Basic Questions – Great Treatise on the Regular Principles of the Six Origins* (*Sù Wèn – Liù Yuán Zhèng Jì Dà Lùn*) stated, "What is the treatment method for severe depression?" "Constrained wood is treated by out-thrusting, fire constraint is treated by effusion, constrained earth is treated by despoliation, constrained metal is treated by discharge, and constrained water is treated by regulation. This is to regulate the qi. For excess, regulate with the medicinal it fears. This is called drainage."

The five constraints reflect an excess of movement in the qi of heaven and earth, and can cause qi stagnation in human body, thus resulting in various diseases. For example, depressed wood is characterized by pain in the stomach duct and heart, distention and fullness of the rib-sides, dysphagia, and tinnitus, dizziness, an inability to recognize people, and frequent stroke; most of these symptoms are associated with the spleen and liver.

Depressed earth is characterized by distention and fullness in the area of the heart and abdomen, rumbling intestines, frequent diarrhea, and possibly heart pain, distention of the rib-sides, vomiting, downpour diarrhea, sudden turmoil (cholera), rheum and puffy swelling; most of these symptoms are associated with the spleen and stomach.

Metal constraint is characterized by coughing and counterflow, distention of the heart region and rib-sides that affects the lesser abdomen, and a dry throat; most of these symptoms are associated with the lung.

Water constraint is characterized by cold contracting, heart pain, lumbar pain, a lack of ease in bending and stretching due to inhibition of large joints; most symptoms are associated with the kidney.

Fire constraint is characterized by sores, swollen welling-abscesses, bone pain, warm malaria, frenetic movement of hot blood, red eyes and heart heat; most symptoms are associated with the heart.

In this chapter, the term "constraint/depression" is brought up many times in several contexts. For example, "its related disease is heat constraint", "qi constraint with middle burner fullness", and "depressed qi has to be regulated". In these cases, the constraint is related to binding and inhibition of the movement of qi.

The Inner Classic also contains quite a few statements regarding conditions that are associated with emotional states.

For example, *The Basic Questions – Treatise on Pain* (*Sù Wèn – Jǔ Tòng Lùn*) states, "When there is pensiveness, there will be reservation of the heart and returning of the spirit; the upright qi lodges without moving, therefore the qi binds."

The Spiritual Pivot The Spiritual Pivot – the Spirit (*Líng Shū – Běn Shén*) states, "For those with anxiety and worry, qi is blocked and is unable to move."

The Basic Questions – Treatise on Sickness (*Sù Wèn – Běn Bìng Lùn*) states, "When people have anxiety, worry, pensiveness and preoccupation, the heart will become damaged." Also, "When people rage, qi counterflows to the upper and is unable to move downwards; this will damage the liver."

This relationship of extreme emotional states to the movements of the qi dynamic form the foundation of disease theory as related to the emotions, and this idea continues to guide Chinese medical practices in the present day.

The disease term *xiè yì* (解㑊) also initially appears several times in *The Inner Classic*.

The Basic Questions – Qi and Manifestations of Healthy Persons (*Sù Wèn – Píng Rén Qì Xiàng Lùn*) states, "Moderate and rough pulses at the cubit position reflect *xiè yì*."

The Basic Questions – Essentials of Needling (*Sù Wèn – Cì Yào Lùn*) states, "When the marrow is damaged it will gradually dry up, and the shins will become sore; one will feel fatigue and an unwillingness to move."

Chapter 2
The History of Depressive Disorder Theory in Chinese Medicine

The Grand Chinese Medical Dictionary (Zhōng Guó Yī Xué Dà Cí Diǎn) also listed this term and provided corresponding treatment methods to address "weariness, anxiety and vague discomfort".

The clinical presentation of *xiè yì* is closely related to depressive disorders in modern medicine, and is also commonly seen in psychiatry and medical practice where it presents as conditions such as fibromyalgia.

The Ming Dynasty physician Li Chan concluded that the chief manifestations, etiologies, and treatment principles for the disease category of *xiè yì* are as follows:

"*Xiè* refers to dispersion of the flesh, and *yì* refers to sinews failing to leash the bones. The condition may appear similar to cold or heat conditions, but it is neither. Manifestations include dispersion of bones and joints of the four limbs, fatigue, vexing pain, and no pleasure in eating. This can be caused by damage from excessive drinking, a direct strike of dampness, contraction of wind-cold, over-indulgence in sexual activities, or menstrual irregularities in women. Treatment should free the qi and blood and course the interstices. Regulate with medicinals appropriate for internal damage and external contraction."

Physician Shen Jin-ao pointed out that the root condition of *xiè yì* is caused by liver and kidney deficiency, saying that what Li Chan had discussed were only referring to the accompanying conditions.

He stated: "Discussing it from the perspective of the root condition, this is a case of extreme deficiency taxation; discussing it from the perspective of the accompanying condition, this pathology is a divergent branch of deficiency taxation."

More significantly, he pointed out that this disease can manifest with emotional symptoms: "When there is liver deficiency, the sinews become soft, slack, and have no strength to leash the bones; this results in dissipating of the flesh all over the body. When there is kidney deficiency, the bones become wilted, tired, and unable to strengthen themselves; this causes sluggishness and a predomination of joint fatigue all over the body. If it is so, then a person will present with weariness and anxiety."

Subsequently, most physicians inherited the concept from *The Inner Classic*, and have considered the root cause of constraint patterns to be a disharmony of qi and blood in the five viscera. Tang and Song Dynasty physicians tended to consider "constraint/depression" more as being related to the pathomechanisms of visceral diseases. Associated conditions include qi glomus, phlegm-damp, food accumulation, and irregular emotional presentations.

In medical texts like the *Treatise on Cold Damage* (Shāng Hán Lùn), *Essentials of the Golden Cabinet* (Jīn Guì Yào Lüè), *The Pulse Classic* (Mài Jīng), *Treatise on the Origins and Manifestations of Various Diseases* (Zhū Bìng Yuán Hòu Lùn), *Important Formulas Worth a Thousand Gold Pieces for Emergency* (Bèi Jí Qiān Jīn Yào Fāng), *Arcane Essentials from the Imperial Library* (Wài Tái Mì Yào) and *Comprehensive Recording of Divine Assistance* (Shèng Jì Zǒng Lù), the pathomechanism and patterns of constraint were discussed in sections on miscellaneous diseases of the five viscera, but they were not listed as separate conditions.

According to Zhang Zhong-jing's six-channel theory in the *Treatise on Cold Damage*, shaoyang is the pivot, also standing in an exterior-interior relationship with jueyin; its qi has the functions of coursing and draining. The ascending, descending, exiting and entering movements of the qi dynamic, and the transportation and transformation of fluids all depend on the coursing, draining, and orderly reaching of the liver and gallbladder. Once the liver and gallbladder contract pathological factors, the pivot function will be affected and this functional impingement gives rise to various presentations. For instance, the spleen and stomach can become affected, resulting in "silence with no desire to eat". Enduring qi constraint can transform into fire that scorches yin and harasses the heart; common manifestations include fullness in the chest and rib-sides and heart vexation.

Zhang Zhong-jing followed the principle of "treating depressed wood with out-thrusting" and invented the liver-coursing method with the well known formula *Xiǎo Chái Hú Tāng* (Minor Bupleurum Decoction). This formula is effective in opening constraint/depression of the liver and gallbladder, freeing the six bowels, quieting the five viscera, calming yin and yang, and regulating qi and blood. This was an innovative treatment for constraint/depression, and remains a classic formula that is still considered as clinically effective.

Chapter 2
The History of Depressive Disorder Theory in Chinese Medicine

The *Essentials of the Golden Cabinet* records two conditions that are closely related to emotions in women: plum-pit qi and visceral agitation. The corresponding formulas *Bàn Xià Hòu Pò Tāng* (Pinellia and Officinal Magnolia Bark Decoction) and *Gān Mài Dà Zǎo Tāng* (Licorice, Wheat and Jujube Decoction) are both still in clinical use.

The *Treatise on the Origins and Manifestations of Various Diseases* states, "The condition of binding qi is engendered from anxiety and pensiveness. There is accumulation of the heart and stoppage of the spirit; qi lodges without moving, therefore it binds internally." This statement is derivative of the perspective found in *The Inner Classic* which has also had a great influence on subsequent generations.

The *Important Formulas Worth a Thousand Gold Pieces for Emergency* describes symptoms and treatment methods for post-partum psychological disorders. In the section on gynecological formulas, *Zhú Yè Tāng* (Lophatherum Decoction) is listed for the treatment of "persistent vexation and oppression in the heart after labor", and *Dàn Zhú Rú Tāng* (Bamboo Shavings Decoction) for "postpartum deficiency vexation, headache, shortage of qi, and persistent vexation and oppression in the heart". The treatment principles and methods of clearing deficiency heat while nourishing qi and blood still inspire contemporary practitioners when treating postpartum depression.

In the twelfth volume, in a section on the gallbladder, the text states, "Those who suffer from gallbladder diseases present with frequent sighing, a bitter mouth, vomiting abiding fluids, a rippling sensation below the heart as if one were getting arrested, uneasiness in the throat, and frequent spitting. The disease is located in foot *shaoyang*." This is very similar to the symptoms of anxiety depression. The text considers the evil to be located in the gallbladder, with the counterflow as related to the stomach. Corresponding formulas such as *Suān Zǎo Tāng* (Sour Jujube Decoction) are also provided.

During the Jin and Yuan Dynasties, the theory of constraint was developed from a variety of angles. Although the theory had become mature, there was still some disagreement on the concept of what constituted a constraint pattern. Zhu Zhen-heng (Zhu Dan-xi) stated, "If qi and blood flow in harmony, none of the ten thousand diseases will be engendered; as soon as there is constraint, all diseases can be engendered." He set aside a specific indication for the constraint pattern in order to distinguish it from other conditions, and also divided constraint into six types: qi, dampness, heat, phlegm, blood, and food constraint. This was the first research specifically examining the pathomechanisms of constraint.

Zhu Zhen-heng created *Yuè Jú Wán* (Constraint-Resolving Pill) declaring that the chief medicinals were *cāng zhú* (Rhizoma Atractylodis) and *chuān xiōng* (Rhizoma Chuanxiong) because they act to "resolve all constraints, and may be added to various formulas according to the pattern." His theoretical approach and ideas about pattern differentiation and treatment have remained very durable and continue to be used by many physicians.

In the *Discourse on Tracing Back to the Medical Classics* (*Yī Jīng Sù Huí Jí*), Wang Lü brilliantly expanded on the traditional concept of the five constraints. However, as he pointed out, "Diseases commonly arise from constraint. Constraint refers to stagnation and stoppage. This can be caused by being overwhelmed, or by root qi being constrained with no overwhelming factor; it is not all caused by changing of the five phases. Thus, the methods of out-thrusting, effusion, despoliation, drainage and regulation can be expanded and supplemented as well."

This idea was key to understanding the constraint pattern, which involves the pathomechanism of stagnation and stoppage. It also expands on the corresponding treatments based on five phase theory in *The Inner Classic* to a broader spectrum, pointing out that since the causes are not limited to the five phases, corresponding treatments must vary as well.

During the Ming Dynasty, Yu Tuan developed a theory based on *The Basic Questions* and *Teachings of [Zhu] Dan-xi* (*Dān Xī Xīn Fǎ*). In his work *The Orthodox Tradition of Medicine* (*Yī Xué Zhèng Zhuàn*) he discusses constraint patterns as a broad concept with etiologies including emotions,

Chapter 2
The History of Depressive Disorder Theory in Chinese Medicine

external pathological factors and even diet. He stated, "Constraint of the seven emotions or invasion of cold and heat can lead to constraint of the nine qi. Invasion of rain dampness or a gathering of alcoholic liquids can lead to diseases of rheum retention and damp constraint." This puts the primary emphasis on emotional causes. However, what he referred to as "constraint" was still not yet characterized by signs of low self-esteem or emotional frustration.

During this time period the focus of constraint gradually shifted to conditions caused by emotional disorders, although the external causative factors were still included. In his *The Complete Compendium of Ancient and Modern Medical Works* (Gǔ Jīn Yī Tǒng Dà Quán), Xu Chun-fu pointed out "Constraint is binding caused by constraint of the seven emotions. Enduring constraint can transform into a variety of diseases."

Zhang Jie-bin's treatise on constraint patterns in *The Complete Works of [Zhang] Jing-yue* (Jǐng Yuè Quán Shū) is quite comprehensive. Explained here are the relationships between the "five constraints" from *The Yellow Emperors Inner Classic* (Huáng Dì Nèi Jīng) and Zhu Dan-xi's "six constraints", stating that "all diseases caused by qi and blood disharmony may be called 'constraint'" and that "constraint of the five qi can be seen in all conditions; this is 'disease leading to constraint'. Depression of the emotions is always related to the heart; this is 'constraint leading to disease'". Thus Chinese medical theory started to separate constraint/depression as a pathomechanism related to the qi dynamic on the one hand, and as a condition characterized by ungratified emotions on the other.

Zhang Jing-yue pointed out that constraint could be caused by the six excesses and the six emotions. He clarified the definition of constraint patterns, distinguished three types of emotional depression which relate to anger, pensiveness, and anxiety, analyzing their pathological location, pathomechanism and treatment, and summarizing a group of effective formulas.

Another Ming Dynasty physician, Zhao Xian-ke stated, "The five rules in *The Yellow Emperors Inner Classic* refer to constraint caused by overwhelming qi of the five phases. It does not have to be constraint as in anxiety and depression. Anxiety is one of the diseases associated with the seven emotions, but anxiety is part of constraint also." He was indicating that emotional depression is only one part of the overall constraint pattern. Additionally, according to the theory of mutual engenderment, restraint, overwhelming and rebellion among the five phases, Zhao Xian-ke thought that the five phases can serve as etiologies for constraint among one another, and that wood constraint is the most common cause of all disease. "When wood is depressed, fire will be depressed with it as well. Also, constraint of fire can cause constraint of earth, which can lead to constraint of metal and result in constraint of water."

Therefore, as stated in the *Key Link of Medicine* (*Yī Guàn*), "all constraints may be attributed to the liver". Since wood engenders fire, wood constraint will cause fire depressed within the wood; also, when *shaoyang* fails to extend and move effectively, it can easily move downwards to restrain spleen-earth causing a dual disease of metal and water. Zhao Xian-ke concluded, "I treat wood constraint with one formula, and all constraints can be cured; that formula is *Xiāo Yáo Sǎn* (Free Wanderer Powder)." This method can "replace" and "be modified with" the other five treatments.

Zhao Xian-ke developed the theory of the pathomechanism of the constraint pattern by revealing the internal relationship among the five constraints, and also by pointing out that qi constraint is primarily caused by an inhibited qi dynamic of the liver. The composition of *Xiāo Yáo Sǎn* (Free Wanderer Powder) acts more effectively than *Yuè Jú Wán* (Constraint-Resolving Pill) in the treatment of constraint originating in the liver.

In the Ming Dynasty text *Black Pearl from Red Waters* (*Chì Shuǐ Xuán Zhū*), Sun Yi-kui states, "When a person with congenital deficiency encounters a personal frustration, there will be a dizzy head and blurred vision, fatigue, sinew wilting, and rapid breathing like that seen in a deficiency pattern. Focus primarily on opening the constraint and normalizing qi, and then the qi condition will resolve spontaneously."

Chapter 2
The History of Depressive Disorder Theory in Chinese Medicine

Qing Dynasty physician Shen Jin-ao in his work *Shen's Books on Respecting Life* (*Shěn Shì Zūn Shēng Shū*) also stated, "All constraints are diseases related to visceral qi. The root cause is excessively deep pensiveness combined with weak visceral qi. That is how the diseases of the six constraints are engendered." This clearly explains the emotional and constitutional aspects of constraint's onset. Regarding the pathomechanisms, he says, "When there is anxious constraint, the upbearing, downbearing, and transformative functions do not fulfill their roles. The constraint can involve qi or blood, and the condition thus occurs."

Physicians in Qing Dynasty had also developed etiologies and pathomechanisms of constraint based on clinical experience. In pattern differentiation, deficiency, excess, and the progress of the disease were often distinguished. Treatment methods matured during this period as well.

Ye Gui was one of the most important figures in this development. In *Case Records as a Guide to Clinical Practice* (*Lín Zhèng Zhǐ Nán Yī Àn*), he concluded that "the majority of constraint is related to the seven emotions", and "constraint first damages the qi aspect, over a period of time it will affect the blood aspect, then it develops into a severe condition of constraint-taxation". The heart, spleen, liver and gallbladder can all be affected. He also mentioned more than once that the patient needs to be content and gratified, and that "simply applying herbs and minerals will not bring observable effects". This psychological treatment principle is still important even today.

Qing Dynasty author Lin Pei-qin also pointed out in his work *Categorized Patterns with Clear-cut Treatments* (*Lèi Zhèng Zhì Cái*) that enduring constraint can affect the blood, damage visceral yin and transform from excess to deficiency, and that simply dispersing and dissipating would not result in effective treatment.

The development of the theory of constraint patterns reached its peak in the Qing Dynasty. In his *Non-retention Collection* (*Bù Jū Jí*), Wu Cheng summed up the theories of previous scholars, saying, "The discussions in *The Yellow Emperors Inner Classic* focused primarily on the overwhelming and retaliation relationships among the five phases, so there is constraint of the five qi. Zhu Dan-xi extended this and developed the six constraints of qi, blood, damp, heat, food and phlegm. Physician Zhao extended it again; stating that conditions of wind damage, cold damage, summerheat warmth, seasonal epidemic and external contractions could all be viewed as constraint. I also now extend it one more time; all diseases related to the seven emotions, five minds, taxation damage and accumulated food are all ascribed to constraint."

This, once again, is "constraint" in its broadest sense, which refers to "non-resolution of the evil" and "stagnation and stoppage". Etiologies such as external contraction and internal damage can all be referred to as constraint. This is neither an independent condition nor a symptom, but rather includes all patterns manifesting with stagnation of the qi dynamic and abnormal transportation of qi, blood and fluids. The five constraints from *The Yellow Emperors Inner Classic* and Zhu Dan-xi's six constraints both belong to this category. However, ever since the Ming Dynasty, medical literature has primarily focused on emotional constraint.

There is another condition referred to as *bēi dié* (卑慄, lit. low self-esteem and fear) which is similar to depression. The *Standards for Diagnosis and Treatment* (*Zhèng Zhì Zhǔn Shéng*) states, "Glomus blockage with no desire to eat, a frequent sense of guilt, a preference for being in dark places or leaning behind the door, becoming frightened and hiding upon seeing people, and appearing to be losing one's mind reflect the condition of *bēi dié*. The cause is blood insufficiency."

Many statements regarding heart palpitations and fearful throbbing may also contain descriptions of depressive status. This is consistent with the fact that anxious, neurotic and depressive patients often present with tachycardia.

Constraint as a disease is related to and yet different from depression

Chapter 2
The History of Depressive Disorder Theory in Chinese Medicine

patterns in a narrow sense. Depression disease refers to an emotionally constrained status. The mild case is equivalent to a depression pattern with constrained emotion, and the severe case may manifest with symptoms similar to that of withdrawal disease, which refers to a more severe emotional condition characterized by frustration, a blank affect, feeble-mindedness, deranged speech, and an unwillingness to move. Even in Western psychiatric medicine it remains difficult to differentiate depressive disorder from schizophrenia in some cases. Therefore, in modern Chinese internal medicine, depression/constraint disorder is only used as a reference for pattern differentiation and treatment of neurasthenia, hysteria, anxiety neurosis, reactive psychosis and menopausal syndrome; for more severe mood disorders, the disease category of withdrawal and mania is most often used as a reference model for treatment.

Contemporarily, textbooks and reference books on Chinese internal medicine describe the constraint pattern (sometimes referred to as depression disease) as "a type of condition caused by constrained qi dynamic characterized by restlessness, fullness and oppression in the chest, distending pain in the rib-sides, irascibility, a tendency to weep, or a sensation of an foreign object blocking the throat". The constraint in this case is completely different from the broader traditional sense. The key to the pathomechanism of emotional constraint is stoppage of the qi dynamic. The visceral location of the pathology depends upon where the qi is blocked. Understanding emotional constraint can help us understand the physical manifestations of psychological conditions, and help to resolve masked depression.

Chapter 3
Five Spirits and the Brain

In this chapter we will discuss the five spirits of Chinese medicine, and their association with the brain-spirit. In keeping with the Taoist saying "the belt that fits is the one that we do not notice" the quality and functions of the spirits are best displayed when we examine their dysfunctional states. Because the brain-spirit is, as the heart spirit was regarded traditionally, both an independent idea and an aggregate of the other spirits; anything that compromises the five spirits will also be reflected in the brain-spirit. Also introduced in this chapter are the corresponding basic principles for managing these conditions. Since most of these conditions will be multi-pattern problems with relatively complex issues, it is important to keep sight of the basic functional nature of the various aspects of the spirit so as to selectively treat the patterns that will most likely resolve the main complaint.

The historical literature of Chinese medicine contains a great number of discussions regarding the brain and its influence on human consciousness. Chinese medical textbooks often introduce ideas such as "The heart governs the spirit-light" as well as "The brain governs the spirit-light". The term spirit-light, *shen ming* 神明, indicates a wide range of concepts, but for the purposes of this text it mainly reflects the idea of consciousness and mental function. Although such expressions may seem to be somewhat abstract, numerous explanations and elaborations have appeared throughout the ages. Although the role of the brain and its association with consciousness had been explored somewhat metaphorically by earlier Taoist meditation texts, Ming Dynasty author Li Shi-zhen is regarded as one of the first mainstream authors to incorporate the brain into the theory of consciousness.

Li wrote, "The brain is the house of the original spirit", and Qing Dynasty physician Wang Qing-ren also put forward somewhat controversial ideas for the time by stating that "The brain governs memory" and "Intelligence and memory rely on the brain instead of the heart". These concepts are obviously relevant to modern clinical practice, and thus warrant further discussion.

The relationship of the five organs to their five respective spirits is explained as "one has five viscera that transform the five qi to engender joy, anger, sorrow, anxiety, and fear". Excesses and deficiencies of yin and yang influence the condition and activities of the viscera and bowels

Chapter 3
Five Spirits and the Brain

and their five spirits, while, conversely, emotional excesses from external stimuli can affect organ function. Traditionally, the heart governs all of these activities, because the spirit of the heart is regarded as the master of the other spirits. We posit that if one gives first place to the brain as the seat of consciousness, it is also logical that the brain also has a respective spirit which would play a role in the coordination of the other viscera-spirits. This brain-spirit would supplement the traditional role of the heart-spirit, but not replace it entirely.

The brain-spirit influences and governs the activities of the viscera and bowels and qi and blood via their five viscera-spirits. However, the normality or abnormality of mental activities can also be a reflection of the condition of the organs or the state of qi and blood. The brain-spirit and the five viscera-spirits integrate to form a "brain-spirit interaction process", where a cooperative relationship develops between the brain-spirit and the viscera-spirits, the spinal cord, and the qi and blood of the five viscera. This coordination regulates yin and yang, and out of this coordination a mental activity dominated by the brain-spirit is formed. The implication of this is that while disorders of the brain-spirit cause functional disorders, functional disorders of this system can also cause mental illness.

Although the brain is categorized as one of the extraordinary bowel-organs, it does have a close association with the five viscera. In *The Yellow Emperor's Inner Classic* (*Huáng Dì Nèi Jīng*), mental activities are associated with the five viscera and six bowels and other vital activities. *The Basic Questions – Treatise Explaining the Five Qi* (*Sù Wèn – Xuān Míng Wǔ Qì Piān*) states, "The heart stores the spirit, the lung stores the corporeal soul, the liver stores the ethereal soul, the spleen stores intention, and the kidney stores mind."

Each of the five viscera stores a specific aspect of spirit, but all of them are manifestations of the brain-spirit as associated with a specific viscus or bowel organ. All five spirits are governed by the brain, with the relationship between the five spirits and the brain being similar to that of a national and regional government. The brain and spinal cord communicate with the heart and other parts of body through the channels and blood vessels.

The Secret Records of the Brocade Sack (*Jǐn Náng Mì Lù*) states that "The brain is the house of the original spirit, governs the five spirits, and thus regulates the viscera and bowels, yin and yang, the four extremities, and the hundred bones", and also that "The brain plots the outline, the viscera and bowels give the details, and the body puts it into effect".

Simply put, the implication here is that the role of the heart-spirit, the spirit that dominates the other visceral spirits, can be easily aligned with the idea of a spirit that is related to the brain, allowing the Chinese medical paradigm to incorporate the Western clinical understanding of the brain as the seat of mental activity and biological regulation. While this does not eliminate the role of the heart-spirit nor invalidate heart-spirit related treatments, it does allow for the possibility of treatments based around both physical pathological processes in the brain, as well as for creating a novel aspect of spirit not affiliated with the regular viscera. This spirit may be addressed to add a new dimension to the treatment of mental-emotional disorders. Since the viscus associated with the brain-spirit does not have any clear traditional function outside of the accumulations of essence as the "sea of marrow", treatment that focuses on the brain organ are generally those that address possible deficiencies of essence due to taxation of the brain-spirit through mental illness, or other more physical causes.

Heart – *Shen*

As one of the five viscera, the major functions of the heart are to govern blood and the vessels, and to store the spirit, or shen. "The heart governs the blood and vessels" refers to the heart's function of promoting and regulating the movement of blood within the vessels. The brain, the brain-spirit, the viscera and bowels, and the limbs and bones all depend upon the moisture and nourishment provided by heart-blood in order to function properly.

The heart-spirit is a major component of the brain-spirit interaction system. The heart is associated with fire and is yang in function. The brain is also described as a delicate organ; it cannot function without proper nourishment of heart-blood and full, unobstructed blood vessels. Heart qi and heart yang provide the warmth required to maintain the free flow of blood within the vessels that provide nourishment to the brain.

The physiological characteristics of the spirit are dependent on the

Chapter 3
Five Spirits and the Brain

physiological characteristics of the heart. Heart-blood is the material basis for the heart-spirit. As stated in *The Spiritual Pivot – the Engendering and Interaction of Ying and Wei* (*Líng Shū – Yíng Wèi Shēng Huì*), "Blood is spiritual qi." When heart-blood is abundant, spirit is generated and fostered, and the mind is confident and clear. The yang qi of the heart stimulates the heartbeat, warms and circulates within the blood vessels, and inspires the mind. The heart-spirit is pure and bright, and healthy heart yang is required to provide it with stimulation and energy. Heart yin, however, calms and contains the mind to prevent it from becoming restless. With such coordination of heart yin and heart yang, the mind remains tranquil, neither over-excited nor depressed. If yang qi of the heart becomes deficient, this leads to insufficient warmth and stimulation that leads to poor memory and mental exhaustion. If heart yin is deficient, the lack of cooling can cause agitation and "deficiency-type stimulation".

The heart-spirit is closely associated with a person's emotions; it is also said that the heart naturally aspires to happiness. *The Basic Questions – Great Treatise on the Correspondences and Manifestation of Yin and Yang* (*Sù Wèn – Yīn Yáng Yìng Xiàng Dà Lùn*) states, "Within the organs this is the heart, and among the minds this is joy."

Joy is usually a positive reaction to external stimulation, with joy and delight being also beneficial for the heart function of governing blood and vessels, because these emotions act to enliven the heart and stimulate qi. *The Basic Questions – Treatise on Pain* (*Sù Wèn – Jǔ Tòng Lùn*) states, "When there is joy, the mind is harmonized, qi flows freely, and ying and wei remain unobstructed."

Joy is usually beneficial for health, but there are exceptional cases; if one is overjoyed beyond the extent that one can bear, either through sudden shock or chronic over-excitement, heart qi becomes dissipated and the spirit fails to be contained. Such disharmony of the heart-spirit can also lead to the onset of disease.

The Spiritual Pivot – the Spirit (*Líng Shū – Běn Shén*) states, "For those with joy and delight, the spirit becomes dissipated and fails to remain stored", and the *Revised Popular Guide to 'Treatise on Cold Damage'* (*Chóng Dìng Tōng Sú Shāng Hán Lùn*) also states, "Joy and delight in excess will dissipate essence and spirit, and the spirit fails to keep its composure; this is taxation damaging the heart".

With excessive mental activity, (perhaps as in mania-phase bipolar disorders, etc.) a person might at first become overjoyed and delighted, only later to become depressed and despondent. Clinical practice shows that not only excessive joy, but also any other excessive emotion can impair the heart-spirit.

Brain-spirit and Heart-spirit in Depression

The brain-spirit is the original spirit, thus governing the other viscera-spirits acting within the body. The heart is the commander of blood and vessels, and it also acts to store the spirit.

As indicated in the theories of channels and collaterals, "A branch of the hand *shaoyin* heart channel goes upwards along the throat, and this is connected to the eye tie". The "eye tie" is a structure usually equated with the optic chiasmus. In Chinese medicine, it is associated with the liver channel in its capacity to govern vision, but also with the center of the brain as the channel emerges from the crown of the head.

The brain and the heart are also connected by channels, with the brain and brain-spirit both nourished by blood circulation as provided by the heart organ. However, further exploration will be required to thoroughly understand how the heart-spirit specifically associates with the brain-spirit. Now that we have presented an understanding of the connections between the brain, brain-spirit and the heart, we can continue by examining the brain-spirit and its relationship with the pathological factors normally associated with depression disease.

(1) INSUFFICIENCY

Palpitations and fearful throbbing, timidity, and frequent unhappiness are common symptoms in many depressive disorder patients, usually caused by insufficiencies of heart qi, heart blood and/or heart yin. Other manifestations may include persistent palpitations, susceptibility to fright, dream disorders, deficiency agitation, loss-of-luxuriance of the flesh, irregular defecation, a pale tongue, and deep and fine pulses. Women may also have pale and scant menses.

If heart blood is unable to sufficiently nourish the brain-spirit, there may be symptoms of impaired memory, dizziness and vertigo, mental fatigue, timidity, trance-like states, sadness, persistent weeping, and

Chapter 3
Five Spirits and the Brain

paranoia; in severe cases the patient may become uncommunicative with no desire for food or drink. The common feature of these symptoms is that blood fails to nourish the heart and brain, and with that failure the original spirit is compromised. These highly variable emotional states reflect the coordinating function of the heart-spirit over all of the emotions: timidity reflects the weakness of qi in the heart that accompanies heart blood vacuity; sadness and persistent crying reflect the intimate relationship of heart and lung as manifested through the formation of *zong qi* (the qi of the chest that drives the action of the heart and lungs); paranoia is a derangement of the spirit where perception of the world as it is becomes lost. Since the heart is traditionally associated with the tongue and speech, when severely compromised, speech is affected and the patient can become withdrawn. The brain-spirit shares all of these attributes of the heart-spirit, and is also affected by a compromised blood supply in a similar way. Because depression often attacks the lifting aspect of the qi dynamic, the clear yang is frequently compromised; when the clear is not upraised, then blood is not produced, leading to deficiency.

With hyperactive fire due to insufficient heart yin, there may also be restlessness, insomnia, dream disorders, anxiety, dry mouth, heat in the center of the palms and soles, and night sweats. Since heart blood and yin stabilizes the spirit, it is also common for these patients to experience anxiety along with their depression, or restlessness induced by the resulting instability. Treatment here should emphasize the nourishing of heart yin and heart blood.

As noted above, insufficiency of heart blood is also generally accompanied by an insufficiency of heart qi, where symptoms would include palpitations and shortness of breath exacerbated by physical activity, spontaneous sweating, mental and physical fatigue, and a hollow distressed feeling in the chest. Treatment in these cases emphasizes supplementation of both qi and blood. In more extreme cases, such as heart failure patients with depression, one can observe a deficiency of heart yang with symptoms of persistent low moods, extreme sadness, loss of interest, and palpitations with a hollow feeling in the chest. As the deficient heart yang fails to inspire and motivate the spirit, the sadness characteristic of these cases is marked by a deep despondency and hopelessness.

(2) FIRE AND HEAT

The heart is the organ associated with fire. When the five emotions become inhibited, the resulting constraint can transform into pathological fire, causing heart fire to become hyperactive. As the heart-spirit becomes disturbed, symptoms may include continuous laughter, restlessness, aggrandizing and exaggeration of reality, and over-excitement with a compulsion to talk. These circumstances also present themselves when a constraint/depressive disorder is converting into a manic disorder. These manifestations reflect the normal qualities of the heart, joy and laughter, aspiration and speech in an exaggerated form. Since the spirit's nature is light and mobile, it is buoyed up by fire and its motion becomes aggravated.

Hyperactive heat of both heart and liver is usually initiated by heart fire, although it may also result from constrained liver qi transforming into fire. In any event, as fire of the heart and liver flows upward to disturb the brain-spirit, a wide variety of conditions may result, most typically manifesting with rash actions, anger and rage. The corresponding treatment principle of clearing heat and draining fire from the heart and liver is a commonly applied treatment principle in Chinese medical psychiatry.

The heart and kidney are the foundation of the qi dynamic. Mental stress and emotional disorders may initiate pathogenic fire that damages yin, where constraint and excessive rumination may also consume heart yin. With deficient heart yin, yang cannot be contained, and this leads to heart fire flaming upward or hyperactive heart yang with non-interaction of heart and kidney. This results in depression accompanied by insomnia, palpitations, irritability, anxiety, impaired memory, and spermatorrhea. These are manifestations of the agitated heart fire harassing the spirit above. Since the heart fire is not descending, the ministerial fire of the kidney is unregulated; this upsets the essence within the lower burner sometimes leading to involuntary seminal emission. An insufficiency of heart yin is most common, but in other cases where yin-blood is insufficient, the heart, as the child-organ, will steal from the mother-organ, the liver. This leads to an insufficiency of liver blood and malnourishment of the liver. In that case, the patient becomes extremely sensitive, where even slight emotional stimulation can lead to qi stagnation and symptoms of depression. The mechanism of this pathology is related to the liver's governing of emotional experience; since the liver regulates the opening and closing of the pathways of the body in response to the movement of qi (emotion), when liver yin or blood is deficient, this function becomes hyperactive in response to the slightest upset.

(3) Phlegm and Blood Stasis

Turbid phlegm disturbing the heart is another typical pattern associated with depression and brain-spirit disease. Any of the following patterns may lead to the formation of phlegm which can disturb the heart:

1) Spleen dampness and phlegm accumulation
2) Dual deficiency of heart and kidney
3) Dual deficiency of spleen and kidney
4) Stasis and stagnation slowing the movement of fluids with phlegm congealing.

In these circumstances where clear yang fails to ascend and turbid yin fails to descend, normal qi transformation becomes weakened; the essence of food and drink is transformed into turbid phlegm which may also cloud the brain. Because the nature of the brain is light and mobile, dampness act to inhibit it, and inhibition of the brain-spirit results in mental dysfunction with symptoms of sluggishness, depression, apathy, and lassitude along with physical symptoms of dampness like weak extremities, loss of appetite, vomiting, nausea, abdominal fullness and oppression, and a pale tongue with a greasy coating. If turbid phlegm combines with constrained qi and transforms into fire, there will also be symptoms of panic, irritation, and insomnia. These patterns are more difficult to resolve because of the tenacious nature of pathogenic phlegm and dampness.

With chronic depression, the qi dynamic is persistently constrained and the circulation of blood becomes inhibited, resulting in patterns of blood stasis that will eventually obstruct the brain collaterals and further inhibit the brain-spirit. When constraint and stasis occur together and interact as both cause and effect, a vicious cycle is formed. Furthermore, blood stasis may also generate pathogenic heat of its own, further damaging yin and blood. Depressive disorders accompanied by cardiac diseases are usually manifestations of static blood or phlegm oppressing the spirit.

(4) Qi Deficiency

Qi deficiency of the heart and lung and/or insufficiency of spirit-qi may also cause disorders of the brain-spirit. There may be sadness and a desire to weep, low mood, depression and unhappiness, shortness of breath and low energy, spontaneous sweating, a pale tongue and weak pulses.

Dual deficiency of heart and spleen can lead to depression as the resulting insufficiency of qi and blood leads to malnourishment of the brain-spirit. Patients with chronic conditions may also display symptoms of internal cold and dampness with stagnation of turbid phlegm. In diagnosis and treatment, all of these various factors must be considered.

To summarize, any functional disorder of the heart may cause insufficiency patterns of heart qi or heart blood, hyperactive heart-fire, restlessness of the heart-spirit, pathogenic phlegm disturbing the heart, deficiency of both heart and spleen, or non-interaction of heart and kidney. However, the patterns of hyperactive heart-fire and pathogenic phlegm disturbing the heart are more common in acute episodes of depressive disorder.

Lung – *Po*

The spirit of the lung is called the po, or corporeal soul. *The Spiritual Pivot – the Spirit* (*Líng Shū – Běn Shén*) states, "That which exits and enters along with the essence is called the corporeal soul".

The corporeal soul is not only part of the mind and consciousness, but is also associated with the instinctive senses and movement. *The Classified Classic* (*Lèi Jīng*) states, "The senses and consciousness of babies as well as their body movements are the creativity and intelligence of the corporeal soul", and also "The function of the corporeal soul is to move and to act; all aches and itchiness are felt because of it". According to the five viscera-spirit theory, movement and perception are both associated with the lung and corporeal soul, and abnormalities within this sphere of influence would include sensory disturbances and dyskinesia.

Chapter 3
Five Spirits and the Brain

The Lung and Depression

The lung governs the qi of the body, linking it with all the vessels; being in the uppermost part of the torso in the area above the diaphragm it is considered as relatively pure and associated with heaven, also known as the "florid canopy", a term with describes its capacity as a sort of umbrella for the heart (the canopy over the emperor was also called the "florid canopy") as well as the shape of the organ, which is often compared to an inverted flower.

Precepts for Physicians (*Yī Mén Fǎ Lǜ*) states, "The qi of the human body receives orders from the lung; when the lung qi is clear and depurated, the qi of the entire body will become obedient and move in order." In patients with depression, disorder of the lung-corporeal soul results in sadness and weeping, generally associated with qi deficiency. In terms of physical symptoms of the lung associated with depression, sighing, yawning and shallow breathing or a weak voice would all reflect the debility or inhibition of lung qi resulting from a failure of the qi dynamic. The voice and the mechanism of breathing are supported by the qi of the lung, so when they are weak, this reflects a weakness of lung qi; yawning and sighing are natural efforts to restore deep breathing caused by stagnation, and if they are frequent, this reflects an inhibition of the qi dynamic. All are common physical symptoms in depression.

The normal lung qi function of ascending, dispersion, purification, and descending are the fundamental mechanisms for qi movement within the human body. However, the corporeal soul is the lung function as manifested in mental activities as well as a manifestation of the brain-spirit as associated with the lung. In Chinese medical theory, the lung governs qi, and the sound associated with the lung is crying. Excessive sorrow and grief are emotions which may impair lung qi and cause shortness of breath. Conversely, a deficiency or a functional disorder of lung qi may cause one to become more vulnerable to negative external stimulation and to more easily feel sorrow and grief.

The Basic Questions – Treatise on Pain (*Sù Wèn – Jǔ Tòng Lùn*) states, "Sorrow scatters qi, sorrow causes tension of the heart collaterals, the pulmonary lobes lift and stretch, the upper burner is obstructed so that *ying qi* and *wei qi* can not be dispersed, heat accumulates within, and thus qi is scattered", and also, "Sorrow in excess impairs the lung and heart causing a sudden deficiency of original qi followed by collapse".

If the lung fails to manage, regulate, or diffuse, the qi dynamic is affected and this in turn causes inhibition and constraint of the brain-spirit. In other cases, mental depression results in a disorder of the qi dynamic which then affects the lung. In clinical practice, patients who are crying frequently as part of their symptomatic picture can be effectively treated by managing patterns that affect the lung.

The lung can contribute to the engendering of both turbid and intangible phlegm, both of which may inhibit or disturb the brain-spirit to cause emotional states such as depression. Internal phlegm turbidity obstructs the qi dynamic and this may also disturb the brain collaterals, or accumulate and transform into pathogenic fire. Phlegm causes qi constraint, which in turn leads to the formation of more phlegm. In these cases, treatments that only regulate and soothe the liver are not going to be effective. Phlegm-resolving, qi-regulating, and lung-diffusing medicinals should also be applied.

For symptoms of constraint or depression disease such as fullness and oppression of chest and rib-sides with frequent sighing, *băi hé* (Bulbus Lilii) should be added; for symptoms such as a sad facial expression and weeping, or when other treatments are ineffective, *zǐ wăn* (Radix et Rhizoma Asteris) and *kuăn dōng* (Flos Farfarae) should be added to diffuse the lung. Simple regulation of liver qi will not guarantee normal lung descending, and at times it must be directly stimulated.

The lung and large intestine stand in an interior-exterior relationship, so when lung qi becomes blocked due to patterns of constraint, a functional disorder of the large intestine may also appear. In those with depression, constipation is a common symptom, but when the normal function of lung qi is restored, large intestine function will often return to normal. However, if untreated, disorder of the large intestine can lead to further impairment of the qi dynamic, forming a vicious cycle. The converse is also true, meaning that the lung qi and brain-spirit can both become inhibited by retention of the stool. To improve communication between the lung and large intestine, treatment for these cases should include medicinals that diffuse the lung and regulate qi such as *xìng rén* (Semen Armeniacae Amarum) and *jié gĕng* (Radix Platycodonis).

Chapter 3
Five Spirits and the Brain

Furthermore, the liver and lung may be concurrently affected. In these cases, liver constraint with qi stagnation can transform into fire which will then invade and impair the lung. Therefore, in addition to soothing the liver to relieve constraint and descend counterflow qi, treatment should aim to restore the lung's purifying and descending functions while also clearing and discharging lung heat. If these patterns have endured and do not respond to treatment, they can also be addressed with medicinals that moisten and dispel dry phlegm. Phlegm will not always manifest obviously, but it can still inhibit the effectiveness of qi regulating medicinals.

Spleen – Yi

The spleen stores intention and intelligence. *Yi*, or intention, is mainly associated with thoughts and memory involving consciousness, thinking, consideration, and recollection. As qi, blood, and fluids are transformed by the spleen and stomach, the material basis of the brain-spirit is formed; spleen qi also nourishes the marrow of the brain and brain-spirit, and intention is a manifestation of this process. Splenic function also includes the governing of transportation and transformation, ascending of the clear yang, and the spreading of essence-qi. The result of this is that intention and the spleen can be symptomatically involved with what we call "overthinking", which reflects a persistent or iterative thought pattern.

Such brooding or rumination can be thought of as a mental manifestation of the failure of the spleen to upraise and distribute its products, one of which is thought; thoughts become stagnated and fail to move. As these relationships are invariably reciprocal, damage to the physical aspects of spleen function can damage the mind of the spleen and vice versa. The classical sayings discuss the spirit as associated with the spleen by calling it intention, and also state that excessive thinking damages the spleen. In that case, the free movement of qi will also become compromised, and thus the more general intellectual functions are affected as well.

The Classified Classic – Volume Fifteen (*Lèi Jīng – Juàn Shí Wǔ*) states, "It is said that that unreleased distress of the spleen impairs intention, the spleen governs middle qi, and that vitality is unable to function if middle qi is inhibited; this results in constraint and distress". Conversely, the *Essentials of the Medical Classics* (*Yī Jīng Jīng Yì*) states that "If the intention is in harmony, the post-natal spleen has no illness."

The Spleen and Depression

The spleen and stomach are the foundation of the acquired essence, which is also essential for maintaining nourishment of the brain-spirit. Factors such as emotional depression, inhibition of the brain-spirit, and rumination with qi binding may inhibit the movement of spleen and stomach qi. On the other hand, disordered ascending and descending or stagnation may also affect the qi dynamic of the other organs, including the brain-spirit. Primarily, spleen and stomach deficiency cause an inability to provide sufficient qi and blood to nourish the brain-spirit, but spleen qi deficiency also leads to impaired transportation and transformation which can result an engendering of turbid phlegm that obstructs the brain collaterals. In some cases, phlegm constraint transforms into pathogenic fire flaring upward to disturb the brain-spirit.

The above-mentioned patterns fall under the category of spleen-intention associated depression, are all are commonly seen in clinical practice. In fact, regulating the qi dynamic of the spleen and stomach is a fundamental treatment principle in the prevention and treatment of depression disease.

The Treatise on Diseases, Patterns, and Formulas Related to the Unification of the Three Etiologies – Patterns and Treatment of the Seven Qi (Sān Yīn Jí Yī Bìng Zhèng Fāng Lùn – Qī Qì Zhèng Zhì) states, "Rumination impairs the spleen, and qi is unable to flow. Accumulation in middle of the stomach cavity results in an inability to eat and drink with abdominal distention and fullness, and tiredness and idleness of the limbs. Thus the classic said: rumination causes qi binding".

When the spleen functions properly, the supply of essence is sufficient for maintaining and nourishing the brain-spirit and the five viscera-spirits. If splenic transportation fails, the essence from food and drink will be insufficient to nourish the brain-spirit and the five viscera-spirits. The resulting deficiency and weakness of the brain-spirit and the five viscera-spirits will compromise the qi dynamic, which then leads to constrained qi movement and disordered mental activity. Spleen-related patterns such as congestion of the qi dynamic and inhibition of the brain-spirit can lead to a depressed mood which may develop further into a depressive disorder.

Chapter 3
Five Spirits and the Brain

In other cases where the spleen-intention is confined, there will be a dull or sad facial expression, fear of strangers, timidity, reticence, a lack of physical strength, and lassitude. These symptoms are similar to those of depressive and manic disorders.

Spleen-*yi* depression has two principal manifestations: psychological and physical. The first aspect involves depression symptoms such as worry, sadness, weeping, mental disturbance, restless sleep, severe palpitations, and fatigue. These reflect the inhibition of spleen qi, which in turn fails to supply the lung (leading to manifestations of sadness) and heart (with manifestations of insomnia and palpitations). Diagnostically, it is important to differentiate fatigue associated with qi stagnation, which responds positively to exercise, from spleen deficiency failing to engender new qi (where activity leads to a deeper fatigue). The other physical symptoms primarily involve the digestive system including poor appetite, a decreased ability to smell and taste, nausea, acid reflux, aversion to food or difficulties in eating, failure to store food in the stomach, and vomiting after eating, though some or all of these can be seen in cases where liver stagnation is the dominant pattern.

Other manifestations may include hypertonicity of the rib-sides, obstruction of the diaphragm and throat, abdominal distention with difficult defecation, a heavy head, and fatigued limbs. Treatment principles here include ascending the clear, descending the turbid, and freeing the six bowels.

Liver – *Hun*

The spirit of the liver is called the hun, or ethereal soul. *The Spiritual Pivot – the Spirit* (*Líng Shū – Běn Shén*) states, "That which comes and goes with the spirit is called the ethereal soul." and also, "The liver stores blood, and blood is the residence of the ethereal soul".

Furthermore, the *Wondrous Lantern for Peering into the Origin and Development of Miscellaneous Diseases* (*Zá Bìng Yuán Líu Xī Zhú*) states, "The images seen in dreams are associated with the ethereal soul of the liver", and the *Treatise on Blood Syndromes* (*Xuě Zhèng Lùn*) also states, "If blood fails to nourish the liver, fire can harass the ethereal soul to cause dream emission and insomnia".

It is also said that "The liver governs the making of strategies." When the liver and gallbladder are functioning properly, the mind is clear with an ability to make sound judgments and decisions. When they are impaired one may become indecisive, anxious, and restless because the liver governs strategy and the gallbladder governs decision-making. The physiological characteristics of the liver in storing blood and governing the free flow of qi clearly influence the activities of the brain-spirit, and this theory is critical in guiding the diagnosis, differentiation and treatment in the clinical practices of Chinese medical psychiatry.

Useful metaphorical understanding of this aspect of the spirit can be had if we consider planning in relationship with the idea of vision, which is dominated by the liver. Dreams, plans and aspirations all reflect an ability to visualize the potential future. When the liver's qi is frustrated by qi stagnation and depression, or muddled by dampness or oppression from other forms of stagnation, the ability of the liver to direct and manage this aspect of its function is compromised. The gallbladder and liver are also associated with judgment, and the gallbladder with bravery (which can be thought of as the force to carry out a plan). When these are weak or stagnated, planning and progress towards goals is stymied and plans and visions of the future can become dissociated from what is real.

The Liver and Depression

Constrained liver qi is frequently the core pathomechanism and etiology of depression, therefore, regulating liver qi and blood and soothing the liver are critical in the treatment of most if not all cases of depression. From the perspective of etiology, it is clear that frustration of hopes and plans is directly related to liver qi constraint.

However, the ethereal soul can become restless when the liver is dysfunctional, leading to confusion and tension, poor judgment and self-control, fright, insomnia and sleep disorders, excessive dreaming, sleepwalking and sleep talking, and hallucinations. With a deficiency of liver blood, the normal functioning of brain-spirit may become inhibited, also resulting in a loss of emotional control.

The Spiritual Pivot – the Spirit (*Líng Shū – Běn Shén*) states, "If there is sorrow of the liver affecting the center, there will be damage to the ethereal soul; damage to the ethereal soul causes mania and a loss of essence".

In liver associated depression, hypofunction of the liver as associated

Chapter 3
Five Spirits and the Brain

with patterns of insufficient liver qi and liver yang are frequently ignored. Insufficient spirit, inhibition of emotion, and low moods are also frequently overlooked. When the lack of functional movement is addressed, the brain-spirit will return to normal and depression will be relieved spontaneously. Therefore, for chronic depression caused by inhibition of the brain-spirit, supplementing qi and warming yang is an essential treatment principle. These types of cases will present with mental fatigue, depressed mood, no strength to speak, slow speech, a lack of strength, cold limbs, somnolence, a loss of motivation, no interest in previously enjoyable activities, a pale tongue, and slow weak pulses. In the West, it seems that liver qi and yang deficiency patterns have become conflated with qi and yang deficiency of the spleen and kidney; it is important to discern the differences in these patterns during the diagnostic process. In treatment, yang or qi should be supplemented in a general way while also making sure to also re-establish the upward movement of the qi dynamic.

"The liver governs free coursing" means that the liver also governs the ascending and dynamic movement of qi. This gives it the capacity to regulate the qi dynamic and promote the circulation of qi, blood, and body fluids. When liver qi is functioning normally, clear yang carries blood to the brain to provide nourishment for the brain-spirit, but mental stress or negative stimulation may cause stagnation of liver qi where qi and blood fail to nourish the brain-spirit. Liver constraint may cause liver qi to counterflow and invade spleen-earth, leading to patterns of liver constraint with spleen deficiency. This is also one of the most common clinical patterns associated with depression disease.

Excess liver qi can lead to ascending qi counterflow and an upward flaming of liver fire which disturbs the brain, with blood sometimes accompanying the counterflow qi. In other cases, the chaotic qi and blood may carry dampness and turbid phlegm upward to obstruct the collaterals and confound the brain. This pattern can lead to mental depression as well as other physical conditions.

In the long term, these conditions damage yin and cause yin deficiency of the heart, liver and kidney. The main patterns include upward flaming of heart-fire, non-interaction of the heart and kidney, dual yin deficiency of the liver and kidney, and insufficient nourishment of the brain-

spirit. Manifestations here include dizziness, a distending feeling in the head, vertigo, headache, a feeling of heat in the head and face, tinnitus, insomnia, agitation, anger, unstable moods, or even madness and rage.

The formation of blood constraint and subsequent blood stasis is also very much associated with the liver. Inhibition, constraint, or stagnation of liver qi causes a slowing of blood circulation where blood stasis is more easily formed. Qi stagnation and static blood will always be present simultaneously because blood stasis usually develops from qi stagnation to some degree.

However, qi stagnation is not the only factor; other associated patterns include blood deficiency, dual qi deficiency of the heart and spleen, and dual qi and yang deficiency of the liver and kidney which leads to internal cold congealing and obstructed blood vessels. In most cases, soothing the liver, regulating qi and activating blood are still the basic principles of treatment. Stasis becomes more significant in chronic conditions where blood-invigorating formulas are often the best choice; however, keep in mind that a variety of relatively complicated patterns will appear in clinical practice.

Kidney – *Zhi*

The spirit of the kidney is called *zhi*. Often translated as "mind", or "will", this is the faculty that allows for keen senses, skills, intelligence, wisdom, and creativity. *The Basic Questions – Treatise on the Secret Scriptures of the Chamber of Spiritual Orchids (Sù Wèn – Líng Lán Mì Diǎn Lùn)* states, "The kidney holds office of labor, whence ingenuity emanates".

Therefore, when kidney essence is abundant, the sea of marrow is full and the brain-spirit is vigorous. *The Basic Questions – Treatise on the Nature of Life in the Distant Past (Sù Wèn – Shàng Gǔ Tiān Zhēn Lùn)* states, "The kidney governs water, receives essence from the five viscera and six bowels, and stores it".

Fear is the emotion associated with the kidney. *The Basic Questions – Great Treatise on the Correspondences and Manifestation of Yin and Yang (Sù Wèn – Yīn Yáng Yìng Xiàng Dà Lùn)* states, "The mind of the kidney is fear", and *The Spiritual Pivot – Channels and Vessels (Líng Shū – Jīng Mài Piān)* states, "Insufficient qi of the foot *shaoyin* kidney channel leads to susceptibly to fear; one feels apprehensive at heart as if he is about to be

Chapter 3
Five Spirits and the Brain

arrested", and also "Fear that remains unresolved will cause damage to the essence".

These passages show how excessive fear damages the essence-qi of the viscera, also causing disorders of the qi dynamic which not only impair the kidney, but also all other organs including the brain.

Any long term illnesses involving the kidney or chronic psychological weakness can result in an insufficiency of *zhi*. The main symptoms of kidney-*zhi* disorder are dizziness, a lack of willpower, and poor memory, understanding, and concentration. Willpower, concentration, and memory all rely on the consolidating strength of the kidney, while dizziness reflects a vacuity of the brain's essence.

Kidney yin deficiency manifestations include tinnitus, restlessness and mania, a preference for darkness and a dislike of light, a fear of seeing people, sweating at the vertex, insomnia, and other symptoms of essence deficiency such as confusion, forgetfulness, and sluggishness. The kidney governs bones and marrow, and due to its link with the brain, there may also be a hollow feeling in the head, declining intelligence, and poor memory (especially short-term), and also character changes such as increasingly selfish behavior.

The Kidney and Depression

The symptoms of kidney-*zhi* depressive disorder are various, the most significant being brain-related symptoms, and these patterns will always involve multiple organs. For example, with kidney yin deficiency, kidney-water is insufficient to contain liver-wood, resulting in yang hyperactivity symptoms such as headache, a distending feeling of the head, cloudiness, and tinnitus. Some patients report a burning sensation at the vertex. When insufficiency of both heart and kidney affect the heart-spirit, manifestations include insomnia, excessive dreaming, palpitations, discomposure, and irritation.

The heart and kidney together form the foundation of the qi dynamic, and the kidney is the driving force; their complementary functions are also based on the mutual rooting of yin and yang. When kidney yang is activated, fire ascends and water descends to unite and harmonize.

On the surface, the brain is linked with the kidney through the governing vessel and the foot *taiyang* bladder channel, and among all the organs, the kidney is well-paired with brain. The "brain – governing vessel – kidney" axis is the foundation for all the human vital activities. The transportation of essential qi within the body, the ascending and descending of yin and yang, and all physiological activities are dominated by this axis.

In the diagnosis of depression, all of the following relationships should be considered:

① The relationship of kidney yin to heart yin, liver yin and liver blood.

② The relationship of kidney qi and kidney yang to the liver and spleen.

③ How the qi dynamic of the kidney influences brain-spirit function.

Therefore, insufficiency of kidney essence is a critical factor in the pathomechanisms of depression and chronic depression, with different mental symptoms according to the specific pathomechanism. Chronic cases present with decreased memory, difficulty concentrating, lassitude, no strength to speak, timidity, and a susceptibly to fear. In severe cases, there may be a lack of motivation, retardation of thought, a lack of intention, low libido, a tendency to lie down and curl up, a dull anguished facial expression, and a pale white or bluish-yellow complexion.

The heart and kidney together are the foundation of the qi dynamic, with the kidney being the driving force. Qing Dynasty physician Li Zhong-zi stated, "The ascending of water actually relies on the rising of fire qi; the descending of fire relies on the moisture from water-damp". This statement also demonstrates the mutual rooting of yin and yang.

With insufficient kidney yin, the heart and kidney will fail to interact, the heart-spirit cannot be contained, and heart fire will flame upward to disturb the brain-spirit, manifesting with symptoms such as insomnia, forgetfulness, and even seminal emission. Although these symptoms are caused by heart-fire, treatment here should focus on nourishing kidney yin to promote the ascending kidney water in order to calm heart fire and settle the spirit.

In clinical practice, chronic depression may also present with symptoms of low mood, insomnia, amnesia, as well as cold limbs and body. This is due to insufficient kidney yang failing to uplift water. Deficiency fire then goes astray and disturbs the spirit-light. The treatment here is to warm kidney yang.

Chapter 3
Five Spirits and the Brain

When kidney yang is deficient and life gate fire declines, spleen-earth will not be warmed and a dual deficiency of spleen and kidney yang will result. In this case, the foundations of both congenital and acquired constitutions are insufficient, and the brain-spirit will become too weak to function properly. Because of the decline in heart-fire and spleen-earth, clear yang is unable to ascend and turbid yin is unable to descend. The brain lacks nourishment and is also disturbed by turbid yin where phlegm, dampness and turbidity will cloud the brain and brain-spirit. This potentially results in slow and confused thinking and a general lack of concentration. Another characteristic of kidney yang deficiency-related depression is a loss of will to live, and decreased libido.

In some cases, chronic liver constraint and spleen deficiency impairs kidney qi. Treatment here should focus on supplementing spleen and kidney and warming yang, while also resolving phlegm and resolving constraint.

Pharmaceutical medications for treating mental diseases tend to damage liver and kidney yin, and also the original qi of both kidney and spleen. Common side effects of antipsychotic drugs and antidepressants also include sexual dysfunction and menstrual disorders. Frequently, doctors will mistakenly focus on the symptoms of low mood, chest oppression, and insomnia, and treat these patients by simply soothing the liver, regulating qi, clearing heat, and calming the mind. However, psychological problems involving sexual function (such as impotence, seminal emission, and premature ejaculation) and menstruation not only can cause depression, but are also key internal factors when the disease is transforming from an excess to a deficiency pattern. The signs of relative deficiency should be monitored and assessed on a regular basis, because over time, all depression patterns will become deficiency conditions when improperly treated.

The Brain-Spirit

In the study and practice of Chinese medicine, the concept of the five viscera and their five "spirits" has taken an increasingly major role within differential diagnosis. Although the predominant idea in Western medicine is that the brain governs consciousness, theories involving the brain-spirit and heart-spirit can both be applied in clinic. We also believe that an appropriate hybrid model can be created by proposing a "brain-spirit interaction process" that would explain the phenomenon of human mental activity and emotion, also serving as a guide to clinical diagnosis and treatment within the realm of Chinese medical psychotherapy.

Brain function is dynamic and extensive in many respects. As the communication center of the human body, the brain controls vital functions while receiving feedback from the internal organs. The brain stores the spirit, controls the mind, and governs over all other viscera-spirits. The brain is in charge of thought, intelligence, memory, and also sensations, desires, ideation, and movement. By influencing the mind, emotion, behavior, and the five viscera organ spirits, the brain also influences the qi and blood and yin and yang of the five viscera. In such circumstances, the "brain-spirit interaction process" is a functional system directly associated with human physiology.

Qing Dynasty physician Tang Rong-chuan stated, "Marrow is engendered from kidney essence; when essence is sufficient, marrow is produced. Marrow is in the bones; when marrow is produced the bones are strong and thus one is able to labor while possessing superior talent and strength. Essence gives birth to the spirit; when essence is sufficient, the spirit is strong and ingenuity will exist naturally.

The generation and early development of the brain marrow depends on the pre-natal essence, while nourishment from post-natal essence is also necessary for its growth and continuing function. *The Basic Questions – Treatise on the Engenderment of Five Viscera* (*Sù Wèn – Wǔ Zàng Shēng Chéng Piān*) states, "The fluids of the five grains combine to form a paste that percolates into the bone cavities and supplements the brain marrow." The formation, growth and functioning of brain marrow relies on the rarified essence of food and drink as well as from the nourishment provided by qi, blood, and body fluids.

1. The Brain and Consciousness

The spirit provides an external life to human mental activities, consciousness, and thinking, where the five spirits involve different reactions of the human brain to external objective experience. Human emotions have a direct influence on the mind, consciousness and thinking, and when considered as a group, they are indivisible and so collectively

Chapter 3
Five Spirits and the Brain

referred to as the spirit, or spirits.

The original spirit is the name for the spirit that dwells within the brain; this spirit is congenital and also the source of the viscera-spirits. The quote, "The brain is the house of the original spirit" comes from *The Grand Compendium of Materia Medica – Flos Magnoliae* (*Běn Cǎo Gāng Mù – Xīn Yí Tiáo*), which also states, "The qi of the nose is connected to heaven. Heaven is the head and the lung. The lung opens at the nose, and the *yangming* stomach channel circulates around the nose and goes upward. The brain is the house of original spirit, and the nose is the orifice of the life gate. When a person lacks middle qi, clear yang fails to ascend, the head inclines, and the nine orifices become inhibited."

The material basis for consciousness is essence-qi (meaning postnatal essence together with qi in the organs and fluids, etc.) and blood. The spirit comes from this essence-qi, and also reflects brain function. The brain is the organ that dominates the functioning of the spirit, and is also the material basis for mental activities, emotions, and thinking. Vital activities of mentation, consciousness, and wisdom all originate from the brain.

The *Correction of Errors in Medical Works* (*Yī Lín Gǎi Cuò*), Wang Qingren suggested that the brain is directly connected with the sense organs: "The two ears are connected to the brain, and the sound being heard goes to the brain. The two eye ties are like threads originating from the brain, and the image being seen goes to the brain. The nose is connected to the brain, and all aromas go to the brain."

Memory is governed by the brain. In the *Essentials of Materia Medica – Flos Magnoliae* (*Běn Cǎo Bèi Yào – Xīn Yí Tiáo*), Qing Dynasty physician Wang Ang stated, "A person's memory is all within the brain. Forgetfulness among children is related to an unfulfilled brain; forgetfulness among the elderly is related to the brain gradually becoming vacant."

2. Inclinations and Aversions

The brain-spirit is tightly integrated with the viscera and bowels by channels, collaterals and the qi dynamic. These unite the entire body, qi, and mind with the material basis of qi and blood and yin and yang. From the viewpoint of traditional Chinese medicine, the five viscera each have respective likes and dislikes. For example, the spleen prefers dryness and is averse to dampness, and the brain is no exception. It is said that the brain is an organ of both extreme clarity and extreme yang. The qi, blood, and clear yang of the five viscera and six bowels are transported upward to the brain marrow, and in this state, the brain-spirit functions smoothly to exercise an influence over the entire body. The brain is also a place of clarity, which has little tolerance for impurities. If pathogenic factors originating from the viscera and bowels reach the brain, inhibition and dysfunction of the brain-spirit will result. While the head is extreme yang, the essence is effectively extreme yin, and this serves to ground and nourish the brain; it is also pure in nature and cannot tolerate impurity, so physical damage or degradation of its nature through the presence of phlegm or blood stasis will create substantial problems.

(1) Calm and Restlessness

The brain-spirit is clear and refined. It requires calmness to function properly, to sense, to think clearly with stable emotions, and to respond appropriately to external stimulation. In order to properly move the qi and blood of the organs and body parts, the brain-spirit needs to have a "calm residence".

Deficiency of qi and blood, disorders of the qi dynamic, external pathogenic factors, and extreme emotions can all disrupt the harmony and balance of body, qi, and mind. When the spirit is disturbed and the brain-spirit becomes restless, the result is mental confusion, illogical thinking, erroneous perception, and emotional disturbances. These behaviors also lead to disorders of the viscera and bowels and the qi dynamic, also forming a vicious cycle.

The *Standards for Diagnosis and Treatment – General Introduction* (*Zhèng Zhì Zhǔn Shéng – Zǒng Lùn*) states, "With quietness, the spirit is stored; with agitation, it disperses and expires. Quietness is the substance of water, and agitation is the function of fire. Therefore, with a quiet personality, the heart can be preserved in the center, but when the emotions are disturbed, the heart becomes lost in the outside world."

(2) Free Activity vs. Inhibition and Constraint

The brain and the brain-spirit dominate the entire human body,

Chapter 3
Five Spirits and the Brain

provided that the brain-spirit is not constrained. In traditional Chinese medicine, the liver is critical to the qi dynamic and to governing the free flow of qi; with proper functioning, the brain-spirit also works smoothly to exercise influence over the entire body.

When the circulation of qi and blood is smooth and unobstructed, the clear qi of the viscera and bowels ascend and turbid qi descends. Under such circumstances, instructions from the brain-spirit are able to reach the viscera and bowels, orifices, and all other body parts. If the qi dynamic is disturbed for any reason, qi and blood fails to flow upward. Qi dynamic disorders of ascending and descending, and also the inward and outward flow of qi can also cause constraint that will affect the brain. Without the proper functioning of the brain and the brain-spirit, other disorders further worsen and so begin a series of deteriorating patterns associated with the brain-spirit.

(3) Coolness, Dryness and Heat

The mind dwells within the brain, which is located at the topmost part of the body; thus the brain is referred to as the chief of all yang. The governing vessel also governs the yang of the entire body by joining with the yang qi of the three foot yang channels that reach the head. Since yang qi is hot in nature, it thus desires coolness and is averse to excess dryness and heat. With appropriate coolness, the brain-spirit remains clear and stimulated, the emotions are calm and stable, and the qi dynamic of the viscera and bowels is in order. Confusion of the brain-spirit, emotional disorders, and abnormal behaviors can occur when the mind is over stimulated or disturbed by pathogenic heat including excess heat in liver channel, ascendant hyperactivity of liver yang, *yangming* heat, or external pathogenic heat associated with warm diseases.

(4) Softness and Moistening

The brain-spirit is said to be averse to harshness, and prefers the qualities of softness and moistening. The yang of the brain and the brain-spirit needs to be complemented by the relative yin of qi and blood. Therefore, nourishment from qi and blood of the organs is critical for the brain and the brain-spirit. Without softness and moistening, the brain and brain-spirit functions become distorted and harsh, manifesting with symptoms like convulsive spasms, mental cloudiness, perverse emotions, and abnormal behaviors.

Softness and moistening of the brain relies on the nourishment provided by yin-blood, thus also greatly affected by heart blood, liver yin, and kidney essence. If heart blood, liver yin and kidney essence are in abundance, the brain and brain-spirit will have sufficient nourishment.

With multiple deficiencies, the clinical condition is generally worse. These typically include dual deficiencies of yin and blood, heart and spleen, qi and blood, spleen and kidney, or a disconnection between heart and kidney; any of these may lead to insufficient moistening and nourishment of the brain-spirit. Any of the above factors may also interact to become the main pathomechanism of a brain-spirit disease.

In summation, the brain-spirit is in many ways a modification of the heart-spirit that is more familiar in the practice of Chinese medicine. Its requirements and characteristics are different primarily in its close relationship with the essence, and its position in the head. The manifestation of thought and emotional process in the body from the earliest writings about the mind in Chinese thought, particularly Mencius, emphasize the role of the heart, but also with the term essence-spirit (*jingshen* 精神), a pairing that we again find here with the "sea of marrow" as providing a ground for the spirit. The brain-spirit, as with the heart spirit, encompasses and manages the other spirits, whose presence is largely known only through their dysfunction. While this text proposes some novel treatments based around the concept of the brain-spirit, the general concepts regarding management of spirit disorders are also intact. The only substantial difference is that with the brain-spirit, there is another possible location for the illness to manifest and persist, and these persistent manifestations can be effectively reduced and eliminated with many of the methods provided in this text.

Chapter 4
Etiology and Pathomechanism

As part of nature and human society, individuals are constantly influenced by their interactions with any number of social, cultural, and environmental factors. From a holistic viewpoint, depression is a systemic disease characterized by abnormal moods and emotions, generally associated with patterns of qi constraint and inhibition of the brain-spirit. There is no single causative factor, the pathomechanism cannot be limited to any single organ or organ system, and there are many possible etiologies. The principal symptom is not limited to depressed moods, and the main pattern is not only limited to liver constraint with qi stagnation. This condition cannot be treated effectively with any single therapy, medication, or system.

Etiology

The etiology of depressive disorders involves the internal and external factors that result in inhibition of the qi dynamic, functional disorders of the viscera and bowels, qi and blood disorders, inhibition of brain-spirit, and emotional depression. The main causative factors are summarized as **follows:**

1. Emotional Disorders

Depressive disorders can result from any impairment associated the seven emotions. Emotional states also reflect the functional status of the brain-spirit, the five viscera, and qi and blood. Normal emotional activity relies on proper organ function as well as the essential qi and yin and yang of the internal organs; emotion can also be viewed as a normal reaction of the brain-spirit and the five viscera-spirits to external stimuli. Mental activities and emotion will manifest in accordance with the stimulation provided by the external environment. The emotional constitution of an individual will vary from one person to another, also affected by environmental factors, age, culture of origin, and personal values.

Extreme or prolonged emotional states can impair organ function, disrupt the balance of qi, blood, yin, and yang, and thus lead to physical disease. Depression disease can also result from this sort of gradual erosion. Persistent and extreme stimulation will exacerbate the emotions of sorrow, anxiety and anger. Among the emotions, these three are the most pathogenic in that they can impair their related organs while also

Chapter 4
Etiology and Pathomechanism

causing constraint and stagnation of the qi dynamic. Let us now examine how emotional movements specifically affect organ function.

Anger: Anger overwhelms the function of the liver. When the liver fails to course freely, patterns of liver qi stagnation and a general inhibition of the qi dynamic will result.

Unfulfilled Desires, Anxiety, and Rumination: These emotional states typically cause qi to bind and dissipate. Over time they can damage the spleen and lung, leading to splenic transportation failure and impaired effusion and downbearing of the lung; both can have a negative impact on the brain-spirit. In clinical practice, chronic or latent depressive disorders usually fall under this category. This scenario is consistent in those patients that initially present with symptoms of acute depression based on the previous model, and then, as liver constraint progressively damages the spleen, the manifestations of this pattern will appear.

Fright and Fear: Fright and fear impair and consume kidney qi. When the kidney fails to support the liver and spleen, they become progressively weaker; the result can also involve inhibition of the brain-spirit and the onset of depression disease.

Multiple Emotions: Emotional patterns involving several organs are obviously harder to diagnose than those which only impact one organ. While it is actually uncommon that a patient would present with a single pathology, there will generally be an element of continuity that will point to one specific aspect of the emotional situation. It is important to realize that extreme emotional states do not always manifest consistently, and while it is informative to gather information about a "precipitating event", other presenting emotional states should not be discounted even when they appear to be inconsistent with the initial cause. Most patterns will transform over time, and for this reason, causative emotional factors and the actual diagnosis may seem to be greatly incongruent, especially in chronic cases.

Some cases of depression are not a result of any specific emotional stimulus because other more primary pathologies can also manifest with emotional disorders as an accompanying symptom. In any case, an inhibition of emotion can be characterized as the initial stage of a depressive disorder, often caused by a combination of psychological and constitutional factors. In such cases, the emotional state can be viewed as a causative factor, with the constitutional issue contributing as an internal factor.

2. Constitutional Factors and Internal Origins

Physiological function and psychological activities are a combination of the inherited and acquired, involving both nature and nurture. Factors affecting the individual constitution are many; these include innate endowment, physical environment, emotional environment, age, gender, diet, lifestyle, and medical factors such as medication or illness. However, some depression cases will have no apparent emotional cause associated with the personal history or environment, and in such cases, the cause would be more associated with the individual constitution as an internal factor. In traditional Chinese medicine, personality traits such as boldness or timidity, susceptibly to fright, rumination, worry, or even a tendency to be over-delighted are all regarded as manifestations of the brain-spirit and five viscera-spirits, and also a reflection of the state of qi and blood function in the five viscera.

3. Iatrogenic Factors

Iatrogenic or medically induced factors should not be ignored in the diagnosis and treatment of depression. Traditional Chinese medicine has long been aware that the inappropriate use of medicinals can cause mental disorders. In modern times, many pharmaceuticals have been shown to induce a low mood similar to those of depression; psychotic symptoms may also appear in severe cases. For example, we should look carefully at those patients prescribed with digitalis, barbiturates, ethanol, amphetamines, opiates and ampicillin. In the development of many common diseases such as cardiovascular and cerebrovascular diseases, vitamin deficiency, endocrine disorders, and cancer, some patients may display symptoms of mental depression that interact with the primary disease. These factors should all be taken into consideration.

Because of the differences in the nature and degree of the negative

Chapter 4
Etiology and Pathomechanism

stimulus, and the constitutional differences in patients, liver constraint often influences the viscera and bowels in different ways to result in distinctly different presentations. Some cases are caused by persistent negative emotional stimuli and a failure to fulfill one's desires and plans.

When fear is the main cause, deficiency of the kidney-mind and impairment of kidney qi may consume the original spirit. This eventually results in a pattern of dual deficiency of the liver and kidney and essence insufficiency. As liver qi becomes inhibited and the liver functions of ascending and dispersion are impaired, malnourishment of the brain-spirit will manifest with a low mood and listlessness.

As emotional factors cause qi and blood disharmony and inhibition of the qi dynamic that impair the viscera and bowels, qi constraint is usually the first pattern that manifests, often followed by patterns of food constraint, phlegm constraint, fire constraint, heat constraint, and blood constraint. These cases are initially of an excess nature, but as upright qi is consumed, complex patterns of deficiency and excess will appear. Eventually, patterns of deficiency will become more predominant.

The pathological locations involve primarily the brain and liver, but the spleen, heart, kidney, gallbladder, and lung may also become affected.

The most common patterns include:

1) Liver constraint with phlegm stagnation
2) Liver constraint with qi stagnation
3) Qi stagnation and static blood
4) Dual yin deficiency of the liver and kidney
5) Liver constraint with spleen deficiency

In some cases, depression appears concurrently with other conditions. If the patient suffers with a chronic disease, depression may develop as a result of persistent frustration, sadness, anger, or anxiety. These emotions may be related to the illness itself or financial stress, interpersonal relationships, and other factors related to the chronic disease. When the pathology of the primary disease directly inhibits or damages the movement of qi and blood or yin and yang of the viscera and bowels, depression can also result.

Pathological products such as phlegm and static blood may obstruct the brain collaterals and brain marrow (or, in a more traditional sense, the heart orifices) also leading to dysfunction of the brain-spirit. Phlegm retention and blood stasis may obstruct the qi dynamic and cause chronic low moods and depression.

Depression cases in these categories may be accompanied by:
1) Debilitation of heart yang
2) Insufficiency of qi and blood
3) Yin deficiency of lung and kidney
4) Decline of the brain-spirit (in the elderly or weak)
5) Cancer, tumors or masses
6) Decline of kidney qi.

Sometimes depression is secondary to other brain-spirit diseases as well as to menstrual or postpartum conditions. In clinical practice, depression is often intertwined with the original disease, making it difficult to clearly differentiate. Depression worsens when the primary disease worsens, and vice versa. This kind of vicious cycle makes diagnosis and treatment more difficult. Concurrent patterns are inextricably linked to one another and cannot be treated in isolation, so a proper diagnosis and treatment must take into account all coexisting pathologies.

Pathomechanisms

1. Qi Constraint

Qi constraint is the core pathomechanism of depression, especially when caused by emotional factors, with liver constraint and qi stagnation as the primary pathomechanisms. Other pathomechanisms are usually a progression of qi constraint patterns, the major exception being those cases primarily associated with deficiency. The qi dynamic influences all aspects of physiology, and qi movement disorders play a decisive role in pathology.

Again, the root of qi constraint as a pathomechanism usually involves binding constraint of liver qi, but patterns of qi deficiency, phlegm-damp obstructing, heat and fire constraint, food stagnation, and blood stasis can also affect the qi dynamic. In any case, the fundamental treatment principle here is to regulate qi.

Chapter 4
Etiology and Pathomechanism

(1) Clinical Manifestations

Symptoms of qi constraint associated with the liver include distending fullness of rib-sides, the back, the waist, or the shoulder and scapular region. Other manifestations include chest tightness, a sensation of a foreign body in the throat, abdominal distension, poor appetite, belching, nausea, reduced food intake, painful distension of lower abdomen, painful swelling of the breasts, and menstrual disorders in women and problems with ejaculation and urination in men.

(2) Prognosis

One of the possible outcomes is spontaneous recovery by self-regulation, although the qi dynamic may also be restored by psychotherapy, medication, or other interventions. Another possible outcome is the worsening of qi stagnation which will impair the circulation of blood and fluid distribution. This may result in the formation of blood stasis, internal dampness, phlegm accumulation, and fluid retention.

Other associated patterns may include:

1) Liver constraint and spleen deficiency
2) Liver-stomach disharmony
3) Non-interaction of heart and kidney
4) Splenic failure of transportation
5) Impaired diffusion and downbearing of the lung
6) Stagnation of phlegm and fluid
7) Constraint of fire and heat resulting in fluids transforming into phlegm
8) Phlegm binding with fire
9) Phlegm-turbidity confounding the heart
10) Liver constraint and phlegm binding
11) Qi stagnation and static blood
12) Upward flaming of liver fire
13) Hyperactivity of liver yang
14) Hyperactivity of heart fire
15) Liver and kidney yin deficiency.

Qi constraint may also transform into heat, phlegm, or fire constraint as described below:

2. Heat (Fire) Constraint

When internal heat and fire are associated with depression, the pathomechanism initially involves an underlying pattern of qi constraint. Because qi is yang in nature, qi constraint patterns often transform into internal fire when left untreated. Those with yang excess or yin deficiency constitutions are especially prone to the development of pathogenic internal heat.

In most cases, patterns of constrained heat are initially associated with the liver. However, hyperactive fire may also result from patterns of heart and kidney yin deficiency, liver qi invading the spleen, or phlegm accumulation. Any of these may also combine with static blood. Western pharmaceuticals often aggravate existing patterns of internal fire and heat, and as drug toxicity accumulates, this may itself become a pathogenic factor.

Excess *yangming* heat is commonly involved with subsequent damage to yin-fluids. Fire patterns can appear in any stage of depression, and the corresponding treatment principles are to clear heat, nourish yin, and purge *yangming* heat.

3. Phlegm Constraint

Phlegm constraint manifests with low spirits, fatigue, somnolence, nausea, stuffiness, and depression. Phlegm constraint is also a common pathomechanism in cases of depression disease because phlegm is a contributing factor which allows qi constraint to transform into other pathomechanisms. This occurrence marks a turning point in the condition where a complex pattern of deficiency and excess will appear; these conditions are more difficult to treat.

Phlegm constraint can be caused by qi constraint or an insufficiency of yang qi. Viscera and bowel patterns may involve liver-wood invading spleen-earth which leads to spleen deficiency with splenic failure to transform water-damp; thus the saying "The spleen is the source of phlegm formation". Phlegm can also form as a result of damp-turbidity caused by an improper diet and non-transformation of food.

Chapter 4
Etiology and Pathomechanism

4. Static Blood

Blood stasis can result from knocks and falls, bleeding, qi stagnation, qi deficiency, and blood-cold or blood-heat impairing the blood. In clinical practice, the main symptoms include localized pain, abdominal masses, bleeding (especially from the vagina), abdominal distention, a dusky purple tongue with stasis speckles or macula, and wiry or rough pulses.

The main causes of bleeding include:
1) External injury
2) Spleen failing to control blood
3) Liver failing to store blood
4) Blood-heat
5) Hyperactive liver yang
6) Sudden swelling of the vessels.

Blood that has left the channels will obstruct the vessels, including the brain collaterals. When qi and blood cannot circulate normally and the brain collaterals are obstructed, depression may also result. When blood stasis overwhelms the heart, abnormal behaviors such as raving, delirious speech, and mania may occur.

5. Phlegm-fire

Constrained qi can transform to fire which condenses fluids into phlegm while also consuming yin. In some cases, fire is as result of phlegm accumulation; disorders of fluid distribution cause fluid retention and phlegm formation that obstructs the free flow of qi and over a period of time, internal heat and fire will become generated.

Patterns of phlegm binding with fire can cause damage anywhere in the body. When phlegm-fire confounds the brain and obstructs the brain-spirit, inhibition of the brain-spirit and depression disease will result. Symptoms include low mood, insomnia, forgetfulness, irritability, angry outbursts, and impulsiveness. It is also important to understand that phlegm-fire can also combine and interact with patterns of internal wind.

6. Deficiency Patterns

Deficiency patterns can also serve as a main pathomechanism in depression cases. Ming Dynasty physician Sun Yi-kui discussed deficiency-type depression in the *Black Pearl from Red Waters – Categories of Depression* (*Chì Shuǐ Xuán Zhū – Yù Mén*): "For people with deficiency-type constitutions, any displeasure can lead to dizziness, blurred vision, low spirits, sinew wilting, and rapid breathing; this resembles the manifestations of deficiency patterns. Treatment should primarily open constraint and normalize qi, and the qi disease will resolve spontaneously."

Deficiencies of qi and yang, especially kidney yang, frequently cause fluid retention and phlegm accumulation that will inhibit the brain-spirit. With essence deficiency, there will be insufficient nourishment for the brain and marrow; this causes the brain-spirit to lose its foundation.

Deficiency caused by constraint is another common pathomechanism. For *shaoyin* yang constraint patterns, *Sì Nì Sǎn* (Counterflow Cold Powder) can be prescribed to soothe the liver and regulate qi.

Chapter 5
Zang-fu Patterns and Treatment

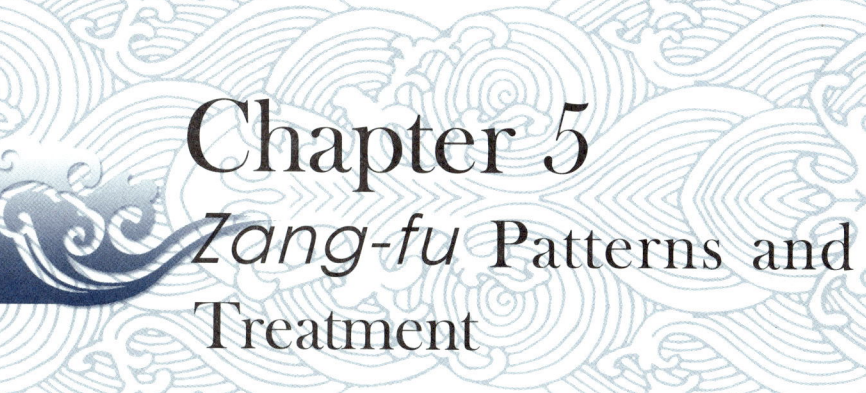

Etiology

Depression can result from stress, persistent mental stimulation, or duress related to marriage, finances, work, or study. When stressors manifest beyond the body's ability to manage, irregular emotions will first begin to affect the liver and its ability to regulate the qi dynamic. Constrained liver qi fails to course and drain, orderly reaching fails and the qi dynamic becomes inhibited, further disrupting the normal movement of qi. Liver dysfunction in this case leads to the physical and emotional inhibition characteristic of depression disease.

Pathomechanism

The early symptoms of depression are said to "begin by emerging in the liver" and low spirits are the main manifestation. Constrained liver-wood can also damage spleen-earth, and intention is stored in the spleen; therefore, signs of depression are often accompanied by spleen-stomach symptoms as well as over-thinking and rumination.

During the initial stage of depression, excess patterns are most predominant as liver qi constraint often transforms into heat. Fire by nature flames upward where it can also combine with heart fire to cause heart vexation, irascibility, agitation and sleeplessness. During the initial or middle stages of illness, exuberant heart fire can scorch the lung and affect the corporeal soul to cause frequent weeping, sorrow, and even suicidal tendencies. Over time, enduring patterns of liver qi constraint may result in the five-phase pattern of "the child stealing the mother's qi" where irregularities of qi, yin, and yang of the liver also impact the kidney. The kidney-mind is thus affected, also resulting in malnourishment of the brain-spirit. Manifestations include poor memory, no interest in previously enjoyable activities, and even suicidal tendencies. Relatively acute symptoms such as these usually occur among those patients with chronic conditions or predominant deficiency patterns.

Clinical Guidelines

1. Pattern Characteristics

Low spirits, worry, anxiety, unstable moods, irascibility, no interest in previously enjoyable activities, no strength to speak or move, pessimism, despair, guilt, poor memory, seminal emission, impotence, a tendency to lie down, sleeplessness, torpid intake, no appetite, and possible suicidal tendencies.

2. Pathological Location

The pathology of depression is primarily related to irregularities of brain-spirit, although the five main viscera are also affected to some degree. While there are similarities, the clinical symptoms will manifest somewhat differently depending upon which particular organ is affected.

When the liver is primarily involved, manifestations include unstable moods, vexation, agitation, irascibility, distending fullness of the chest and rib-sides, frequent vomiting, reticence, no appetite, anxiety, fidgetiness, and low spirits.

When the heart is primarily involved, manifestations include constrained emotions, over-thinking, abstraction of the spirit, palpitations, susceptibility to fright, sleeplessness, profuse dreaming, and difficulty falling asleep with a tendency to wake up easily in fright.

When the spleen is primarily involved, manifestations include anxiety, heaviness of the extremities, torpid intake, loose stools, abdominal distention, constipation, difficulty falling asleep, waking up early, susceptibility to fright, emaciation, a bright white facial complexion, fatigue, laziness, and suicidal ideation with no will to carry it out.

When the lung is primarily involved, manifestations include shortness of breath, no strength to speak, sighing with an inability to catch one's breath, sorrow and weeping.

When the kidney is primarily involved, manifestations include a substantial decline in memory, no strength to speak or move about, a tendency to lie down, a general lack of interest, no faith in the worth of a life or career, sighing, frequent suicidal ideation and behaviors, low libido, impotence, seminal emission, and cold limbs. This presentation is especially common among the elderly and in cases of long-term depression.

3. Pathological Characteristics

Generally speaking, depression disease involves deficiency as the root, with excess manifestations as the branch. The initial stage may be of short duration and with a predominantly excess presentation; the middle stage may display mixed patterns of deficiency and excess. In the late or chronic stage there can also be excess within deficiency, but the deficiency pattern is generally more predominant. The pathological locations associated with the early and middle stages usually involve the liver, heart, spleen and lung; the late stage generally affects the spleen and kidney. The most commonly seen excess patterns are qi stagnation, phlegm exuberance, and blood stasis, and root deficiencies will involve depletions of qi, blood, and fluids.

Pattern Differentiation and Treatment

1. Mild Depressive Disorder

Patients with mild depressive disorder usually fail to attend to the illness in the early stages. Some patients may be strongly cognizant of their physical discomfort and low appetite, yet physical examination is often unremarkable.

(1) LIVER CONSTRAINT AND QI STAGNATION

Manifestations: mood swings, anxiety, restlessness, sleeplessness, frequent sighing, irascibility, heart vexation, worry, sorrow, a red tongue with a white slimy coating, and wiry pulses. Urination and defecation are often normal.

Accompanying signs and symptoms may include stomach-duct discomfort, distending fullness of the chest and rib-sides, reduced appetite, torpid intake, nausea, vomiting; also menstrual irregularities, menstrual pain, or amenorrhea among women.

Principles: course the liver, resolve constraint, regulate the brain-spirit.

Formula: Modified *Chái Hú Shū Gān Sǎn* (Bupleurum Liver-Soothing Powder)

柴胡	*chái hú*	6g	Radix Bupleuri
郁金	*yù jīn*	30g	Radix Curcumae
香附	*xiāng fù*	10g	Rhizoma Cyperi

Chapter 5
Zang-fu Patterns and Treatment

白芍	bái sháo	30g	Radix Paeoniae Alba
青皮	qīng pí	10g	Pericarpium Citri Reticulatae Viride
陈皮	chén pí	10g	Pericarpium Citri Reticulatae
法半夏	fǎ bàn xià	10g	Rhizoma Pinelliae Praeparatum
砂仁	shā rén	10g	Fructus Amomi
栀子	zhī zǐ	10g	Fructus Gardeniae
牡丹皮	mǔ dān pí	10g	Cortex Moutan
炙甘草	zhì gān cǎo	6g	Radix et Rhizoma Glycyrrhizae Praeparata cum Melle
生石膏	shēng shí gāo	30–60g	Gypsum Fibrosum Cruda (decocted first)
天竺黄	tiān zhú huáng	15g	Concretio Silicea Bambusae

Modifications:

➤ For predominant heat patterns manifesting with a bitter taste in the mouth and dry bound stools, add *dà huáng* (Radix et Rhizoma Rhei) 10g and *lóng dǎn cǎo* (Radix et Rhizoma Gentianae) 6–10g to drain heat and free the bowels.

➤ For liver qi invading the spleen with manifestions of scurrying pain in the rib-sides, clamoring stomach, belching, and acid reflux or vomiting add *suō luó zǐ* (Semen Aesculi) 30g, *wǎ léng zǐ* (Concha Arcae) 20g and *chuān liàn zǐ* (Fructus Toosendan); with red eyes, add *jú huā* (Flos Chrysanthemi) 15g, *bái jí lí* (Fructus Tribuli) 30g and *gōu téng* (Ramulus Uncariae Cum Uncis) 30g.

➤ For liver yang hyperactivity with manifestions of dizziness, blurred vision and tinnitus, add *shēng shí jué míng* (Concha Haliotidis, raw) 30g, *cí shí* (Magnetitum) 30–60g, and *zhēn zhū mǔ* (Concha Margaritiferae Usta) 30g.

(2) LIVER CONSTRAINT WITH PHLEGM BINDING

Manifestations: low spirits, frequent irascibility, no strength to move or speak, no feeling of pleasure, reduced sleep, vexation, agitation, poor memory, slow responses, self criticism and self-reproach, fright, fear, reduced appetite, torpid intake, dry stools, frequent turbid urine, a red tongue with a slimy white coating, and wiry slippery pulses.

Accompanying symptoms may include distending fullness and

scurrying pain in the chest, rib-sides and stomach duct, frequent belching and vomiting, palpitations, fearful throbbing, dizziness, and blurred vision.

Principles: course the liver, sweep phlegm, arouse the brain, calm the spirit.

Formula: Modified *Wēn Dǎn Tāng* (Gallbladder-Warming Decoction)

茯苓	*fú líng*	30g	Poria
法半夏	*fǎ bàn xià*	10g	Rhizoma Pinelliae Praeparatum
黄芩	*huáng qín*	10g	Radix Scutellariae
胆南星	*dǎn nán xīng*	10g	Arisaema cum Bile
竹茹	*zhú rú*	6g	Caulis Bambusae in Taenia
陈皮	*chén pí*	10g	Pericarpium Citri Reticulatae
炒枳壳	*chǎo zhǐ qiào*	10g	Fructus Aurantii (stir-fried)
郁金	*yù jīn*	30g	Radix Curcumae
栀子	*zhī zǐ*	10g	Fructus Gardeniae
石菖蒲	*shí chāng pú*	6g	Rhizoma Acori Tatarinowii
甘草	*gān cǎo*	10g	Radix et Rhizoma Glycyrrhizae

Modifications:

➤ With vexation, agitation, and irascibility, add *shēng shí gāo* (Gypsum Fibrosum Cruda, decocted first) 80–300g, *cí shí* (Magnetitum, decocted first) 30–60g, and *zhēn zhū mǔ* (Concha Margaritiferae Usta, decocted first) 30g.

➤ With a red tongue and a yellow slimy coating, add *huáng lián* (Rhizoma Coptidis) 12g and *pèi lán* (Herba Eupatorii) 12g.

➤ With poor appetite, add *shén qū* (Massa Medicata Fermentata) 12g and *chǎo mài yá* (Fructus Hordei Germinatus, stir-fried) 30g.

➤ With dry stools, add *niú xī* (Radix Achyranthis Bidentatae) 30g, *dà huáng* (Radix et Rhizoma Rhei) 15g, and *lái fú zǐ* (Semen Raphani) 30g.

(3) Qi Stagnation and Blood Stasis

Manifestations: vexation, agitation, decreased sleep with profuse dreaming, headache, dizziness, low spirits, frequent sighing, forgetfulness, somnolence, palpitations, dry stools, a red tongue with purple spots, stasis

Chapter 5
Zang-fu Patterns and Treatment

macules and a white slimy coating.

Accompanying symptoms may include no pleasure in eating, generalized discomfort, slow movements and speech, fixed staring, occasional auditory hallucinations; among women there can be menstrual irregularities, breast distention, and generally intermittent manifestations.

Principles: rectify qi, resolve phlegm, clear the brain, calm the spirit.

Formula:

Modified *Xuè Fǔ Zhú Yū Tāng* （Blood Stasis Expelling Decoction）

柴胡	chái hú	6g	Radix Bupleuri
郁金	yù jīn	30g	Radix Curcumae
炒枳壳	chǎo zhǐ qiào	10g	Fructus Aurantii (stir-fried)
当归	dāng guī	15g	Radix Angelicae Sinensis
川芎	chuān xiōng	20g	Rhizoma Chuanxiong
赤芍	chì sháo	30g	Radix Paeoniae Rubra
桃仁	táo rén	10g	Semen Persicae
红花	hóng huā	10g	Flos Carthami
牛膝	niú xī	30g	Radix Achyranthis Bidentatae
茯苓	fú líng	30g	Poria
生地	shēng dì	30g	Radix Rehmanniae
香附	xiāng fù	10g	Rhizoma Cyperi
大黄	dà huáng	10g	Radix et Rhizoma Rhei (preserved in liquor)

Modifications:

➢ With fidgetiness and heart vexation, add *zhī zǐ* (Fructus Gardeniae) 12g, *xuán shēn* (Radix Scrophulariae) 30g and *mài mén dōng* (Radix Ophiopogonis) 30g.

➢ With sleeplessness, add *chǎo zǎo rén* (Semen Ziziphi Spinosae, stir-fried) 30–80g.

➢ With amenorrhea, add *é zhú* (Rhizoma Curcumae) 15g, *zé lán* (Herba Lycopi) 30g and *chuān niú xī* (Radix Cyathulae) 30g.

➢ With stomach duct oppression and poor appetite, add *chǎo shān zhā* (Fructus Crataegi, stir-fried) 10g and *shén qū* (Massa Medicata Fermentata) 15g.

(4) Heart and Liver Heat Ascending

Manifestations: unstable moods, vexation, agitation, impulsive behavior, fear, suspicion, despair, an eagerness to be cured, sleeplessness, red face and eyes, intense facial expressions, a preference for cold drinks, constipation, turbid urine, a red tongue with a yellow slimy coating, and wiry rapid pulses.

Accompanying symptoms may include frequent sweating and frequent dream-disturbed sleep.

Principles: clear heart heat, drain the liver, open the orifices, calm the spirit.

Formula: Modified *Sì Huáng Zhī Zǐ Tāng* (Four Yellows and Gardenia Decoction)

黄连	*huáng lián*	10g	Rhizoma Coptidis
黄芩	*huáng qín*	10g	Radix Scutellariae
黄柏	*huáng bǎi*	10g	Cortex Phellodendri Chinensis
大黄	*dà huáng*	10g	Radix et Rhizoma Rhei (preserved in liquor)
栀子	*zhī zǐ*	10g	Fructus Gardeniae
生石膏	*shēng shí gāo*	30-80g	Gypsum Fibrosum Cruda (decocted first)
磁石	*cí shí*	30g	Magnetitum (decocted first)
牛膝	*niú xī*	30g	Radix Achyranthis Bidentatae
炒枣仁	*chǎo zǎo rén*	30g	Semen Ziziphi Spinosae (stir-fried)
钩藤	*gōu téng*	30g	Ramulus Uncariae Cum Uncis

Modifications:
- With thirst and a preference for cold drinks, use *shēng shí gāo* (Gypsum Fibrosum Cruda, decocted first) 180–380g and add *zhī mǔ* (Rhizoma Anemarrhenae) 12g.
- With a red tongue and a slimy coating, add *huáng lián* (Rhizoma Coptidis) 12g, *pèi lán* (Herba Eupatorii) 12g and *shén qū* (Massa Medicata Fermentata) 15g.
- With dry stools and constipation, add *shēng dà huáng* (Radix et Rhizoma Rhei, raw) 15g, and *máng xiāo* (Natrii Sulfas).

When appearing in otherwise healthy people, etiologies of the four

Chapter 5
Zang-fu Patterns and Treatment

preceding patterns usually share the following characteristics:

1) Unexpected death of a family member, death of a spouse, or children
2) Natural or man-made disasters
3) Marital difficulties
4) Unexpected financial problems
5) Severe difficulty with one's social circle

Patients with mild depression are still able to work and maintain their social lives, but they occasionally experience low spirits and deeply pensive thoughts and anxiety when alone. They are fully aware of their condition, are willing to change, and want to resolve their condition.

Special attention should be paid to patients presenting with exuberant heat in the heart and liver because the volatile nature of heat causes both the pathomechanism and progression of the disease to become very changeable; the condition can change drastically within days. In these cases, add medicinals with stronger sedative functions while also clearing and draining evil heat from the heart, liver and stomach.

In this type of case, hallucinations may not appear at the onset, however, the condition can become drastically aggravated when effulgent heat disturbs the brain-spirit; hallucinations and violent self-damaging or suicidal behaviors may appear. This pattern is characteristic of younger people and is relatively rare among the elderly. With this type of patient, the physician also needs to emphasize to the family the importance of taking all medications on schedule.

2. Moderate Depressive Disorder

With delayed or improper treatment, the initial condition can often become more severe. With moderate depressive disorder, although an awareness of the subjective symptoms remains, the patient's activities in daily living, work, and social life are generally affected, usually accompanied by self-reproach and self-blame to different degrees. Severe depression can be almost completely debilitating.

Commonly seen patterns include the following:

65

(1) Heart and Spleen Dual Deficiency

Manifestations: enduring disease, low spirits, uneasiness, anxiety, worry, oppression, sleeplessness, profuse dreaming, poor appetite, torpid intake, fright, palpitations, fearful throbbing, emaciation, a bright white facial complexion, shortness of breath, laconic speech, a tendency to lie down, fatigue, lack of strength, irregular defecation or loose stools, a pale red tongue with a white coating, and fine sunken pulses.

Accompanying signs and symptoms may include distending fullness of the stomach duct, generalized scurrying pain, over-thinking, spontaneous sweating, night sweats, heart vexation, irascibility, self-reproach, and suicidal tendencies without a strong will to act on them.

Principles: supplement heart and spleen, nourish the brain, calm the spirit.

Formula: Modified *Sì Jūn Zǐ Tāng* (Four Gentlemen Decoction)

党参	dǎng shēn	15g	Radix Codonopsis
炒白术	chǎo bái zhú	15g	Rhizoma Atractylodis Macrocephalae (mix-fried)
茯苓	fú líng	30g	Poria
炙甘草	zhì gān cǎo	6g	Radix et Rhizoma Glycyrrhizae Praeparata cum Melle
麦门冬	mài mén dōng	30g	Radix Ophiopogonis
百合	bǎi hé	30g	Bulbus Lilii
当归	dāng guī	15g	Radix Angelicae Sinensis
炒枣仁	chǎo zǎo rén	30g	Semen Ziziphi Spinosae (stir-fried)
天竺黄	tiān zhú huáng	15g	Concretio Silicea Bambusae
郁金	yù jīn	30g	Radix Curcumae
石菖蒲	shí chāng pú	6g	Rhizoma Acori Tatarinowii
女贞子	nǚ zhēn zǐ	30g	Fructus Ligustri Lucidi
神曲	shén qū	15g	Massa Medicata Fermentata

Modifications:
- With loose stools and frequent urination, add *bǔ gǔ zhī* (Fructus Psoraleae) 30g, *yì zhì rén* (Fructus Alpiniae Oxyphyllae) 15g, and *dà zǎo* (Fructus Jujubae) 10g.
- With frequent weeping, add *bǎi hé* (Bulbus Lilii) 60g.

Chapter 5
Zang-fu Patterns and Treatment

- ➢ With severe insomnia, add *chǎo zǎo rén* (Semen Ziziphi Spinosae, stir-fried) 30–80g, *hé huān pí* (Cortex Albiziae) 30g, and *yuǎn zhì* (Radix Polygalae) 10g.
- ➢ With poor memory, add *tù sī zǐ* (Semen Cuscutae) 30g and *shān zhū yú* (Fructus Corni) 15g.
- ➢ With low libido, add *tù sī zǐ* (Semen Cuscutae) 60g and *xiān líng pí* (Herba Epimedii) 15g.

(2) Liver Constraint with Spleen Deficiency

Manifestations: low spirits, difficulty falling asleep and being easily awakened, profuse nightmares, a tendency to become lost in thought, over-thinking, an inability to focus, pessimism, despair, an inability to decide whether to live or die, a bright white facial complexion, emaciation, lack of strength, fatigue, lassitude, a tendency to lie down, loose stools, a pale red tongue with a white coating, and fine wiry pulses.

Accompanying signs and symptoms may include decreased appetite, distending fullness of the stomach duct, scurrying pain in the chest and rib-sides, and low libido.

Principles: course the liver, fortify the spleen, nourish the brain, calm the spirit.

Formula: Modified *Yuè Jú Wán* (Constraint-Resolving Pill)

苍术	cāng zhú	30g	Rhizoma Atractylodis
香附	xiāng fù	10g	Rhizoma Cyperi
川芎	chuān xiōng	20g	Rhizoma Chuanxiong
神曲	shén qū	15g	Massa Medicata Fermentata
栀子	zhī zǐ	10g	Fructus Gardeniae
太子参	tài zǐ shēn	30g	Radix Pseudostellariae
茯苓	fú líng	30g	Poria
大枣	dà zǎo	10g	Fructus Jujubae
郁金	yù jīn	30g	Radix Curcumae
炒枣仁	chǎo zǎo rén	30g	Semen Ziziphi Spinosae (stir-fried)

Modifications:
- ➢ Use no more than 60g *fú líng* (Poria).
- ➢ With palpitations and flusteredness, add *tài zǐ shēn* (Radix

Pseudostellariae) 30g, *mài mén dōng* (Radix Ophiopogonis) 30g and *wǔ wèi zǐ* (Fructus Schisandrae Chinensis) 12g.

➤ With loose stools, add *bǔ gǔ zhī* (Fructus Psoraleae) 30g and *huái shān yào* (Rhizoma Dioscoreae) 30g.

➤ With kidney depletion and low libido, add *dù zhòng* (Cortex Eucommiae) 30g, *tù sī zǐ* (Semen Cuscutae) 60g and *shān zhū yú* (Fructus Corni) 15g.

(3) LIVER AND KIDNEY YIN DEFICIENCY

Manifestations: low spirits, no interest in previously enjoyable activities, pessimism, despair, anxiety, worry, frequent sighing, fatigue, disquieted heart-spirit, frequent sobbing, distraction, poor memory, a disinclination to speak or move, spontaneous sweating, night sweats, vexing heat in the five hearts, impotence, seminal emission, irregular defecation, a pale red tongue with a white coating, and fine wiry pulses.

Accompanying signs and symptoms may include cold extremities, frequent sweating, decreased appetite, dizziness and blurred vision, tinnitus, oversensitivity and suspicion.

Principles: supplement liver and kidney, nourish the brain, calm the spirit.

Formula: *Qù Yù Yì Nǎo Tāng* (Depression-Eliminating Brain-Benefiting Decoction)

菊花	*jú huā*	15g	Flos Chrysanthemi
白芍	*bái sháo*	30g	Radix Paeoniae Alba
白蒺藜	*bái jí lí*	30g	Fructus Tribuli
玄参	*xuán shēn*	30g	Radix Scrophulariae
生地	*shēng dì*	30g	Radix Rehmanniae
麦门冬	*mài mén dōng*	30g	Radix Ophiopogonis
女贞子	*nǚ zhēn zǐ*	30g	Fructus Ligustri Lucidi
枸杞子	*gǒu qǐ zǐ*	30g	Fructus Lycii
炒枣仁	*chǎo zǎo rén*	30g	Semen Ziziphi Spinosae (stir-fried)
柏子仁	*bǎi zǐ rén*	30g	Semen Platycladi

Modifications:
➤ With low libido, add *xiān líng pí* (Herba Epimedii) and *xiān máo*

Chapter 5
Zang-fu Patterns and Treatment

(Rhizoma Curculiginis) 30g each.

➢ With heat in the heart of palms and soles and night sweats, add *qīng hāo* (Herba Artemisiae Annuae) 15g, *dì gǔ pí* (Cortex Lycii) 30g and *biē jiǎ* (Carapax Trionycis) 15g.

➢ With aching limp lumbus and knees, add *dù zhòng* (Cortex Eucommiae) 30g and *bǔ gǔ zhī* (Fructus Psoraleae) 30g.

➢ With a pale facial complexion, add *dāng guī* (Radix Angelicae Sinensis) 15g, *ē jiāo* (Colla Corii Asini) 15g and *dà zǎo* (Fructus Jujubae) 10g.

(4) Spleen and Kidney Dual Deficiency with Failure to Nourish the Brain

Manifestations: low spirits, pessimism, weak limbs, lack of strength, a tendency to lie down, decreased focus and memory, no interest in previously enjoyable activities, fear of communicating, a pale red tongue with a thin white coating, and fine sunken pulses.

Accompanying signs and symptoms may include decreased appetite, frightening dreams, heart throbbing and sudden fright caused by loud noises, a lusterless facial complexion, and dizziness.

Principles: supplement liver and kidney, nourish the brain, calm the spirit.

Formula: *Yì Zhì Xǐng Shén Tāng* (Intelligence-Benefiting Spirit-Awakening Decoction)

菊花	jú huā	15g	Flos Chrysanthemi
川芎	chuān xiōng	30g	Rhizoma Chuanxiong
丹参	dān shēn	30g	Radix et Rhizoma Salviae Miltiorrhizae
葛根	gé gēn	15g	Radix Puerariae Lobatae
党参	dǎng shēn	15g	Radix Codonopsis
茯苓	fú líng	30g	Poria
白术	bái zhú	15g	Rhizoma Atractylodis Macrocephalae
枸杞子	gǒu qǐ zǐ	15g	Fructus Lycii
菟丝子	tù sī zǐ	30g	Semen Cuscutae
女贞子	nǚ zhēn zǐ	30g	Fructus Ligustri Lucidi
山茱萸	shān zhū yú	30g	Fructus Corni

五味子	wǔ wèi zǐ	10g	Fructus Schisandrae Chinensis
炒枣仁	chǎo zǎo rén	30g	Semen Ziziphi Spinosae (stir-fried)
大枣	dà zǎo	10g	Fructus Jujubae

Modifications:
- With kidney yang deficiency, add *xiān líng pí* (Herba Epimedii) 12g and *xiān máo* (Rhizoma Curculiginis) 6g.
- With aching cold lumbus and knees, add *bǔ gǔ zhī* (Fructus Psoraleae) 30g and *guī jiǎ* (Carapax et Plastrum Testudinis) 15g.
- With frequent urination, add *yì zhì rén* (Fructus Alpiniae Oxyphyllae) 15g and *bā jǐ tiān* (Radix Morindae Officinalis) 10g.
- With shortness of breath, add *shēng huáng qí* (Radix Astragali raw) 30–60g.

(5) Lung and Kidney Dual Deficiency

Manifestations: enduring disease, sadness and weeping, anxiety, worry, frequent sighing, fear, suspicion, weeping that causes incontinence, frequent urination at night, low spirits, shortness of breath, reticence, a pale red tongue with a white coating, and sunken fine weak pulses.

Accompanying signs and symptoms may include a lack of pleasure in eating, distending fullness after forced eating, distraction, poor memory, and a reduced ability to calculate.

Principles: supplement lung and kidney, nourish the brain-spirit.

Formula: *Yì Qì Bǎi Hé Tāng* (Qi-Benefiting Lily Bulb Decoction)

生黄芪	shēng huáng qí	30g	Radix Astragali raw
百合	bǎi hé	30g	Bulbus Lilii
沙参	shā shēn	30g	Radix Adenophorae
麦门冬	mài mén dōng	30g	Radix Ophiopogonis
大枣	dà zǎo	10g	Fructus Jujubae
紫菀	zǐ wǎn	15g	Radix et Rhizoma Asteris
枸杞子	gǒu qǐ zǐ	15g	Fructus Lycii
菟丝子	tù sī zǐ	30g	Semen Cuscutae
巴戟天	bā jǐ tiān	15g	Radix Morindae Officinalis
龟甲	guī jiǎ	10g	Carapax et Plastrum Testudinis

Chapter 5
Zang-fu Patterns and Treatment

山茱萸	*shān zhū yú*	15g	Fructus Corni
炒枣仁	*chǎo zǎo rén*	30g	Semen Ziziphi Spinosae (stir-fried)
神曲	*shén qū*	15g	Massa Medicata Fermentata

Modifications:

➤ With spontaneous sweating and night sweats, add *wǔ wèi zǐ* (Fructus Schisandrae Chinensis) 12g, *dì gǔ pí* (Cortex Lycii) 30g and *fú xiǎo mài* (Fructus Tritici Levis) 30g.

➤ With heat in the palms and soles, add *qīng hāo* (Herba Artemisiae Annuae) 15g and *biē jiǎ* (Carapax Trionycis) 15g.

➤ With dizziness and blurred vision, add *bái sháo* (Radix Paeoniae Alba) 30g and *shēng mǔ lì* (Concha Ostreae Cruda, decocted first) 30g.

➤ With loose stools, add *chǎo bái zhú* (Rhizoma Atractylodis Macrocephalae, stir-fried) 10g, *shān yào* (Rhizoma Dioscoreae) 30g and *dǎng shēn* (Radix Codonopsis) 15g.

The five patterns described above are also seen in patients with mild depressive disorder. In general, according to the protracted nature of the condition, these patients will present with different degrees of yin-humor damage and dysfunction of the spirits of the five viscera. Enduring yin deficiency can eventually damage yang qi which results in a decreased libido and very low spirits. Such a patient will present with pessimism, despair, or even suicidal tendencies.

For all of these patterns, it is important to engender yang qi by securing the root and benefiting the kidney. *Tù sī zǐ* (Semen Cuscutae), *nǚ zhēn zǐ* (Fructus Ligustri Lucidi), *wǔ wèi zǐ* (Fructus Schisandrae Chinensis), *xiān líng pí* (Herba Epimedii), *biē jiǎ* (Carapax Trionycis) and *guī jiǎ* (Carapax et Plastrum Testudinis) are essential medicinals for astringing and nourishing yin to form a substantial basis for yang. Pay special attention to elderly patients suffering with incontinence; medicinals that strengthen kidney yang are especially helpful in thee cases.

When applying supplementation, medicinals that disperse and conduct should also be added in appropriate amounts. For example, *shén qū* (Massa Medicata Fermentata) 12g and *mài yá* (Fructus Hordei Germinatus) 30g can be added in order to supplement without cloying.

In general, supplementing medicinals and those which nourish yin should be added or removed from the basic formula on a monthly basis. These would include *dāng guī* (Radix Angelicae Sinensis) 10g, *dān shēn* (Radix et Rhizoma Salviae Miltiorrhizae) 30g, *bái sháo* (Radix Paeoniae Alba) 30g and *chì sháo* (Radix Paeoniae Rubra) 30g.

3. Major Depressive Disorder

This severe depressive condition is characterized by a prolonged disease course with various symptoms including: low spirits, pessimism, world-weariness, unsociability, suicidal or self-damaging tendencies, and secretly planning suicide. With careful observation and early diagnosis, the condition can be managed effectively.

Commonly seen patterns include the following:

(1) Phlegm-fire Mingle and Fume, Rushing upwards to Obscure the Brain-spirit

This pattern is commonly seen in young and middle-aged people, and may have a sudden and unexpected triggering event; however the patient will generally have a history of phlegm heat retention that is exacerbated by sudden depressing or disruptive changes. The course of disease can be quite short.

Signs and Symptoms: red face and eyes, sudden violent anger, staring angrily without speaking, extreme vigilance and nervousness about their surroundings, sleeplessness, self-damaging behaviors such as banging one's head against the wall, constipation, turbid urine, and a yellow thick slimy tongue coating.

Other signs may include long periods without eating followed by occasional binge eating, anxiety, worry, reticence, and a tendency to become lost in thought.

Treatment Principles: flush phlegm, drain heat, clear the brain, awaken the spirit.

Formula: *Huō Tán Qīng Nǎo Tāng* (Phlegm-Flushing Brain-Clearing Formula)

菊花	jú huā	15g	Flos Chrysanthemi
川芎	chuān xiōng	20g	Rhizoma Chuanxiong

Chapter 5
Zang-fu Patterns and Treatment

丹参	dān shēn	30g	Radix et Rhizoma Salviae Miltiorrhizae
生石膏	shēng shí gāo	30-80g	Gypsum Fibrosum Cruda (decocted first)
磁石	cí shí	30g	Magnetitum (decocted first)
生龙齿	shēng lóng chǐ	30g	Dens Draconis (raw, decocted first)
牡蛎	mǔ lì	30g	Concha Ostreae (raw, decocted first)
黄连	huáng lián	10g	Rhizoma Coptidis
黄芩	huáng qín	10g	Radix Scutellariae
青皮	qīng pí	10g	Pericarpium Citri Reticulatae Viride
陈皮	chén pí	10g	Pericarpium Citri Reticulatae
栀子	zhī zǐ	10g	Fructus Gardeniae
牛膝	niú xī	30g	Radix Achyranthis Bidentatae
佩兰	pèi lán	10g	Herba Eupatorii
天竺黄	tiān zhú huáng	10g	Concretio Silicea Bambusae
莱菔子	lái fú zǐ	30g	Semen Raphani
大黄	dà huáng	10g	Radix et Rhizoma Rhei (preserved in liquor)
玄明粉	xuán míng fěn	3-6g	Natrii Sulfas Exsiccatus

Modifications:

➢ With exuberant phlegm, add *Qīng Xīn Gǔn Tán Wán* (Heart-Clearing Phlegm-Rolling Pill), 1 pill, twice daily.

➢ With amenorrhea, add *táo rén* (Semen Persicae) 20g and *hóng huā* (Flos Carthami) 15g.

➢ With insomnia, add *chǎo suān zǎo rén* (Semen Ziziphi Spinosae, stir-fried) 60g and *hǔ pò* (Succinum, powdered and infused) 3g.

(2) Liver-stomach Disharmony with Irregularity of the Brain-spirit

Characterized by sudden onset and a short disease course with a generally obvious cause.

Signs and Symptoms: unstable mood, anxiety, fear, uneasiness, sleeplessness, pessimism, a sense that life is not worth living, a willingness to suicide if the condition is not resolved, disharmony of the intestines and stomach, generalized scurrying pain, dizziness and blurred vision, defecation several times daily with loose stools, possible fecal incontinence, a pale red tongue with a white coating, and wiry fine pulses.

Other signs may include a severely bad disposition, a reluctance to eat or move, and obvious despair.

Treatment Principles: course the liver, harmonize the stomach, nourish the brain, calm the spirit.

Formula:

Shū Gān Hé Wèi Yǐn (Liver-Coursing Stomach-Harmonizing Beverage)

生黄芪	*shēng huáng qí*	30g	Radix Astragali raw
太子参	*tài zǐ shēn*	30g	Radix Pseudostellariae
炒白术	*chǎo bái zhú*	15g	Rhizoma Atractylodis Macrocephalae (stir-fried)
草豆蔻	*cǎo dòu kòu*	10g	Semen Alpiniae Katsumadai
砂仁	*shā rén*	10g	Fructus Amomi
延胡索	*yán hú suǒ*	15g	Rhizoma Corydalis
白芍	*bái sháo*	30g	Radix Paeoniae Alba
怀山药	*huái shān yào*	30g	Rhizoma Dioscoreae
枸杞子	*gǒu qǐ zǐ*	15g	Fructus Lycii
菟丝子	*tù sī zǐ*	30g	Semen Cuscutae
补骨脂	*bǔ gǔ zhī*	15g	Fructus Psoraleae
石菖蒲	*shí chāng pú*	6g	Rhizoma Acori Tatarinowii
香橼	*xiāng yuán*	15g	Fructus Citri
佛手	*fó shǒu*	10g	Fructus Citri Sarcodactylis
炒枣仁	*chǎo zǎo rén*	30g	Semen Ziziphi Spinosae (stir-fried)
炙甘草	*zhì gān cǎo*	6g	Radix et Rhizoma Glycyrrhizae Praeparata cum Melle

Modifications:

➤ With sorrow and desire to weep, add *bǎi hé* (Bulbus Lilii) 60g and *shā shēn* (Radix Adenophorae) 30g.

➤ With unstable moods, add *shēng shí jué míng* (Concha Haliotidis raw) and *cí shí* (Magnetitum) 30g respectively.

(3) **KIDNEY YANG DEPLETION WITH IRREGULARITY OF THE BRAIN-SPIRIT**

Signs and Symptoms: a prolonged course of disease, low spirits,

Chapter 5
Zang-fu Patterns and Treatment

decreased libido, frequent nocturnal seminal emission and premature ejaculation, impotence, a cold sensation in the scrotum, aching coldness of the lumbar spine and knees, cold extremities, aversion to cold, no pleasure in eating, fifth-watch diarrhea, epigastric discomfort, frequent long voidings of clear urine, a pale red tongue with no coating, and sunken fine weak pulses.

Other symptoms may include fatigue, lack of strength, a strong sense of personal powerlessness, struggling with life, no desire to see family or acquaintances, and a desire for quiet and solitude.

Treatment Principles: secure the kidney, strengthen yang, supplement the brain, benefit the spirit.

Formula: Modified *Yòu Guī Wán*（Right-Restoring Pill）

熟地黄	shú dì huáng	15g	Radix Rehmanniae Praeparata
山茱萸	shān zhū yú	15g	Fructus Corni
杜仲	dù zhòng	15g	Cortex Eucommiae
怀山药	huái shān yào	30g	Rhizoma Dioscoreae
枸杞子	gǒu qǐ zǐ	15g	Fructus Lycii
菟丝子	tù sī zǐ	30g	Semen Cuscutae
鹿角胶	lù jiǎo jiāo	10g	Colla Cornus Cervi
仙茅	xiān máo	10g	Rhizoma Curculiginis
仙灵脾	xiān líng pí	15g	Herba Epimedii
巴戟天	bā jǐ tiān	15g	Radix Morindae Officinalis

Modifications:

➤ With genital cold, add *zhì fù zǐ* (Radix Aconiti Lateralis Praeparata) 3g and *ròu guì* (Cortex Cinnamomi) 3g to warm the kidney and invigorate yang.

➤ With frequent urination, add *bǔ gǔ zhī* (Fructus Psoraleae) 30g and *yì zhì rén* (Fructus Alpiniae Oxyphyllae) 30g.

(4) QI AND BLOOD DUAL DEFICIENCY WITH BRAIN-SPIRIT DAMAGE

Commonly seen in elderly patients with a prolonged course of disease; physical symptoms are commonly present.

Signs and Symptoms: low spirits, extreme pessimism, struggling with life, tendency to self injury, no desire to seek medical help or counseling, a tendency to lie down, emaciation, cold extremities, slow speech, constipation, frequent dribbling urination, a frequent desire to urinate, a pale red tongue with no coating, and sunken fine weak pulses. In women, there can be vaginal flatulence or discomfort of the genital region and anus.

Other symptoms may include a dull facial expression, reticence, no pleasure in eating, sleeplessness, and excessive rumination.

Treatment Principles: supplement qi and blood, engender marrow, nourish the brain.

Formula: Modified *Bā Zhēn Tāng*（Eight Gem Decoction）

生晒参	shēng shài shēn	3g	Radix et Rhizoma Ginseng Cruda
五味子	wǔ wèi zǐ	10g	Fructus Schisandrae Chinensis
麦门冬	mài mén dōng	30g	Radix Ophiopogonis
熟地黄	shú dì huáng	15g	Radix Rehmanniae Praeparata
当归	dāng guī	15g	Radix Angelicae Sinensis
川芎	chuān xiōng	20g	Rhizoma Chuanxiong
白芍	bái sháo	30g	Radix Paeoniae Alba
枸杞子	gǒu qǐ zǐ	15g	Fructus Lycii
菟丝子	tù sī zǐ	60g	Semen Cuscutae
女贞子	nǚ zhēn zǐ	30g	Fructus Ligustri Lucidi
何首乌	hé shǒu wū	30g	Radix Polygoni Multiflori
鹿茸	lù róng	3g	Cornu Cervi Pantotrichum
巴戟天	bā jǐ tiān	15g	Radix Morindae Officinalis
龟甲	guī jiǎ	10g	Carapax et Plastrum Testudinis
鳖甲	biē jiǎ	10g	Carapax Trionycis

Modifications:

➤ With shortness of breath, add *shēng huáng qí* (Radix Astragali raw) 60g.
➤ With dry bound stool, add *huǒ má rén* (Fructus Cannabis) 15 – 30g.
➤ With frequent urination, add *bǔ gǔ zhī* (Fructus Psoraleae) 30g and *yì zhì rén* (Fructus Alpiniae Oxyphyllae) 15g.

Commentary

The onset of major depressive disorder can be either acute or slow.

Chapter 5
Zang-fu Patterns and Treatment

During the initial stage, hospitalization is often best for the patient, and a personal caretaker may be required. There are two possible causes for this stage of depression. One involves a prolonged period of relatively mild depression with unexpected incidents or emotional upsets such as relationship problems among young people; the other cause involves a constitutional weakness combined with prolonged physical ailments; most common among elderly patients who have lost their will to live.

Chapter 6
Acupuncture and Moxibustion

Acupuncture and moxibustion acts to regulate and adjust the body without producing toxicity or side effects in most cases; in fact, acupuncture is often employed to reduce the side effects of other treatment methods. Furthermore, these treatment methods have been shown as especially effective in the treatment of depressive disorders. Because the main symptom of low moods can often be quickly resolved with acupuncture alone, these methods are often employed as an initial intervention in mild to moderate cases of depression. However, acupuncture and moxibustion are also quite effective as part of a long-term treatment plan.

Main Objectives

In the treatment of depression, acupuncture and moxibustion mainly aim to regulate the brain-spirit and soothe the liver while also relieving the associated somatic symptoms.

1. The *Du* Channel

The *du* channel acts to govern the yang qi of the entire body; also referred to as the "sea of all yang channels". This key function plays an important role in regulating pathological changes that involve the channels. The *du* channel "arises from the lowest polar point and travels internally within the spine, then arriving at DU 16 (*fēng fǔ*); it then enters into and homes within the brain". "A channel governs and treats the areas that it traverses and reaches", so as the *du* channel travels to the vertex, it also links deeply inside the brain which makes this channel especially useful in the treatment of mental-emotional conditions. Because the *du* channel also functions to regulate physiological processes in general, it can indirectly calm the mind and brain simply by restoring normal *zang-fu* organ function. "When yin is at peace and yang is contained, the essence-spirit is also regulated".

Modern research shows that stimulating the *du* channel with electro-acupuncture (EA) can significantly increase 5-HT neuron activity within the raphe nuclei, and increase the content of 5-HT in the substantia nigra and hypothalamus. Such therapy has been shown to improve blood circulation within the brain, increase the antioxidant capacity of brain tissues, and improve memory.

Chapter 6
Acupuncture and Moxibustion

DU 20 (*bǎi huì*) is the convergent point of the three hand and foot yang channels, the *du* channel, and the foot *jueyin* liver channel. The point is located on the vertex of head where all channels and vessels in the body are said to converge. Needling DU 20 (*bǎi huì*) acts to regulate the qi of all the channels, adjust and supplement middle qi, raise yang to treat qi collapse, awaken the brain, and open the orifices. Du 20 (*bǎi huì*) is an essential point for regulating the emotions and calming the mind.

The Great Compendium of Acupuncture and Moxibustion – Attending Function of the Points of the Du Channel (*Zhēn Jiǔ Dà Chéng – Dū Mài Jīng Xuè Zhǔ Zhì*) states that DU 20 (*bǎi huì*) can be used to treat "anguish, fear palpitations and forgetfulness, a lack of mental energy…heaviness of the head, nasal congestion, headache, dizziness, and impaired taste".

Sì Shén Cōng (四神聪) is also located at the vertex region. This group of points can effectively regulate the emotions, and are also frequently used for mental and emotional conditions. *Sì Shén Cōng* can also relieve insomnia.

DU 24 (*shén tíng*) is located at the anterior aspect of the head. This point marks the convergence of the *du* channel with the foot *taiyang* and foot *yangming* channels, also known as "the point where consciousness resides". Its main function is to calm the mind and open the orifices. *The Great Compendium of Acupuncture and Moxibustion states* that DU 24 (*shén tíng*) can treat "fearful throbbing, palpitations, and sleeplessness".

Yìn Táng (印堂) is an extra point located on the *du* channel at the forehead. Similar in function to DU 24 (*shén tíng*), it acts to awaken and regulate the spirit. In clinical practice, DU 20 (*bǎi huì*) is often combined with *yìn táng* and treated with EA. To prevent "point fatigue", DU 20 (*bǎi huì*) or *Sì shén cōng* can be paired with either DU 24 (*shén tíng*) or *yìn táng* and treated alternately.

SI 3 (*hòu xī*) is the wood-stream point of the hand *taiyang* small intestine channel, a confluent point of the eight extra channels, and links with the *du* channel. The small intestine channel is interior-exteriorly related to the heart channel, so SI 3 (*hòu xī*) is also used to regulate qi in the heart channel and calm the mind. It also acts to regulate the *du* channel, and is frequently paired with PC 6 (*nèi guān*) which links with the *yinwei* channel.

2. Soothing the Liver and Regulating Qi

The principle of soothing the liver and regulating qi is the most commonly used acupuncture and moxibustion therapy for depressive disorders, but not the only one. Proper treatment should be based on pattern differentiation, with the entire clinical presentation taken into consideration.

Emotional inhibition is a primary cause of depressive disorder, thus the general emphasis on qi regulation. The liver governs the free flow of qi, and therefore, to regulate qi, points on liver channel are among the first choices. The foot *jueyin* liver channel joins the *du* channel at the vertex, and for this reason it also has a close relationship with the brain.

LV 3 (*tài chōng*) is the *shu*-stream/earth point and *yuan*-source point of the foot *jueyin* liver channel. "For diseases of the five *zang*-organs, one should select the twelve source points".

LV 3 (*tài chōng*) acts to resolve liver qi constraint, soothe the liver, and discharge heat.

LV 3 is often combined with LI 4 (*hé gǔ*), commonly known as the "four gates". This pair of points can calm the mind, soothe the liver, and extinguish wind.

LV 3 combined with DU 20 (*bǎi huì*) and LV 2 (*xíng jiān*) with KI 3 (*tài xī*) treat headaches caused by hyperactive liver yang.

LV 3 with RN 12 (*zhōng wǎn*), SP 9 (*yīn líng quán*), and *yìn táng* treats dizziness caused by wind-yang disturbing the head.

LV 3 with HT 7 (*shén mén*), PC 8 (*láo gōng*), DU 26 (*shuǐ gōu*) and ST 40 (*fēng lóng*) treats anxiety caused by phlegm-fire disturbing the mind.

LV 3 with LV 14 (*qī mén*) and GB 24 (*rì yuè*) treats rib-side pain.

LV 3 with RN 13 (*shàng wǎn*), GB 34 (*yáng líng quán*), PC 6 (*nèi guān*), ST 34 (*liáng qiū*) and HT 7 (*shén mén*) treats vomiting caused by liver qi invading the spleen and stomach.

LV 3 (*tài chōng*) with SP 6 (*sān yīn jiāo*), SP 10 (*xuè hǎi*) and RN 4 (*guān yuán*) treats irregular menstruation caused by liver constraint.

LV 3 with SJ 3 (*zhōng zhǔ*), GB 43 (*xiá xī*), RN 23 (*lián quán*) and GB 20 (*fēng chí*) treats pain in the pharynx caused by liver fire.

Chapter 6
Acupuncture and Moxibustion

LV 2 (*xíng jiān*) is the *ying*-spring/water point of the foot *jueyin* liver channel. *Ying*-spring points are commonly used to treat fever, while LV 2 (*xíng jiān*) also acts to discharge liver fire, soothe the liver and relieve constraint, and treat disorders of the head and eyes.

LV 2 with GB 44 (*zú qiào yīn*), GB 20 (*fēng chí*), and HT 7 (*shén mén*) treats insomnia caused by liver-fire disturbing the mind.

LV 2 with *yìn táng*, GB 34 (*yáng líng quán*), GB 20 (*fēng chí*), and *tài yáng* (太阳) treats dizziness caused by internal wind and heat stirring the liver and gallbladder.

LV 2 with RN 6 (*qì hǎi*), LV 3 (*tài chōng*), SP 6 (*sān yīn jiāo*) and GB 34 (*yáng líng quán*) treats dysmenorrhea caused by liver constraint with qi stagnation.

LV 14 (*qī mén*) is the front-*mu* point of the liver channel and marks the area where the foot *jueyin* channel spreads to the rib-sides and links internally with the liver. LV 14 (*qī mén*) is also where the foot *taiyin* and *yin wei* channel join.

LV 14 with GB 34 (*yáng líng quán*), PC 6 (*nèi guān*), SP 4 (*gōng sūn*) and LV 2 (*xíng jiān*) treats stomach pain and acid reflux caused by liver constraint.

LV 14 with BL 18 (*gān shù*), LV 3 (*tài chōng*), ST 36 (*zú sān lǐ*), ST 25 (*tiān shū*) and RN 12 (*zhōng wǎn*) treats diarrhea caused by liver constraint and spleen deficiency.

LV 14 with GB 34 (*yáng líng quán*), RN 10 (*xià wǎn*), ST 21 (*liáng mén*) and ST 36 (*zú sān lǐ*) treats hunger with no desire for food.

In addition to liver channel points, other channel points can also be used to regulate liver qi.

BL 18 (*gān shù*) is the back-*shu* point of the liver. It soothes and emolliates the liver, relieves constraint, discharges heat, and nourishes blood.

BL 19 (*dǎn shù*) is the back-*shu* point of the gallbladder. It soothes the liver, promotes gallbladder function, nourishes yin, clears heat, harmonizes the stomach, and descends rebellious qi.

GB 40 (*qiū xū*) is the *yuan*-source point of the foot *shaoyang* gallbladder channel. It soothes the liver, promotes gallbladder function, regulates qi and relieves constraint, rejuvenates the brain, and calms the mind.

GB 34 (*yáng líng quán*) is the *he*-sea point of the gallbladder channel and the influential meeting point of the sinews. It soothes the liver and regulates qi, clears heat and eliminates dampness, sedates and calms the mind, harmonizes the stomach, and controls vomiting.

For liver constraint with phlegm obstructing, add ST 40 (*fēng lóng*), RN 17 (*dàn zhōng*) and PC 6 (*nèi guān*) to relieve the chest, regulate qi, and transform phlegm.

For liver constraint and spleen deficiency, add BL 18 (*gān shù*), BL 20 (*pí shù*), SP 3 (*tài bái*) and SP 6 (*sān yīn jiāo*) to soothe the liver and strengthen the spleen.

For yin deficiency of the liver and kidney add KI 3 (*tài xī*), BL 18 (*gān shù*), BL 23 (*shèn shù*) to nourish both liver and kidney.

For yin deficiency of the heart and kidney, add BL 23 (*shèn shù*), KI 3 (*tài xī*) and DU 4 (*mìng mén*) to supplement the kidney.

3. Flexible Uses of Special Points

Special points include the five transport points, *yuan*-source points, *luo*-connecting points, back-*shu* points, front-*mu* points, *xi*-cleft points, eight influential points, lower *he*-sea points, confluent points of the eight extra vessels, and intersecting points. All of these are points of the fourteen channels with special therapeutic functions, and many of them are essential points in the treatment of depressive disorder.

(1) FIVE TRANSPORT POINTS

Jing-well, *ying*-spring, *shu*-stream, *jing*-river, and *he*-sea points of the yin channels are associated with wood, fire, earth, metal, and water, respectively. Those of the yang channels are associated with metal, water, wood, fire, and earth.

These points can be applied according to the principle "supplement the mother for deficiency, drain the son for excess", according to the individual characteristics of the points and according to pattern differentiation.

Chapter 6
Acupuncture and Moxibustion

(2) Yuan-source Points and *Luo*-connecting Points

Yuan-source points are locations where original qi of the related channel collects. The yuan-source points of the yin channels are the same points as the *shu*-stream points.

Luo-connecting points are where the collaterals part from the channels, and they also act to establish communication between their exteriorly and interiorly paired channels. Therefore they can treat both the channel and its related exterior or interior channel or organ. The phrase "enduring illness enters the collaterals" means that over time, illnesses will generally express themselves with blood stasis that manifests in the channel system collateral vessels. Because *luo* points also influence the *luo* vessels, these points are commonly used for chronic conditions.

1) Yuan-source points and corresponding *luo*-connecting points:
- Lung: LU 9 (*tài yuān*) and LU 7 (*liè quē*)
- Large Intestine: LI 4 (*hé gǔ*) and LI 6 (*piān lì*)
- Stomach: ST 42 (*chōng yáng*) and ST 40 (*fēng lóng*)
- Spleen: SP 3 (*tài bái*) and SP 4 (*gōng sūn*)
- Heart: HT 7 (*shén mén*) and HT 5 (*tōng lǐ*)
- Small Intestine: SI 4 (*wàn gǔ*) and SI 7 (*zhī zhèng*)
- Bladder: BL 64 (*jīng gǔ*) and BL 58 (*fēi yáng*)
- Kidney: KI 3 (*tài xī*) and KI 4 (*dà zhōng*)
- Pericardium: PC 7 (*dà líng*) and PC 6 (*nèi guān*)
- Sanjiao: SJ 4 (*yáng chí*) and SJ 5 (*wài guān*)
- Gallbladder: GB 40 (*qiū xū*) and GB 37 (*guāng míng*)
- Liver: LV 3 (*tài chōng*) and LV 5 (*lí gōu*)

2) Combining channel and point categories

The combining of *yuan*-source points based on channel categories commonly includes *shaoyin* channel points with *shaoyang* points, *taiyin* points with *taiyang*, and *jueyin* points with *yangming*. For example, LV 3 (*tài chōng*) and PC 6 (*nèi guān*) effectively treat the dizziness, vertigo, and irritation associated with liver hyperactivity. This pairing of upper and lower points also promotes communication between the *yangming* and *jueyin* channels.

Yuan-source and *luo*-connecting points are combined according to paired channel relationships to treat an issue of a single channel system; for example, *jueyin* points can be used to help address the mental and emotional effects of *yangming* heat conditions. The combination can also be used to treat channel diseases through the interior-exterior relationship (e.g., heart and small intestine) where pathology of one channel affects its paired channel. For chronic or difficult cases, use the *yuan*-source points. For acute and mild cases and for preventive purposes, use the *luo*-connecting points. For example, the combination of GB 40 (*qiū xū*) and LV 5 (*lí gōu*) is effective for treating conditions affecting the liver and gallbladder channels, and the combination of PC 7 (*dà líng*) and PC 6 (*nèi guān*) can effectively treat palpitations.

Yuan-source and back-*shu* points are generally combined for supplementing the channel and organ system, as they tend to work synergistically. These combinations are most effective for diseases that are yin in nature (interior syndromes, deficiency syndromes, cold syndromes). For example, KI 3 (*tài xī*) and BL 23 (*shèn shù*) can be selected for a wide variety of kidney deficiency patterns.

Yuan-source and *he-sea* or lower *he-sea* points are combined to address mixed cases of accumulation, or excess and deficiency complex patterns.

For example, SP 3 (*tài bái*) and ST 36 (*zú sān lǐ*) are effective for strengthening the spleen and harmonizing the stomach, and for ascending the clear and descending the turbid.

LV 3 (*tài chōng*) and GB 34 (*yáng líng quán*) clear the liver and promote gallbladder function by soothing spleen-earth and inhibiting liver-wood.

LI 4 (*hé gǔ*) and ST 36 (*zú sān lǐ*) are effective for regulating the stomach and intestines, transforming stagnation, relieving distention, and promoting defecation.

LI 4 and LI 11 (*qū chí*) are effective for dispersing wind, dissipating heat, and clearing the upper *jiao*.

LV 3 (*tài chōng*) and ST 36 (*zú sān lǐ*) can be used to soothe the liver and harmonize the stomach.

Chapter 6
Acupuncture and Moxibustion

(3) BACK-*SHU* POINTS AND FRONT-*MU* POINTS

Back-*shu* points are locations where the *yuan qi* generated by the ministerial fire is dispersed to the *zang-fu* organs, but collaterals of the BL channel also enter the brain. Back-*shu* points can be used to regulate the brain-spirit also because qi and blood of the *zang-fu* organs not only communicate with the bladder channel, but also link with the *du* channel.

Back-*shu* points can therefore treat depressive disorders when differentiated on the basis of organ pathology, where supplementation and drainage methods act to regulate the brain-spirit. These points are especially beneficial for chronic cases associated with deficiency. In such cases, after needling points on the front of the body, *shu* points can be needled with relatively short retention, or as a supplement to other channel treatments.

Front-*mu* points are locations where the qi and blood of the *zang-fu* organs irrigate the chest and abdomen, and are also seen as points where yang excess accumulation in an organ is expressed. The location of front-*mu* points also correlate with the anatomical location of the *zang-fu* inside the body, so tenderness here usually indicates an excess pathology of the organ itself, as opposed to the channel.

Zang-fu **organs and their corresponding front-*mu* points:**
1) Large Intestine: ST 25 (*tiān shū*)
2) Lung: LU 1 (*zhōng fǔ*)
3) Small Intestine: RN 4 (*guān yuán*)
4) Heart: RN 14 (*jù quē*)
5) Bladder: RN 3 (*zhōng jí*)
6) Kidney: GB 25 (*jīng mén*)
7) Liver: LV 14 (*qī mén*)
8) Gallbladder: GB 24 (*rì yuè*)
9) Spleen: LV 13 (*zhāng mén*)
10) Stomach: RN 12 (*zhōng wǎn*)
11) Sanjiao: RN 5 (*shí mén*)
12) Pericardium: RN 17 (*dàn zhōng*)

Front-*mu* points are significantly effective for treating diseases of the six bowels, for example, select RN 12 (*zhōng wǎn*) for stomach conditions and GB 24 (*rì yuè*) for gallbladder conditions.

In clinical practice, back-*shu* points can be used for diseases of the five *zang* and diseases of the yin channels, whereas front-*mu* points can be used for diseases of the six bowels and diseases of the yang channels. Back-*shu* points may always be combined with front-*mu* points as a yin-yang combination of front and back. This combination is effective because of the cooperation between the points; their effect can be further enhanced if the combination includes four points with one pair from each of the interior-exterior *zang-fu* channels. For example, BL 18 (*gān shù*) and BL 19 (*dǎn shù*) can be combined with LV 14 (*qī mén*) and GB 24 (*rì yuè*).

Furthermore, front-*mu* and *he*-sea points are often combined for bowel diseases, heat syndromes, and patterns of excess. For example, ST 25 (*tiān shū*) and ST 37 (*shàng jù xū*) are commonly selected for diarrhea and constipation.

(4) THE EIGHT MEETING POINTS

Zang organs: LV 13 (*zhāng mén*)   *Fu* organs: RN 12 (*zhōng wǎn*)
Marrow: GB 39 (*xuán zhōng*)   Sinews: GB 34 (*yáng líng quán*)
Bones: BL 11 (*dà zhù*)   Blood: BL 17 (*gé shù*)
Qi: RN 17 (*dàn zhōng*)   Vessels: LU 9 (*tài yuān*).

LV 13 (*zhāng mén*)—The *zang*-organ meeting point is where the *jueyin* channel, *shaoyang* channel and girdling channels meet. It is also the front-*mu* point of the spleen, so this point can strengthen the spleen, regulate the stomach, relieve distention, harmonize liver and spleen, and benefit the gallbladder. LV 13 (*zhāng mén*) can be used to treat many *zang* diseases, especially those related to the liver and spleen, but also for complex deficiency and excess patterns and situations where the qi dynamic is impaired.

RN 12 (*zhōng wǎn*)—The *fu*-organ meeting point is where the hand *taiyang*, hand *shaoyang*, foot *yangming* and the *ren* channel meet, and its actions include ascending the clear and descending the turbid. It can also free and promote the downward flow of qi of the six bowels, strengthen the spleen and stomach, promote transportation and transformation, supplement middle qi, and calm the mind. The functions of this point mainly focus on treatment of spleen and stomach conditions, but it is also

Chapter 6
Acupuncture and Moxibustion

effective for regulating the six bowels and the *ren* channel.

Depression patients commonly have digestive symptoms caused by deregulation of the qi dynamic such as poor appetite, abdominal distention, and diarrhea. RN 12 (*zhōng wǎn*) can also treat insomnia when associated with stomach disharmony. RN 12 (*zhōng wǎn*) is often combined with LV 13 (*zhāng mén*).

RN 17 (*dàn zhōng*)—The meeting point of qi is also the meeting place of the foot *taiyin*, foot *shaoyin*, hand *taiyang*, and hand *shaoyang* channels. RN 17 (*dàn zhōng*) acts to regulate qi, activate blood, promote the free flow of qi, free the vessels, relieve constraint in the chest, and descend counterflow. It is also effective for treating qi deficiency and qi stagnation, especially when they affect the chest. It is commonly used for excess syndromes, stomach qi counterflow, and binding constraint of liver qi.

BL 17 (*gé shù*)—The meeting point of blood acts to regulate and harmonize blood, and since the point is located on the bladder channel which has branches and collaterals that link to the brain, this point is also effective for brain diseases associated with blood stasis and blood heat.

LU 9 (*tài yuān*)—The meeting point of the vessels is also the *yuan*-source point of the hand *taiyin* channel, and the *shu*-stream-earth point. Because the lung channel links with all vessels, LU 9 (*tài yuān*) can effectively regulate qi, activate blood, and free the vessels. LU 9 (*tài yuān*) is effective for treating qi-related patterns, blood patterns, vessel patterns, and disorders of the *po*.

The Great Compendium of Acupuncture and Moxibustion – Indications of Hand Taiyin Channel and Points (*Zhēn Jiǔ Dà Chéng – Shǒu Tài Yīn Jīng Xuè Zhǔ Zhì*) states that the indications for this point are "chest impediment and qi counterflow, tendency to hiccough, vomiting, coughing, and irritation and oppression with insomnia".

DU 14 (*dà zhuī*)—The meeting point of bone is where the three hand yang channels, three foot yang channels, and the *du* channel meet. However, some believe that the point should be BL 11 (*dà zhù*), which is where the hand and foot *taiyang* and *shaoyang* channels meet. DU 14 (*dà* *zhuī*) has a special therapeutic effect for treating brain diseases because the *du* channel connects with the brain, and also because the *du* channel connects with the kidney, which generates marrow. In clinical practice, DU 14 (*dà zhuī*) is commonly used to activate yang qi, strengthen the brain, and benefit the spirit. It is often needled with supplementation or moxibustion to treat depressive disorders, and, because of its relationship with the yang channels, drainage techniques are also applicable for draining heat from the body.

GB 39 (*xuán zhōng*)—The meeting point of marrow acts to supplement marrow, generate blood, regulate and free the qi dynamic, relax the sinews, and activate the collaterals. GB 39 (*xuán zhōng*) is effective for sinew and bone diseases, cerebrovascular conditions, dizziness, memory loss. It is commonly used as an adjunct point in the treatment of depressive disorders because marrow acts to promote function of the brain-spirit.

GB 34 (*yáng líng quán*)—The meeting point of the sinews is also the lower *he*-sea point of the foot *shaoyang* gallbladder channel. GB 34 (*yáng líng quán*) acts to relax the sinews, activate the collaterals, soothe the liver and regulate qi, calm the mind, clear heat, and eliminate dampness. It is also typically used for conditions associated with the liver and gallbladder.

Pattern Differentiation and Symptomatic Treatment

1. Selecting points according to *zang-fu* patterns

Because depressive disorders are often complex, and also because there is no uniform criteria for pattern differentiation in the Chinese medical community, there are a variety of patterns classifications to consider. The best approach to point selection is to first discern the root, and then to differentiate any secondary symptoms.

Depressive disorder is a state of generally diminished *zang-fu* function, so electro-acupuncture (EA) is frequently used on points of the *du* channel. For example, DU 20 (*bǎi huì*) or *sì shén cōng* with DU 24 (*shén tíng*) or *yìn táng* are frequently applied. Generally speaking, almost all depression-related patterns will also benefit from liver channel points that soothe the

Chapter 6
Acupuncture and Moxibustion

liver and relieve constraint.

Although mental symptoms are the symptomatic focus of depressive disorder, individual constitutional differences and other factors play a large role in the onset and development of the condition. The clinical manifestations are also quite different in many patients, so treatment should be based on clear pattern differentiation with the goal of rebalancing yin and yang.

Typical patterns and basic point combinations:

1) Liver constraint with qi stagnation: LV 3 (*tài chōng*), LV 14 (*qī mén*), PC 6 (*nèi guān*), HT 7 (*shén mén*), RN 12 (*zhōng wăn*), RN 6 (*qì hăi*).

2) Liver constraint with phlegm binding: LV 3 (*tài chōng*), ST 40 (*fēng lóng*), RN 12 (*zhōng wăn*), LI 4 (*hé gŭ*), PC 6 (*nèi guān*).

3) Liver constraint with spleen deficiency: BL 18 (*gān shù*), BL 20 (*pí shù*), SP 3 (*tài bái*), LV 3 (*tài chōng*), ST 36 (*zú sān lĭ*), SP 6 (*sān yīn jiāo*).

4) Disharmony of liver and stomach: LV 14 (*qī mén*), RN 12 (*zhōng wăn*), PC 6 (*nèi guān*), ST 34 (*liáng qiū*), GB 34 (*yáng líng quán*), ST 36 (*zú sān lĭ*).

5) Upward flaming heat of heart and liver: HT 7 (*shén mén*), PC 8 (*láo gōng*), LI 4 (*hé gŭ*), GB 34 (*yáng líng quán*), LV 2 (*xíng jiān*).

6) Qi stagnation with static blood: LV 3 (*tài chōng*), SP 6 (*sān yīn jiāo*), SP 10 (*xuè hăi*), BL 17 (*gé shù*).

7) Phlegm-fire: LI 4 (*hé gŭ*), PC 7 (*dà líng*), ST 40 (*fēng lóng*), ST 44 (*nèi tíng*), LV 3 (*tài chōng*), GB 20 (*fēng chí*), also ST 45 (*lì duì*) and LI 1 (*shāng yáng*), (prick to bleed).

8) Kidney yang deficiency: DU 14 (*dà zhuī*), RN 4 (*guān yuán*), RN 6 (*qì hăi*), DU 4 (*mìng mén*), BL 23 (*shèn shù*), KI 3 (*tài xī*).

9) Liver and kidney yin deficiency: BL 18 (*gān shù*), BL 23 (*shèn shù*), KI 3 (*tài xī*), SP 6 (*sān yīn jiāo*).

10) Lung and kidney dual deficiency: LU 9 (*tài yuān*), RN 4 (*guān yuán*), RN 6 (*qì hăi*), SP 6 (*sān yīn jiāo*), KI 3 (*tài xī*), also BL 13 (*fèi shù*) and BL 23 (*shèn shù*) with moxibustion.

11) Spleen and kidney dual deficiency: moxibustion at RN 4 (*guān yuán*) and RN 6 (*qì hăi*), DU 4 (*mìng mén*), ST 36 (*zú sān lĭ*), SP 6 (*sān yīn jiāo*), SP 3 (*tài bái*), KI 3 (*tài xī*).

12) Heart and spleen dual deficiency: BL 15 (*xīn shù*), BL 20 (*pí shù*), HT 7 (*shén mén*), ST 36 (*zú sān lĭ*), SP 10 (*xuè hăi*), SP 6 (*sān yīn jiāo*).

⑬ Qi and blood deficiency: RN 6 (*qì hǎi*), ST 36 (*zú sān lǐ*), SP 10 (*xuè hǎi*), SP 6 (*sān yīn jiāo*), BL 15 (*xīn shù*), BL 20 (*pí shù*).

For depression patients, electro-acupuncture (EA) is frequently used to stimulate points on the scalp. However, this approach also effectively raises yang qi, and is thus contraindicated for patients with patterns of excessive heat of the heart and liver or hyperactive liver yang. For these patients, manual needle manipulation with appropriate supplementation and draining techniques should be used instead.

For deficient patients, supplementation techniques and moxibustion are usually applied; drainage techniques are used in patients with heat or excess patterns. For those with constraint and stagnation as the main syndrome, supplementation and draining techniques should be used together, or the even technique should be applied. For patients with excessive heat, bloodletting therapy at the *jing*-well points of the affected channel can be used.

2. Accompanying symptoms

Depression may lead to a variety of other clinical manifestations, as many patients display highly individualized patterns. Many of these accompanying symptoms can be difficult to resolve, and they even may become significant enough to affect the course of the main condition. In other cases, patients will have a primary disease with depression developing as a secondary condition; in such cases, treatment of the primary condition would be paramount.

Point combinations for accompanying symptoms:

Amnesia: DU 20 (*bǎi huì*), *sì shén cōng*, GB 13 (*běn shén*), DU 11 (*shén dào*), BL 23 (*shèn shù*).

Profuse dreaming: RN 12 (*zhōng wǎn*), HT 7 (*shén mén*), *yìn táng*, GB 20 (*fēng chí*).

Stupor and sluggishness: DU 26 (*shuǐ gōu*), SP 1 (*yǐn bái*), KI 1 (*yǒng quán*), DU 17 (*nǎo hù*), needle with drainage.

Hallucinations: DU 26 (*shuǐ gōu*), DU 14 (*dà zhuī*), HT 7 (*shén mén*), SP 1 (*yǐn bái*), needle with drainage.

Headache: GB 20 (*fēng chí*), *tài yáng*.

Chapter 6
Acupuncture and Moxibustion

Forehead pain: add DU 23 (*shàng xīng*), ST 8 (*tóu wéi*), BL 2 (*cuán zhú*), LI 4 (*hé gǔ*).

Vertex pain: add DU 20 (*bǎi huì*), DU 23 (*shàng xīng*), DU 19 (*hòu dǐng*), GB 19 (*nǎo kōng*), LV 3 (*tài chōng*).

Occipital pain: add BL 10 (*tiān zhù*), DU 20 (*bǎi huì*), DU 19 (*hòu dǐng*), SI 3 (*hòu xī*).

Migraines: add ST 8 (*tóu wéi*), GB 4 (*hàn yàn*) and SJ 9 (*sì dú*).

Tinnitus: SJ 21 (*ěr mén*), SI 19 (*tīng gōng*), GB 2 (*tīng huì*) and GB 32 (*zhōng dú*). With recent onset, needle GB 43 (*xiá xī*) and GB 8 (*shuài gǔ*) with drainage. For chronic tinnitus, needle DU 20 (*bǎi huì*), BL 23 (*shèn shù*) and KI 6 (*zhào hǎi*) with supplementation.

Auditory hallucinations: SJ 21 (*ěr mén*), SI 19 (*tīng gōng*), GB 2 (*tīng huì*), SJ 17 (*yì fēng*) and GB 32 (*zhōng dú*).

Insomnia: DU 24 (*shén tíng*), *sì shén cōng*, *tài yáng*, *ān mián* (安眠), HT 7 (*shén mén*), KI 3 (*tài xī*) and others; low frequency EA is applicable.

Sleepiness: DU 26 (*shuǐ gōu*), SP 1 (*yǐn bái*) and *wú míng xuè* (ulnar side of the second ring finger knuckle, Wang Le-ting empirical point).

Anxiety: BL 20 (*pí shù*), BL 49 (*yì shè*), DU 16 (*fēng fǔ*), DU 26 (*shuǐ gōu*), SP 5 (*shāng qiū*) and PC 5 (*jiān shǐ*), needle with drainage.

Irritation: HT 7 (*shén mén*), PC 5 (*jiān shǐ*), LV 14 (*qī mén*), LV 3 (*tài chōng*).

Easily crying: BL 13 (*fèi shù*), BL 42 (*pò hù*), DU 20 (*bǎi huì*), LU 9 (*tài yuān*), PC 6 (*nèi guān*).

Easily frightened: HT 8 (*shào fǔ*), PC 6 (*nèi guān*), HT 7 (*shén mén*), KI 3 (*tài xī*).

Unreleased anger: LV 3 (*tài chōng*), KI 3 (*tài xī*), LU 9 (*tài yuān*), HT 7 (*shén mén*), ST 36 (*zú sān lǐ*).

Obsessive compulsion: HT 7 (*shén mén*), LU 9 (*tài yuān*), PC 6 (*nèi guān*), GB 40 (*qiū xū*).

Somatic pain: DU 14 (*dà zhuī*), SI 3 (*hòu xī*), BL 62 (*shēn mài*) and local points.

Rib-side pain: LV 14 (*qī mén*), GB 34 (*yáng líng quán*), LV 2 (*xíng jiān*), PC 6 (*nèi guān*) through to SJ 5 (*wài guān*).

Stiffness and sinew rigidity: DU 14 (*dà zhuī*), SP 1 (*yǐn bái*), GB 39 (*xuán zhōng*), GB 34 (*yáng líng quán*).

Heavy aching limbs: GB 34 (*yáng líng quán*) joining SP 9 (*yīn líng quán*),

LI 11 (*qū chí*), ST 36 (*zú sān lǐ*), RN 12 (*zhōng wǎn*).

Obesity: RN 12 (*zhōng wǎn*), ST 25 (*tiān shū*), PC 6 (*nèi guān*), ST 40 (*fēng lóng*), SP 5 (*shāng qiū*), needle with drainage.

Olfaction disorders: ST 36 (*zú sān lǐ*), LI 4 (*hé gǔ*), LI 20 (*yíng xiāng*) and BL 7 (*tōng tiān*).

Dry mouth: LU 5 (*chǐ zé*), PC 3 (*qū zé*), LI 2 (*èr jiān*), RN 24 (*chéng jiāng*).

Blurred vision: LV 3 (*tài chōng*), SJ 5 (*wài guān*), BL 1 (*jīng míng*), ST 2 (*sì bái*), GB 20 (*fēng chí*).

Abdominal distention and fullness: RN 12 (*zhōng wǎn*), RN 10 (*xià wǎn*), ST 25 (*tiān shū*), ST 36 (*zú sān lǐ*).

Nausea: PC 6 (*nèi guān*), ST 36 (*zú sān lǐ*), SP 4 (*gōng sūn*), RN 10 (*xià wǎn*), RN 6 (*qì hǎi*).

Constipation: BL 25 (*dà cháng shù*), ST 25 (*tiān shū*), SJ 6 (*zhī gōu*), ST 36 (*zú sān lǐ*).

Diarrhea: LV 3 (*tài chōng*), ST 36 (*zú sān lǐ*), SP 6 (*sān yīn jiāo*) and moxibustion at RN 8 (*shén què*).

Seminal emission: KI 3 (*tài xī*), LV 3 (*tài chōng*), needle with supplementation at RN 4 (*guān yuán*) and SP 6 (*sān yīn jiāo*), with drainage at HT 8 (*shào fǔ*).

Enuresis: HT 5 (*tōng lǐ*), KI 4 (*dà zhōng*), or moxibustion at RN 4 (*guān yuán*) and RN 3 (*zhōng jí*).

Urinary retention: RN 3 (*zhōng jí*) with RN 4 (*guān yuán*), KI 5 (*shuǐ quán*), SP 9 (*yīn líng quán*) and HT 7 (*shén mén*).

For excess patterns: add LV 2 (*xíng jiān*) and ST 40 (*fēng lóng*).

For deficiency patterns: add KI 3 (*tài xī*) and BL 23 (*shèn shù*).

3. Electro-acupuncture (EA)

Depressed patients have neurotransmitter imbalances within the central nervous system. Declined 5-HT is a critical factor which affects emotion, appetite, sleep, and endocrine function. There are studies showing that electro-acupuncture can improve the monoaminergic function of the central nervous system and also increase the content of 5-HT, NE, DA in specific locations within the brain.

Scalp EA is often used in the treatment of depression, especially points on the *du* channel. For diminished *zang-fu* function, the excitatory stimuli can help restore the body to a normal physiological state. This effect also

Chapter 6
Acupuncture and Moxibustion

applies to manual stimulation techniques and moxibustion.

Although electro-acupuncture is a highly effective therapy, the effects of antidepressants are significantly faster. However, EA is actually more effective than Western psychiatric drugs for improving cognitive function, relieving anxiety, and in the treatment of somatic symptoms. EA therapy can be applied once daily for 30-60 minutes, 5 days a week.

(1) DU 20 (*bǎi huì*) can be used as the main acupuncture point because it can not only regulate the CNS, but it can also treat hypofunctional conditions in general. Below DU 20 (*bǎi huì*) lies the cortical motor area and the lobulus paracentralis, therefore both acupuncture and medical ECT use this point and adjacent areas. Deep to DU 24 (*shén tíng*) and *yìn táng* is the prefrontal cortex, where the frontal nerve branch of the trigeminal nerve runs in the superficial layer. Below DU 20 (*bǎi huì*) and DU 24 (*shén tíng*) is galea aponeurosis and the cranium, and below *yìn táng* is subcutaneous tissue and the nasal bone.

Electro-acupuncture therapy of DU 20 (*bǎi huì*) and *yìn táng* frequently causes an imbalanced needle sensation, and high frequency EA at *yìn táng* may also cause pain. That being the case, EA is more frequently applied to DU 20 (*bǎi huì*) and DU 24 (*shén tíng*) as an alternative prescription. EA at these points can also improve sleep and cognitive function.

(2) Other commonly used ea point combinations:

LI 4 (*hé gǔ*) and LV 3 (*tài chōng*)
Tài yáng and ST 8 (*tóu wéi*)
DU 24 (*shén tíng*) and DU 26 (*shuǐ gōu*)
Ān mián and GB 20 (*fēng chí*)
DU 20 (*bǎi huì*) and *Sì Shén Cōng*
GB 13 (*běn shén*) and SI 3 (*hòu xī*)
HT 7 (*shén mén*) and LI 4 (*hé gǔ*)
HT 7 (*shén mén*) and PC 6 (*nèi guān*)
HT 7 (*shén mén*) and SP 6 (*sān yīn jiāo*)
ST 40 (*fēng lóng*) and LI 4 (*hé gǔ*)
DU 14 (*dà zhuī*) and DU 12 (*shēn zhù*)

Psychological Guidance

With chronic emotional disturbances, verbal support can be an important aspect of the treatment – *when performed within one's scope of*

practice. Guidance and counseling can help to provide self-esteem, self-awareness, and confidence.

The Spiritual Pivot – Knowledge from the Masters (*Líng Shū – Shī Chuán*) states, "Tell the patient of their weaknesses, speak to them of their goodness, guide them to that which comforts them, and open that which makes them feel bitter".

When giving treatment, a therapeutic environment is also essential. Because depressed patients usually have difficulties feeling at ease, if the environment is noisy or distracting, patients will become anxious and irritated and qi and blood disorders will worsen. Therefore, a quiet space is required, and the time given for treatment should be relatively longer than for typical treatment of internal diseases. At least 30 minutes to one hour per session is required to ensure effectiveness.

[**Editors note:** generally acupuncture treatments in the West are substantially longer than treatments in China; however, Chinese treatments are often applied on a daily basis. In the treatment of disorders of the qi dynamic that are not supported by Chinese medicinal therapy, relatively frequent treatment can be the difference between progress and temporary palliative treatment.]

Compliance and Course of Treatment

Generally, depression is not an acute disease and cannot be quickly resolved. These therapies may have some effect in a relatively short time, but a longer time is required for the body to fully recover and re-establish normal movement within the qi dynamic. If a patient fails to follow the treatment protocol, a relapse is very likely. Daily treatments should be scheduled at the beginning, with five sessions a week in order to establish a strong base; one month constitutes one course of treatment. Depending on the nature of the case, the second course of treatment may include 3 treatments per week. It usually takes 2 or 3 courses to establish effectiveness, but with recurrent depression, the course of treatment should continue for a half year or more.

Chapter 7
Associated Disease Categories

SCHIZOPHRENIA (WITHDRAWAL)

Withdrawal disease is comparable to the Western medical diagnosis of schizophrenia, although it could also encompass aspects of Asperger's spectrum disorders. In withdrawal disease with depressive disorder, the psychiatric and depressive symptoms can manifest spontaneously, or, in the stable stage of schizophrenia, depressive disorder may manifest only with low spirits, pessimism or despair.

Etiology

External factors include liver qi constraint due to chronic disease, unfulfilled desires, or suffering from social discrimination, personal rejection or other emotionally charged events that cause the patient to feel rejected and cut off from society. In students, the heavy burden of study may result in an irregular lifestyle that causes insomnia, profuse dreaming, and an inability to focus. In the middle-aged, a sudden event such as death of a loved one or a major challenge in the workplace can often result in insomnia, pessimism, an aversion to people, and a sense of world-weariness. Elderly people who suffer from chronic physical or mental conditions can also present with low spirits and world-weariness.

General factors include an irregular lifestyle, chronic diseases, long-term medication, and psychiatric medication side-effects that cause pathological changes of qi, blood, phlegm, fire. Internal pathological changes also play an important role in the onset of withdrawal disease with depressive disorder, but this condition may arise when the body's constitutional endurance has decreased, and that condition is compounded by external factors. There is a common saying in Chinese medicine: "For evil to encroach, qi must be deficient."

Pathomechanism

The pathomechanism of this condition characteristically begins with the liver affecting other organs, resulting in a disturbance of the brain. However, the liver will be the primary locus of this disease, with all clinical symptoms first arising due to liver constraint. Sudden psychological stimulation can trigger pathological changes of the brain-spirit system; also, excessive qi, blood, phlegm, fire and stasis can damage different visceral spirits to result in depressive symptoms.

When there is liver qi constraint, the liver loses its function of coursing and draining. The ethereal soul of the liver loses its composure, manifesting with low spirits, pessimism and frequent sighing. Next, as liver qi damages the spleen manifestations include digestive symptoms such as low appetite, obliviousness to hunger and satiety, reflux during or after eating, and distending fullness of the stomach duct and abdomen. In severe cases there can be scurrying pain of the rib-sides that is aggravated by pressure, with pain extending from the throat to the lower abdomen.

Long term liver qi counterflow can also result in "the child stealing the mother's qi" which then affects the function of kidney-mind. This manifests with aching limp lumbus and knees, severely decreased libido, impotence, and decreases in memory, comprehension, and the ability to calculate. When flaming liver fire encounters heart fire, the result is exuberant heart fire and disquieting of the heart-spirit, which manifests with insomnia, profuse dreaming, and heart vexation.

The other type of pathomechanism involves qi constraint, yin or blood deficiency, blood stasis, or phlegm congealing caused by medication. These factors can also result in disturbance of the qi dynamic and manifest with depressive symptoms. No matter what the pathomechanism, the manifestations of low spirits and decreased social skills are all present to different degrees. These are the major criteria for pattern differentiation and treatment of this condition.

Diagnostic Criteria

1. Withdrawal disease

(1) Family history

(2) A timid personality with a recent history of unfulfilled emotions

(3) Constrained or blank facial expression, quiet with no desire to move, feeble-minded behavior or muttering to oneself with deranged speech.

(4) Not caused by poison or fever.

(5) CT and imaging or other diagnostic testing fails to show brain anomalies.

With (3) and (4) present, using (1), (2) and (5) as a reference to confirm the diagnosis.

(Source: *Lín Chuáng Zhōng Yī Nèi Kē Xué* (Chinese Internal Medicine in Clinic), chief editor Wang Yong-yan)

In addition to the above standards, the author also believes that such symptoms should be present for at least one month to make a positive diagnosis.

2. Withdrawal disease with depressive disorder

(1) A history of withdrawal disease

(2) Low spirits, pessimism, world-weariness, sleeplessness, and heart flusteredness

(3) Low appetite, distending fullness in the stomach duct, and generalized scurrying pain

(4) Suicidal tendencies and behaviors

(5) Fear, mental tension, and lack of normal sexual activity

With (1), (2) and (5) present, using (3) and (4) as a reference can confirm the diagnosis.

3. Characteristic Symptoms

(1) Initial Stage

Patients tend to be overlooked during this stage, since the condition develops slowly. Manifestations include reduced talking, distancing people, seeming distracted, decreased passion and ability to work or study, no interest in previously enjoyable activities, and vacant speech.

Other symptoms may include headache, distention or cloudiness of the head, sleeplessness, fatigue, lack of strength, frequent pacing, unstable moods, bizarre thoughts and behaviors, and in severe cases hallucination. One must pay special attention if these symptoms occur among teenagers.

(2) Full Development

In this stage there are complex clinical manifestations; the patient's ability for self care, work and socializing is decreased or completely lost. The pathology is characterized by internally exuberant qi and blood

Chapter 7
Associated Disease Categories

disturbing the brain-spirit, which results in various psychiatric symptoms. Typical patterns include the following:

1) Liver qi stagnation
2) Phlegm binding with heat
3) Qi stagnation and blood stasis
4) Internal heat of the heart, liver, and stomach
5) Pathological *yangming* heat

(3) Advanced Stage

With a prolonged disease course, the upright becomes deficient as evil excess increases. This results in dysfunctions of the heart-spirit, spleen-intention, and kidney-mind with failure to nourish the brain. Typical patterns include the following:

1) Heart-spleen dual deficiency
2) Spleen-kidney dual deficiency
3) Yin deficiency with internal heat
4) Liver-kidney dual deficiency

During the course of withdrawal disease, patients may develop an accompanying depressive disorder regardless of age group or stage. Signs and symptoms include low spirits, feeble-mindedness, decreased talking, a tendency to lie down, self isolation, and decreased socialization.

At any stage, diagnosis and treatment of this disorder requires coordination with psychiatric and mental health professionals who will be able to support the patient and make appropriate interventions should the patient exhibit any potential for harm to themselves or others.

Withdrawal disease with depressive disorder as compared with regular depressive disorder:

1) Withdrawal disease is the root and depressive disorder is the branch.
2) Medical treatment for withdrawal disease should be systematic and consistent; with depressive symptoms, additional short-term symptomatic treatment should be applied.
3) The course of withdrawal disease is long, with a relatively shorter period of depressive disorder.

4) Patients with withdrawal disease may commit suicide while affected by hallucinations or paranoia, whereas with depressive disorder, suicide is most commonly associated with feelings of despair.

For example, a 22 year-old male was diagnosed with schizophrenia. While hallucinating, he thought his friends were telling him to jump out of the fourth floor window because the staff was going to hurt him. The patient jumped and broke his lower limbs. Such behaviors are common in psychiatric wards and not necessarily related to depressive disorder.

Pattern Differentiation and Treatment

(1) HEART AND LIVER HEAT DISTURBING THE BRAIN-SPIRIT

Signs and symptoms: vexation, irascibility, unstable moods, a bitter taste in the mouth, dry mouth, low spirits, pessimism, sleeplessness, profuse dreaming, a red tongue with a yellow slimy coating, and wiry rapid pulses.

Other symptoms may include slow thinking, occasional auditory hallucinations, over-sensitivity, suspicion, patient is cognizant of their condition; with a prolonged disease course the patient's mood may fluctuate between the desire to be cured and a lack of faith in the treatment process. There will be a moderate appetite, and regular urination and defecation.

Treatment Principles: clear the heart, drain the liver, course the gallbladder.

Formula: *Sān Huáng Zhī Zǐ Tāng* (Three Yellows and Gardenia Decoction)

黄连	huáng lián	10g	Rhizoma Coptidis
栀子	zhī zǐ	10g	Fructus Gardeniae
黄芩	huáng qín	10g	Radix Scutellariae
大黄	dà huáng	10g	Radix et Rhizoma Rhei (preserved in liquor)
生石膏	shēng shí gāo	30–80g	Gypsum Fibrosum Cruda (decocted first)
钩藤	gōu téng	30g	Ramulus Uncariae Cum Uncis
牛膝	niú xī	30g	Radix Achyranthis Bidentatae
炒枣仁	chǎo zǎo rén	30g	Semen Ziziphi Spinosae (stir-fried)

Chapter 7
Associated Disease Categories

(2) Liver Qi Constraint with Irregularity of the Brain-spirit

Signs and Symptoms: a history of withdrawal disease with recent distending fullness in the stomach duct, belching, low spirits, a tendency to weep, pessimism, world-weariness, no faith in the treatment process or will to live, a sensation of qi scurrying all over the body, reliance on sleeping pills, a sad affect, emaciation, a red tongue with a white coating, and wiry pulses.

Other symptoms may include partial cognizance, a bland taste in the mouth, fatigue, lack of strength, profuse dreaming, frequent dizziness and distention in the eyes, and no pleasure in eating.

Treatment Principles: course the liver, resolve constraint, nourish the brain, calm the spirit.

Formula: *Shū Yù Tāng* (Liver-Soothing Decoction)

柴胡	*chái hú*	6g	Radix Bupleuri
白芍	*bái sháo*	30g	Radix Paeoniae Alba
香附	*xiāng fù*	10g	Rhizoma Cyperi
天竺黄	*tiān zhú huáng*	15g	Concretio Silicea Bambusae
郁金	*yù jīn*	30g	Radix Curcumae
佛手	*fó shǒu*	15g	Fructus Citri Sarcodactylis
香橼	*xiāng yuán*	15g	Fructus Citri
百合	*bǎi hé*	30g	Bulbus Lilii
炒枣仁	*chǎo zǎo rén*	30g	Semen Ziziphi Spinosae (stir-fried)
神曲	*shén qū*	15g	Massa Medicata Fermentata

(3) Spleen-kidney Dual Deficiency with Failure to Nourish the Brain

Signs and Symptoms: pessimism, frequent feelings of world-weariness, passive in social situations, stomach duct discomfort, aching limp lumbus and knees, decreased appetite, emaciation, distraction, and poor short-term memory.

Other symptoms may include a bright white facial complexion, frequent trembling of the extremities, sleeping lightly and easily aroused, the appearance of chronic illness, shortness of breath, no strength to speak, self isolation, a tendency to lie down and become lost in thought, loose stools, long voidings of clear urine, and fine sunken pulses.

Treatment Principles: supplement the spleen, secure the kidney, nourish the brain-spirit.

Formula: *Qù Dāi Xǐng Nǎo Tāng* (Torpidity-Eliminating Brain-Awakening Decoction)

党参	dǎng shēn	15g	Radix Codonopsis
茯苓	fú líng	30g	Poria
太子参	tài zǐ shēn	30g	Radix Pseudostellariae
枸杞子	gǒu qǐ zǐ	15g	Fructus Lycii
肉苁蓉	ròu cōng róng	30g	Herba Cistanches
巴戟天	bā jǐ tiān	30g	Radix Morindae Officinalis
龟甲	guī jiǎ	10g	Carapax et Plastrum Testudinis
女贞子	nǚ zhēn zǐ	30g	Fructus Ligustri Lucidi
菟丝子	tù sī zǐ	30g	Semen Cuscutae
仙灵脾	xiān líng pí	15g	Herba Epimedii
炒枣仁	chǎo zǎo rén	30g	Semen Ziziphi Spinosae (stir-fried)
神曲	shén qū	15g	Massa Medicata Fermentata

(4) Heart-spleen Dual Deficiency, Kidney Failing to Nourish the Brain

This pattern is commonly seen during the remission stage of withdrawal disease when the patient's ability to work recovers.

Signs and Symptoms: a tendency to become lost in thought, fear of incidents involving family or work life, worry about misery in old age, pessimism, disappointment, world-weariness, emaciation, a desire to end the misery by killing oneself, and sunken fine pulses.

Other symptoms may include fatigue of the extremities, worry, no desire to eat or dietary irregularities, and blank staring.

Treatment Principles: supplement heart and spleen, nourish the brain, calm the spirit.

Formula:

太子参	tài zǐ shēn	30g	Radix Pseudostellariae

Chapter 7
Associated Disease Categories

麦门冬	mài mén dōng	30g	Radix Ophiopogonis
五味子	wǔ wèi zǐ	10g	Fructus Schisandrae Chinensis
茯神	fú shén	15g	Sclerotium Poriae Pararadicis
枸杞子	gǒu qǐ zǐ	15g	Fructus Lycii
女贞子	nǔ zhēn zǐ	30g	Fructus Ligustri Lucidi
菟丝子	tù sī zǐ	30g	Semen Cuscutae
仙灵脾	xiān líng pí	15g	Herba Epimedii
龟甲	guī jiǎ	10g	Carapax et Plastrum Testudinis
赤芍	chì sháo	30g	Radix Paeoniae Rubra
白芍	bái sháo	30g	Radix Paeoniae Alba
肉苁蓉	ròu cōng róng	30g	Herba Cistanches
红花	hóng huā	10g	Flos Carthami
葛根	gé gēn	15g	Radix Puerariae Lobatae

Commentary

Depressive symptoms can occur in any clinical stage of withdrawal disease; however, in most cases they occur during the late stage. Regarding the standard methods of treatment, with liver yin insufficiency, water-benefiting and liver-nourishing methods are recommended. Yang-invigorating medicinals can be added while supplementing yin. Once the yin and yang of the kidney is harmonized, marrow can be engendered, the brain-spirit will be adequately nourished and can be awakened and freed.

INSOMNIA

This condition is characterized by intractable insomnia with accompanying depressive disorder symptoms. It is very frequently encountered in the clinic.

Insomnia with depressive disorder refers to cases where, after the onset of insomnia, the patient starts to develop relatively severe and persistent low spirits, pessimism, despair, and decreased outside activities and socializing. This tends to aggravate the existing insomnia and thus forms a negative cycle. If the primary condition is depressive disorder with insomnia as a main symptom, readers can refer to other more appropriate sections of this chapter.

Etiology

1. Emotional irregularities with inhibition of the qi dynamic transforming into fire. Fire flames upwards to disturb the brain-spirit.

2. Physical conditions resulting in yin and yang imbalances of the five viscera where qi and blood depletion leads to malnourishment the brain.

3. Improper treatment of externally contracted seasonal evils.

Pathomechanism

During the initial stage, over-thinking, anxiety, worry, or sorrow can all lead to qi and blood depletion in the five viscera which in turn fail to nourish the brain-spirit.

Internal phlegm-fire and insufficiency or stagnation of the upright qi can all cause irregularities of the qi dynamic and a disharmony of yin and yang that can affect the brain-spirit.

Prolonged physical conditions with resulting damages to qi and blood, improper treatment of externally contracted seasonal evils, or spleen-stomach disharmonies can all cause disquietude of the brain-spirit which results in sleeplessness. When the brain-spirit is restless it also becomes constrained and stagnated. Additionally, the qi dynamic of the viscera and bowels is already inhibited in these cases, which will naturally lead to a feeling of ungratified emotions and eventually depression. Therefore, in diseases related to the brain-spirit, insomnia and depression are commonly seen together. In this condition, insomnia occurs before the depression and is as such the main symptom, however, it should be noted that the occurrence of depression marks an aggravation of the overall condition.

Location, nature, and prognosis

This condition can involve the heart, liver, spleen, kidney and brain, often manifesting with complex multiple deficiency patterns. Heart-spleen dual deficiency is the predominant expression, but excess patterns like qi stagnation and phlegm-fire are also very common. This condition can last for years without improvement, and eventually leads to spleen-kidney

Chapter 7
Associated Disease Categories

deficiency with brain-spirit depletion. When insomnia is the primary symptom, the emotional states tend to improve after the quality of sleep improves.

Clinical Guidelines

1. Thoroughly understand the patient's history; inquire of the patient and his family or acquaintances in detail regarding the onset, progress and associated symptoms. Primarily focus on the sequence and severity of insomnia and emotional symptoms. Understand all medications the patient is taking.

2. When you have diagnosed a patient with insomnia that leads to depressive disorder, focus on improving the patient's sleep quality while also paying attention for other possible causes of emotional disorder, as they may not be causally related.

3. If the condition persists, then the insomnia may be a manifestation of the depressive disorder. In that case, the treatment should focus on regulating qi. If the depressive disorder is primary, when the depression improves sleep will also improve spontaneously, or at least become easier to treat. Clinically, insomnia is a very common complaint, but in many cases the actual condition is depressive disorder. Both physicians and patients can easily ignore emotional factors even though they are the key to understanding the actual pathomechanism.

4. Long term use of sleeping medications or heavy-settling medicinal formulas to induce sleep can exacerbate qi depression, potentially leading to increased patterns depressed heat and insomnia. If the primary complaint is insomnia, this should be less of a problem, but in primary depression, especially where emotional factors were not taking into account in the diagnosis, this is in fact a common side effect of treatment.

Pattern Differentiation and Treatment

(1) LIVER AND KIDNEY YIN DEFICIENCY

Signs and Symptoms: difficulty falling asleep, sleeplessness or a tendency to sleep lightly, dizziness, blurred vision, vexation, agitation, irascibility, fatigue upon waking, palpitations, heart throbbing, poor memory, distraction, aching limp lumbus and knees, worry, sorrow, pessimism, world-weariness, irregular defecation, frequent urination, a red tongue with a white coating or thin yellow coating, and fine wiry rapid pulses.

Other symptoms may include dietary irregularity, distending fullness of the stomach duct, frequent aching of the rib-sides, sores of the mouth and tongue, limp lower extremities, seminal emission, impotence, and premature ejaculation.

Treatment Principles: nourish the liver and kidney, quiet the spirit, resolve constraint.

Formulas: *Wū Tù Tāng* (Fleeceflower Root and Dodder Seed Decoction)

Qù Yù Xǐng Shén Tāng (Constraint-Eliminating Spirit-Awakening Decoction)

何首乌	hé shǒu wū	15g	Radix Polygoni Multiflori
桑叶	sāng yè	10g	Folium Mori
炒枣仁	chǎo zǎo rén	15g	Semen Ziziphi Spinosae (stir-fried)
菟丝子	tù sī zǐ	15g	Semen Cuscutae
菊花	jú huā	10g	Flos Chrysanthemi
五味子	wǔ wèi zǐ	10g	Fructus Schisandrae Chinensis
桑椹	sāng shèn	15g	Fructus Mori
远志	yuǎn zhì	6g	Radix Polygalae
生龙骨	shēng lóng gǔ	30g	Os Draconis (decocted first)
生牡蛎	shēng mǔ lì	30g	Concha Ostreae Cruda (decocted first)

菊花	jú huā	15g	Flos Chrysanthemi
白芍	bái sháo	30g	Radix Paeoniae Alba
白蒺藜	bái jí lí	30g	Fructus Tribuli
枸杞子	gǒu qǐ zǐ	30g	Fructus Lycii
山茱萸	shān zhū yú	15g	Fructus Corni
女贞子	nǚ zhēn zǐ	30g	Fructus Ligustri Lucidi
菟丝子	tù sī zǐ	30g	Semen Cuscutae
炒枣仁	chǎo zǎo rén	30g	Semen Ziziphi Spinosae (stir-fried)
丹参	dān shēn	30g	Radix et Rhizoma Salviae Miltiorrhizae
肉苁蓉	ròu cōng róng	30g	Herba Cistanches

Chapter 7
Associated Disease Categories

Modifications:

➢ With extremely poor sleep or with no observable effect after taking the formula, increase the dosage of *chǎo zǎo rén* (Semen Ziziphi Spinosae, stir-fried) to 70g, add *hé huān pí* (Cortex Albiziae) 30g and *yè jiāo téng* (Caulis Polygoni Multiflori) 30g.

➢ With thirst, add *shēng shí gāo* (Gypsum Fibrosum Cruda, decocted first) 80g.

➢ With predominant liver-kidney yin deficiency, add *shú dì huáng* (Radix Rehmanniae Praeparata) 20g.

➢ With headache, add *chuān xiōng* (Rhizoma Chuanxiong) 15g.

➢ With dizziness, add *gōu téng* (Ramulus Uncariae Cum Uncis) 30g.

➢ With low appetite, add *chén pí* (Pericarpium Citri Reticulatae) 12g, and *jiāo mài yá* (Fructus Hordei Germinatus Ustus), *jiāo shān zhā* (Fructus Crataegi) and *jiāo shén qū* (Massa Medicata Fermentata Ustus) 30g respectively.

➢ With liver yin insufficiency manifesting with agitation and irascibility, substantially increase the dosage of *bái sháo* (Radix Paeoniae Alba), add *dāng guī* (Radix Angelicae Sinensis) 15g and *shēng dì* (Radix Rehmanniae) 20g.

➢ With spontaneous sweating, add *mǔ dān pí* (Cortex Moutan) 10g and *shēng dì* (Radix Rehmanniae) 30g.

➢ With spleen-stomach qi stagnation accompanied by glomus and oppression of the chest and stomach duct, belching, and slimy tongue fur, add *xiāng fù* (Rhizoma Cyperi) 10g, *fó shǒu* (Fructus Citri Sarcodactylis) 10g and *cāng zhú* (Rhizoma Atractylodis) 15g.

➢ With phlegm-heat, add *zhú rú* (Caulis Bambusae in Taenia) 10g, *guā lóu* (FructusTrichosanthis) 30g, *huáng qín* (Radix Scutellariae) 15g, and *huáng lián* (Rhizoma Coptidis) 15g.

➢ With aching lumbus and limp lower extremities, add *dù zhòng* (Cortex Eucommiae) 15g and *niú xī* (Radix Achyranthis Bidentatae) 30g.

(2) HEART AND SPLEEN DUAL DEFICIENCY

Signs and Symptoms: insomnia, profuse dreaming, tendency to sleep lightly, flusteredness, heart palpitations, shortness of breath, fatigue, lack of strength, a yellowish-white facial complexion, lusterless flesh or emaciation, no pleasure in eating, occasional sensations of tightness in the head, low spirits, no interest in formerly enjoyable activities, laziness, decreased appetite, loose stools, long voidings of clear urine, a pale tongue with a white coating, and fine, sunken, weak pulses.

Other symptoms may include occasional spontaneous sweating, mental vexation and derangement at night, extreme fatigue upon waking in the morning, difficulty thinking, a tendency to lie down, and generalized discomfort.

Treatment Principles: nourish the heart, benefit the spleen, quiet the mind, calm the spirit.

Formula: Modified *Guī Pí Tāng* (Spleen-Restoring Decoction)

生黄芪	shēng huáng qí	15g	Radix Astragali raw
党参	dǎng shēn	15g	Radix Codonopsis
太子参	tài zǐ shēn	30g	Radix Pseudostellariae
炒白术	chǎo bái zhú	15g	Rhizoma Atractylodis Macrocephalae (stir-fried)
茯苓	fú líng	30g	Poria
炒枣仁	chǎo zǎo rén	60g	Semen Ziziphi Spinosae (stir-fried)
当归	dāng guī	12g	Radix Angelicae Sinensis
远志	yuǎn zhì	10g	Radix Polygalae
炙甘草	zhì gān cǎo	10g	Radix et Rhizoma Glycyrrhizae Praeparata cum Melle
神曲	shén qū	15g	Massa Medicata Fermentata
郁金	yù jīn	30g	Radix Curcumae
香附	xiāng fù	10g	Rhizoma Cyperi
佛手	fó shǒu	10g	Fructus Citri Sarcodactylis
枳壳	zhǐ qiào	10g	Fructus Aurantii

Modifications:

➢ With poor sleep, use 30–60g *chǎo zǎo rén* (Semen Ziziphi Spinosae, stir-fried) with additional *yè jiāo téng* (Caulis Polygoni Multiflori) 30g, *hé huān pí* (Cortex Albiziae) 30g, and *wǔ wèi zǐ* (Fructus Schisandrae Chinensis) 30g.

➢ With predominant head discomfort, add *jú huā* (Flos Chrysanthemi) 15g, *dān shēn* (Radix et Rhizoma Salviae Miltiorrhizae) 30g, and *chuān xiōng* (Rhizoma Chuanxiong) 20g.

➢ With chest oppression, add *chái hú* (Radix Bupleuri) 6g, *yù jīn*

Chapter 7
Associated Disease Categories

(Radix Curcumae) 30g, and *bái sháo* (Radix Paeoniae Alba) 30g.

➤ With a slimy tongue coating, add *huò xiāng* (Herba Agastachis) 10g and *pèi lán* (Herba Eupatorii) 10g.

➤ With severe spontaneous sweating, increase the dosage of *shēng huáng qí* (Radix Astragali raw) and *chǎo bái zhú* (Rhizoma Atractylodis Macrocephalae, stir-fried), add *fáng fēng* (Radix Saposhnikoviae) and *fú xiǎo mài* (Fructus Tritici Levis).

(3) Yin Deficiency with Effulgent Fire

Signs and Symptoms: deficiency vexation with sleeplessness, profuse dreaming, flusteredness, heart palpitations, dry mouth with scant fluids, dry eyes, vexing heat in the hearts of palms and soles, spontaneous sweating, night sweats, sores of the mouth and tongue, no pleasure in eating, low spirits, intermittent vexation and agitation, dry stools or irregular defecation, a red tongue with scant fluids and a thin coating, and fine rapid pulses.

Other symptoms may include pessimism, occasional sobbing, fidgetiness, susceptibility to fright, timidity, distraction, poor memory, seminal emission, impotence, premature ejaculation, and an aching limp lumbus and knees.

Treatment Principles: nourish yin, clear heat, calm the brain-spirit.

Formula: Modified *Huáng Lián Ē Jiāo Tāng*（Coptis and Donkey-Hide Gelatin Decoction）

黄连	huáng lián	6g	Rhizoma Coptidis
生地	shēng dì	20g	Radix Rehmanniae
麦门冬	mài mén dōng	20g	Radix Ophiopogonis
青蒿	qīng hāo	10g	Herba Artemisiae Annuae
地骨皮	dì gǔ pí	30g	Cortex Lycii
生石膏	shēng shí gāo	60g	Gypsum Fibrosum Cruda (decocted first)
远志	yuǎn zhì	10g	Radix Polygalae
当归	dāng guī	12g	Radix Angelicae Sinensis
炒枣仁	chǎo zǎo rén	30g	Semen Ziziphi Spinosae (stir-fried)
合欢皮	hé huān pí	30g	Cortex Albiziae
石斛	shí hú	30g	Caulis Dendrobii
鸡子黄	jī zǐ huáng	2 pieces	

Modifications:

➢ With predominant heart-yin deficiency, add *Tiān Wáng Bǔ Xīn Dān* (Celestial Emperor Heart-Supplementing Elixir), 1 pill, twice daily.

➢ With predominant heart-kidney yin deficiency, add *Mài Wèi Dì Huáng Wán* (Ophiopogon and Rehmannia Pill), 1 pill, twice daily.

➢ With effulgent deficiency fire, add *Zhū Shā Ān Shén Wán* (Cinnabar Spirit-Calming Pill), 2 pills at night.

➢ With frequent seminal emission, add *Zhī Bǎi Dì Huáng Wán* (Anemarrhena, Phellodendron and Rehmannia Pill).

➢ With agitation and irascibility, add *shēng shí jué míng* (Concha Haliotidis raw, decocted first) 30g, *cí shí* (Magnetitum) (decocted first) 30g, *gōu téng* (Ramulus Uncariae Cum Uncis) 30g and *zhī zǐ* (Fructus Gardeniae) 10g.

➢ With decreased memory, add *gǒu qǐ zǐ* (Fructus Lycii) 15g, *tù sī zǐ* (Semen Cuscutae) 30g and *zhì biē jiǎ* (Carapax Trionycis, processed) 10g.

(4) STOMACH QI DISHARMONY

Signs and Symptoms: sleeplessness, profuse dreaming, dietary irregularity, discomfort in the chest and rib-sides, distending fullness in the stomach duct, hunger with no desire to eat or fullness upon forced eating, belching, hiccoughing, occasional nausea and vomiting or putrid belching and acid swallowing, extremely smelly stools, constipation, vexation and agitation, disquietude or low spirits, sad facial expressions, no interest in previously enjoyable activities, passiveness, and a red tongue with a dry yellow or slimy yellow coating.

Other symptoms may include dream-disturbed sleep with difficulty getting back to sleep, distention, heaviness and pain in the head, pain of the forehead, a sensation of tightness in the head and nape, and generalized discomfort.

Treatment Principles: harmonize the stomach, quiet the spirit.
Formula: Modified *Bǎo Hé Wán* (Harmony-Preserving Pill)

神曲	*shén qū*	15g	Massa Medicata Fermentata
山楂	*shān zhā*	15g	Fructus Crataegi

Chapter 7
Associated Disease Categories

莱菔子	lái fú zǐ	30g	Semen Raphani
陈皮	chén pí	12g	Pericarpium Citri Reticulatae
半夏	bàn xià	12g	Rhizoma Pinelliae
瓦楞子	wǎ léng zǐ	30g	Concha Arcae
茯苓	fú líng	30g	Poria
连翘	lián qiào	6g	Fructus Forsythiae
槟榔	bīng láng	10g	Semen Arecae
青皮	qīng pí	10g	Pericarpium Citri Reticulatae Viride
香附	xiāng fù	10g	Rhizoma Cyperi
炒枣仁	chǎo zǎo rén	30g	Semen Ziziphi Spinosae (stir-fried)
柏子仁	bǎi zǐ rén	30g	Semen Platycladi
合欢皮	hé huān pí	30g	Cortex Albiziae

Modifications:

➢ With foul-smelling stools, add *jiǔ zhì dà huáng* (Radix et Rhizoma Rhei, preserved in liquor) 15g and *huǒ má rén* (Fructus Cannabis) 30g.

➢ With heart vexation, add *huáng lián* (Rhizoma Coptidis) 10g and *zhī zǐ* (Fructus Gardeniae) 10g.

➢ With abdominal distention and fullness of the chest and rib-sides, add *xiāng fù* (Rhizoma Cyperi) 10g, *xiāng yuán* (Fructus Citri) 15g, *yù jīn* (Radix Curcumae) 30g, and *zhǐ qiào* (Fructus Aurantii) 15g.

➢ With predominant spleen deficiency, add *fú líng* (Poria) 30g.

(5) Phlegm-fire Disturbing the Heart, Harassing the Brain-spirit

Signs and Symptoms: sleeplessness, bitterness in the mouth, nausea and vomiting, glomus and oppression in the chest and stomach duct, heart vexation, vexing heat, susceptibility to fright, low spirits, unstable moods, irascibility, dry stool, a red tongue with a dry yellow or slimy yellow coating, and wiry slippery rapid pulses.

Other symptoms may include profuse dreaming, difficulty falling asleep, reddish-yellow urine, a dry mouth and loss of voice.

Treatment Principles: sweep phlegm, clear fire, calm the spirit.

Formula: Modified *Wēn Dǎn Tāng* (Gallbladder-Warming Decoction)

半夏	bàn xià	10g	Rhizoma Pinelliae
茯苓	fú líng	30g	Poria
橘红	jú hóng	10g	Exocarpium Citri Rubrum
竹茹	zhú rú	6g	Caulis Bambusae in Taenia
枳实	zhǐ shí	10g	Fructus Aurantii Immaturus
炙甘草	zhì gān cǎo	6g	Radix et Rhizoma Glycyrrhizae Praeparata cum Melle
炒枣仁	chǎo zǎo rén	30g	Semen Ziziphi Spinosae (stir-fried)
夜交藤	yè jiāo téng	30g	Caulis Polygoni Multiflori
合欢皮	hé huān pí	30g	Cortex Albiziae
远志	yuǎn zhì	10g	Radix Polygalae
大黄	dà huáng	10g	Radix et Rhizoma Rhei (preserved in liquor)
火麻仁	huǒ má rén	30g	Fructus Cannabis
莱菔子	lái fú zǐ	30g	Semen Raphani
天竺黄	tiān zhú huáng	15g	Concretio Silicea Bambusae
郁金	yù jīn	30g	Radix Curcumae

Modifications:

➢ With predominant vexation and agitation, add *zhī zǐ* (Fructus Gardeniae) 10g and *huáng qín* (Radix Scutellariae) 15g.

➢ With qi stagnation, add *xiāng fù* (Rhizoma Cyperi) 10g, *xiāng yuán* (Fructus Citri) 10g, and *yù jīn* (Radix Curcumae) 15g.

➢ With heart vexation, add *huáng lián* (Rhizoma Coptidis) 15g and *zhī zǐ* (Fructus Gardeniae) 10g.

➢ With vexation, agitation and irascibility, add *shēng shí gāo* (Gypsum Crudum) 80g, *shēng shí jué míng* (Concha Haliotidis Cruda) 30g and *cí shí* (Magnetitum) (decocted first) 30g.

➢ With cloudiness of head and cloudy vision, add *jú huā* (Flos Chrysanthemi) 15g, *bái jí lí* (Fructus Tribuli) 30g, *chuān xiōng* (Rhizoma Chuanxiong) 15g, and *dān shēn* (Radix et Rhizoma Salviae Miltiorrhizae) 15g.

➢ With effulgent liver fire, add *lóng dǎn cǎo* (Radix et Rhizoma Gentianae) 10g and *niú xī* (Radix Achyranthis Bidentatae) 30g.

➢ With severe insomnia, add *hǔ pò miàn* (Succinum, powdered) (not decocted, infused) 6g.

➢ With exuberant phlegm, add *méng shí* (Chlorite-schist) 30g and

Chapter 7
Associated Disease Categories

dǎn nán xīng (Arisaema cum Bile) 10g.

Commentary

Clinically, insomnia can occur as a symptom in a wide variety of physical and mental conditions; in this case, however, the insomnia occurs with no other physical or mental conditions, or, if there are other symptoms, the insomnia is primary. In severe cases, patients may present with total sleeplessness, profuse dreaming after falling asleep, fatigue all day after awakening, low energy, and no pleasure in eating. Over a period of time, the presentation will include low spirits, vexation, agitation, and a gradually decreasing quality of life. Although this will induce pessimism and disappointment, insomnia remains at the core of the pathological process.

The typical causes of insomnia with concurrent depressive disorder can be divided into two categories: The first is sudden emotional stimulation and ungratified emotions that cannot be resolved within a short period of time. The strains of these emotional forces disrupt the qi dynamic and impede normal emotional expression. Thus, because they are stagnant, the five minds transform into fire and insomnia occurs. The nature of this kind of condition is acute, and usually falls into the category of excess. The other is long-term emotional stimulation, usually ascribed to deficiency patterns. The patient suffers from unspeakable sorrow and tends to remain lost in reflective thoughts most of the time.

Typical symptoms include drowsiness, distending sensations of the head, a generalized lack of strength, extreme fatigue especially on waking, vexation, irascibility, no pleasure in eating, low spirits, pessimism, a sad facial expression, and decreased memory and mental focus. Although this condition is considered primarily as insomnia with secondary depression, the pathomechanism is unified in this case and should be treated appropriately.

Typical treatment methods for insomnia involve either tranquilizing with heavy sedation or through nourishing of the the spirit, however, just using large doses of tranquilizing medicinals or only applying heart-nourishing spirit-calming methods may not bring satisfactory results. To treat the root, especially in chronic cases, one must regulate qi and blood, especially the qi dynamic. When differentiating the pattern, pay attention to both the nature and location of the disease, and also the emotional triggers of the condition.

In cases where a patient has already been taking large doses of sedatives for a long period of time and the symptoms remain unresolved, when they seek Chinese medicine treatment, advise the patient to discuss how they should proceed with their physician. Advise them against terminating any pharmaceuticals all at once, and to reduce the dosage gradually while increasing the dosages of spirit-calming medicinals.

In the chronic stage, patients also tend to present with underlying pattetrn of qi and blood stagnation. If initial treatment is ineffective, pay attention to moving qi and blood, resolving possible drug toxicities, and calming and regulating of the viscera and bowels.

Generally speaking, if the patient presents with physical conditions that are related to the insomnia, treatments that improve sleep quality and mood will also help to resolve the physical condition. There is not always a need to address all accompanying physical symptoms by the adding of ingredients to a formula; simply prescribe constraint-opening or spirit-calming medicinals, and be sure that the patient is compliant. At the beginning of treatment, tranquilizing medications can still be utilized, especially if they serve as the only relief the patient has had over a long period of time. However, once there is improvement in the quality and quantity of sleep, the dosages of Western medicine should be reduced to the minimum as soon as possible. At this point, the goal of treatment is to effectively regulate the viscera and bowels with Chinese medicinals alone.

SOMNOLENCE

Somnolence is characterized by falling asleep intermittently and uncontrollably during the daytime. A somnolent patient can be awake and alert and then fall asleep any time. Somnolence with depressive disorder refers to any condition manifesting with primary somnolence and additional symptoms of low spirits, pessimism, despair, and no interest in life. The somnolence is predominant and usually occurs first; secondary depression appears as somnolence erodes quality of life and social relations.

Chapter 7
Associated Disease Categories

Etiology and Pathomechanism

Dietary irregularity with excessive consumption of raw, cold, greasy or sweet foods, external contraction of damp evil, over-thinking, over-indulgence in sexual activities, severe or chronic diseases or blood loss damaging the upright qi of the body, and blood vessel blockage due to head trauma or other factors can all cause malnourishment and constraint of the brain-spirit. When somnolence affects quality of life, the emotions tend to become depressed and pessimistic and depression disease can result.

1. Dietary irregularity, damp-evil external contraction

Spleen-stomach damage due to excessive consumption of raw, cold, greasy and sweet foods and excessive drinking, and contraction of damp evil due to long-term residence in damp places, or excessive exposure to rain can all lead to damp evil accumulating in the middle burner to obstruct the spleen and stomach. This causes impaired splenic transportation and transformation, and internal brewing of phlegm-turbidity. When obstructed by phlegm, clear yang qi will not be effused and fails to nourish the brain spirit, and yin becomes more exuberant; the resulting obstruction of the qi dynamic leaves the body feeling lethargic and heavy. Since the spirit is both undernourished and obstructed, somnolence occurs.

2. Over-thinking and taxation fatigue

Over-thinking and taxation fatigue can damage the heart and spleen. When the spleen and heart are weakened, their function of engendering of qi and blood suffers. When the source of transformation is insufficient, qi and blood become depleted and the brain-spirit becomes dysfunctional. In other cases, the brain-spirit becomes malnourished and somnolence appears due to irregularities of qi, blood, yin and yang resulting from severe or chronic physical conditions, profuse menstrual bleeding, or kidney yin and yang depletion.

3. Other factors

Include blood vessel obstruction due to head trauma, qi and blood derangement due to emotional irregularities, and phlegm-turbidity obstructing the collaterals. These can all lead to constraint of the brain-spirit and result in somnolence.

Pattern Differentiation and Treatment

(1) Dampness Encumbering Spleen-yang, Brain-spirit Loss of Regularity

Signs and Symptoms: somnolence, fatigue, a tendency to lie down, worry, pessimism, despair, heavy sensations in the head and extremities, irregular defecation, a pale tongue with a white slimy or yellow slimy coating, and sunken slippery or soggy slippery pulses.

Other symptoms may include weight gain, profuse dreaming, vexation, and agitation.

Treatment Principles: fortify the spleen, disinhibit dampness, awaken the brain, open orifices, resolve constraint.

Formula:

苍术	cāng zhú	15g	Rhizoma Atractylodis
茯苓	fú líng	30g	Poria
陈皮	chén pí	10g	Pericarpium Citri Reticulatae
青皮	qīng pí	10g	Pericarpium Citri Reticulatae Viride
佩兰	pèi lán	10g	Herba Eupatorii
石菖蒲	shí chāng pú	6g	Rhizoma Acori Tatarinowii
厚朴	hòu pò	10g	Cortex Magnoliae Officinalis
栀子	zhī zǐ	10g	Fructus Gardeniae
生姜	shēng jiāng	6g	Rhizoma Zingiberis Recens
猪苓	zhū líng	10g	Polyporus
焦麦芽	jiāo mài yá	30g	Fructus Hordei Germinatus Ustus
焦山楂	jiāo shān zhā	30g	Fructus Crataegi
焦神曲	jiāo shén qū	30g	Massa Medicata Fermentata Ustus

Modifications:

➢ With vexation and agitation, slimy yellow tongue coating and anguish in the heart, add *bàn xià* (Rhizoma Pinelliae), *zhú rú* (Caulis Bambusae in Taenia) 6g, *huáng qín* (Radix Scutellariae)

Chapter 7
Associated Disease Categories

10g, and *huáng lián* (Rhizoma Coptidis) 10g.

➤ With qi stagnation, add *yù jīn* (Radix Curcumae) 15g, *xiāng fù* (Rhizoma Cyperi) 10g, and *shā rén* (Fructus Amomi) 6g.

(2) KIDNEY YANG DEFICIENCY

Signs and Symptoms: somnolence, fatigue, disinclination to move, low spirits, no interest in life, denial of the condition, pessimism, despair, suicidal thoughts, aversion to cold, cold limbs, aching limp lumbus and knees, listlessness of the spirit, loose stools, poor memory, frequent nighttime urination, a pale tongue with a white coating, and sunken fine weak pulses.

Other symptoms may include low appetite, a bland taste in the mouth, lack of strength in walking, profuse dreaming with a tendency to be easily roused from sleep.

Treatment Principles: warm and supplement kidney yang, nourish the brain, calm the spirit.

Formula:

炮附子	páo fù zǐ	6g	Radix Aconiti Lateralis (blast-fried)
熟地黄	shú dì huáng	10g	Radix Rehmanniae Praeparata
炒山药	chǎo shān yào	15g	Rhizoma Dioscoreae (mix-fried)
山茱萸	shān zhū yú	10g	Fructus Corni
茯苓	fú líng	30g	Poria
泽泻	zé xiè	15g	Rhizoma Alismatis
牡丹皮	mǔ dān pí	15g	Cortex Moutan
仙灵脾	xiān líng pí	15g	Herba Epimedii
菟丝子	tù sī zǐ	15g	Semen Cuscutae

(3) KIDNEY-ESSENCE DEPLETION

Signs and Symptoms: fatigue, a tendency to lie down, intermittent sleeping, slowed thought and reactions, forgetfulness, low spirits, pessimism, despair, no interest in life, timidity, no desire for social interaction, tinnitus or loss of hearing, aching limp lumbus and legs, frequent seminal emission and seminal efflux, a pale tongue with scanty coating, and fine sunken rapid pulses.

Other symptoms may include emaciation, difficulty moving, a low, faint voice, occasional deficiency vexation, and light sleeping

Treatment Principles: benefit the kidney, replenish essence, supplement marrow, fortify the brain.

Formula:

枸杞子	gǒu qǐ zǐ	10g	Fructus Lycii
五味子	wǔ wèi zǐ	10g	Fructus Schisandrae Chinensis
菟丝子	tù sī zǐ	30g	Semen Cuscutae
桑椹	sāng shèn	15g	Fructus Mori
炒山药	chǎo shān yào	15g	Rhizoma Dioscoreae (mix-fried)
山茱萸	shān zhū yú	10g	Fructus Corni
鹿角胶	lù jiǎo jiāo	15g	Colla Cornus Cervi
龟甲	guī jiǎ	10g	Carapax et Plastrum Testudinis
牛膝	niú xī	30g	Radix Achyranthis Bidentatae

Modifications:

➢ With lumbar pain, add *dù zhòng* (Cortex Eucommiae) 15g.

➢ With poor food intake, add *chǎo gǔ yá* (Fructus Setariae Germinatus, mix-fried) and *chǎo mài yá* (Fructus Hordei Germinatus) 10g each.

(4) Heart and Spleen Dual Deficiency

Signs and Symptoms: somnolence, forgetfulness, susceptibility to fright, heart palpitations, shortness of breath, profuse dreaming at night, timidity, no desire to socialize, lassitude, low spirits, pessimism, fatigue of the extremities, bright white facial complexion, reduced food intake, loose stools, spontaneous sweating or sweating at the slightest exertion, a pale tongue with no coating, and fine slow or soggy fine pulses.

Other symptoms may include blank or sad affect, slow speech and reticence, vexing heat in the five hearts, occasional spontaneous sweating, cold night sweats, poor appetite, stomach duct discomfort, and generalized fatigue.

Treatment Principles: supplement heart and spleen, nourish the brain, calm the spirit.

Formula:

Chapter 7
Associated Disease Categories

茯苓	fú líng	30g	Poria
党参	dǎng shēn	15g	Radix Codonopsis
太子参	tài zǐ shēn	30g	Radix Pseudostellariae
炒白术	chǎo bái zhú	15g	Rhizoma Atractylodis Macrocephalae (mix-fried)
炙甘草	zhì gān cǎo	10g	Radix et Rhizoma Glycyrrhizae Praeparata cum Melle
麦门冬	mài mén dōng	30g	Radix Ophiopogonis
五味子	wǔ wèi zǐ	15g	Fructus Schisandrae Chinensis
生黄芪	shēng huáng qí	30g	Radix Astragali raw
大枣	dà zǎo	10g	Fructus Jujubae
炒谷芽	chǎo gǔ yá	15g	Fructus Setariae Germinatus (mix-fried)
炒麦芽	chǎo mài yá	15g	Fructus Hordei Germinatus

Modifications:

➢ With shortness of breath and sweating at the slightest exertion, add *shēng huáng qí* (Radix Astragali raw) 30g and *dà zǎo* (Fructus Jujubae) 10g.

➢ With spontaneous sweating, add *dì gǔ pí* (Cortex Lycii) 15g and *wǔ wèi zǐ* (Fructus Schisandrae Chinensis) 10g.

(5) LIVER-GALLBLADDER DAMP-HEAT

Signs and Symptoms: somnolence with light sleeping, drowsiness and oppression as if drunk or sedated, heaviness of the head, low spirits, unstable mood, vexation, agitation, irascibility, short bursts of rage, bitterness or sliminess in the mouth, yellow or turbid urine, dry stools, a red tongue with yellow or yellow slimy coating, and slippery rapid pulses.

Other symptoms may include fullness in the chest and rib-sides, no pleasure in eating, profuse dreaming, and intermittent sleeping.

Treatment Principles: clear the liver, disinhibit the gallbladder, eliminate dampness, clear the brain.

Formula:

龙胆草	lóng dǎn cǎo	10g	Radix et Rhizoma Gentianae
栀子	zhī zǐ	10g	Fructus Gardeniae
牡丹皮	mǔ dān pí	15g	Cortex Moutan
柴胡	chái hú	6g	Radix Bupleuri

青皮	qīng pí	10g	Pericarpium Citri Reticulatae Viride
陈皮	chén pí	10g	Pericarpium Citri Reticulatae
生地	shēng dì	30g	Radix Rehmanniae
黄芩	huáng qín	10g	Radix Scutellariae
泽泻	zé xiè	10g	Rhizoma Alismatis
车前子	chē qián zǐ	10g	Semen Plantaginis
当归	dāng guī	10g	Radix Angelicae Sinensis
佩兰	pèi lán	10g	Herba Eupatorii
黄连	huáng lián	10g	Rhizoma Coptidis
大黄	dà huáng	10g	Radix et Rhizoma Rhei (preserved in liquor)
莱菔子	lái fú zǐ	30g	Semen Raphani

Modifications:

➤ With agitation and irascibility, add *shēng shí jué míng* (Concha Haliotidis raw) (decocted first) 30g.

➤ With poor appetite, add *chǎo gǔ yá* (Fructus Setariae Germinatus, mix-fried) and *chǎo mài yá* (Fructus Hordei Germinatus) 15g each.

➤ With a slimy thick yellow tongue coating, add *huò xiāng* (Herba Agastachis) 10g.

Commentary

Somnolence with depressive disorder is commonly seen in psychiatric wards. The condition has recently become more common, apparently coinciding with increased obesity due to changing dietary habits in modern lifestyles.

Regarding treatment approaches; experience has shown that if the goal is to adjust the sleeping schedule, antidepressant medications are best taken in the morning. In Chinese medicine, the primary focus is to nourish the heart, fortify the spleen, benefit the kidney and replenish essence. For children, adding a small amount of *xiān líng pí* (Herba Epimedii) and *tù sī zǐ* (Semen Cuscutae) for a short period of time has been proven very effective. Because they can be deleterious to the heart yin and heart blood, orifice-opening medicinals should be used in smaller than standard dosages and over shorter periods of time. The patient should be carefully monitored as dosages are adjusted to avoid potential heart-draining effects.

Acupuncture therapy can also be a useful adjunct treatment method; children have been shown to respond especially quickly when treated for this condition. One very effective empirical combination includes DU 20 (*bǎi huì*), DU 26 (*shuǐ gōu*) and GB 20 (*fēng chí*) and extra points *sì shén cōng*.

POOR MEMORY

Poor memory and forgetfulness is also commonly seen in the psychiatric department. Clinically, the main manifestations include the starting of a sentence or task without finishing and poor short-term memory. If at the same time there is depression disease manifesting with low spirits, pessimism, despair and suicidal ideation, this may be considered as poor memory combined with depression disease. When making a diagnosis, physiological and psychiatric examinations are required in order to rule out mental disorders such as dementia or organic brain disease. Poor memory combined with depressive disorder is commonly seen during the late stages of neurosis and other mental diseases involving brain-spirit taxation with essence damage.

Poor memory and forgetfulness can result from loss of emotional regularity, over-thinking, overindulgence in sexual activities, or malnourishment of the brain-spirit due to blood stagnation or phlegm-damp brewing internally. Congenital mental disability and inherent cognitive deficits are not in this disease category.

Pervasive forgetfulness can cause difficulty in the patient's life and also provide a source of sadness and frustration. This can lead to low spirits, pessimism, despair, and potentially even suicidal ideation. When poor memory and forgetfulness is combined with depressive disorder, it is usually categorized as a deficiency condition, with pathology involving the brain, heart, spleen and kidney. In some cases, there will be patterns of phlegm or static blood disturbing the brain-spirit. Treatment principles include supplementing deficiency, eliminating evil accumulation, fortifying the brain, and resolving constraint.

Etiology

Typical causes include emotional irregularities, over-thinking, and over-indulgence in sexual activities that lead to essence and blood depletion. Static blood and phlegm-turbidity can also complicate the condition.

Pathomechanism

The most commonly encountered pattern involves a dysfunctional relationship of the heart and kidney. A balanced relationship is critical for normal memory function, because perception is governed by the heart, while storage is governed by the kidney. When the pathomechanism involves over-indulgence in sexual activities, emotional irregularities, or over-thinking damaging the heart and spleen, two transformations that are possible. The first is the non-interaction of the heart and kidney due to hyperactive heart fire; the other involves splenic failure of transportation that leads to an insufficiency of kidney essence.

Clinical Guidelines

When depressive disorder is combined with poor memory, a variety of physical conditions can also be involved. This is also a common side effect of long-term antipsychotic and antidepressant use which in many cases can damage the brain-spirit and cause forgetfulness. After determining the location of the disease, first determine whether the nature is deficiency or excess. For deficiency, the primary possibilities are quite broad: qi, blood, yin and yang; for excess, differentiate whether it is qi stagnation, phlegm-turbidity, blood stasis or, more typically, some combination of these. Cases will often involve complex deficiency-excess situations. In these complex cases it is important to balance the treatment according to which causative factor is predominant.

Pattern Differentiation and Treatment

(1) Heart-spleen Dual Deficiency

Signs and Symptoms: forgetfulness, insomnia or profuse dreaming, fatigue, persistent low spirits, sorrow with a desire to weep, a sad facial expression, despair, suicidal ideation, dizziness, heart flusteredness, palpitations, a bright white facial complexion, reduced eating, loose stools, frequent sweating, a pale red tongue with no coating, and fine sunken weak pulses.

Other symptoms may include decreased appetite, stomach duct discomfort, shortness of breath, no strength to speak, anxiety, low self-esteem and self-reproach.

Treatment Principles: supplement the heart and spleen, nourish the brain, calm the spirit.

Formula:

茯苓	fú líng	30g	Poria
生黄芪	shēng huáng qí	30g	Radix Astragali raw
炒白术	chǎo bái zhú	15g	Rhizoma Atractylodis Macrocephalae (stir-fried)
党参	dǎng shēn	15g	Radix Codonopsis
太子参	tài zǐ shēn	30g	Radix Pseudostellariae
当归	dāng guī	15g	Radix Angelicae Sinensis
远志	yuǎn zhì	10g	Radix Polygalae
大枣	dà zǎo	10g	Fructus Jujubae
山茱萸	shān zhū yú	15g	Fructus Corni
炙甘草	zhì gān cǎo	6g	Radix et Rhizoma Glycyrrhizae Praeparata cum Melle
炒枣仁	chǎo zǎo rén	30g	Semen Ziziphi Spinosae (stir-fried)

Modifications:

➢ With loose stools, add *shān yào* (Rhizoma Dioscoreae) 15g and *biǎn dòu* (Semen Lablab Album) 15g.

➢ With reduced eating, add *chǎo mài yá* (Fructus Hordei Germinatus, stir-fried) 10g.

➢ With frequent weeping, add *tài zǐ shēn* (Radix Pseudostellariae) 30g, *bǎi hé* (Bulbus Lilii) 30g and *shā shēn* (Radix Adenophorae) 30g.

➢ With persistent low spirits, *chái hú* (Radix Bupleuri) 6g and *bái sháo* (Radix Paeoniae Alba) 30g can be added.

➢ With predominant qi stagnation, add *xiāng fù* (Rhizoma Cyperi) 10g and *yù jīn* (Radix Curcumae) 15g.

(2) Kidney-essence Depletion

Signs and Symptoms: forgetfulness, low spirits, pessimism, despair, a sad facial expression, suicidal ideation, no interest in life, distraction, hypochondria with a suspicion of suffering from untreatable diseases, dizziness, tinnitus, aching limp lumbus and knees; seminal emission, impotence and premature ejaculation among men, and amenorrhea and infertility among women.

Other symptoms may include fatigue, slow reactions, a tendency to lie down, sleeping lightly with profuse dreaming, a low, faint voice, a blank facial expression, fine sunken weak pulses, and a pale red tongue with a white coating.

Treatment Principles: supplement the kidney, benefit the essence, nourish the brain-spirit.

Formula:

熟地黄	shú dì huáng	15g	Radix Rehmanniae Praeparata
山药	shān yào	15g	Rhizoma Dioscoreae
山茱萸	shān zhū yú	15g	Fructus Corni
茯苓	fú líng	30g	Poria
泽泻	zé xiè	30g	Rhizoma Alismatis
牡丹皮	mǔ dān pí	10g	Cortex Moutan
菟丝子	tù sī zǐ	30g	Semen Cuscutae
女贞子	nǚ zhēn zǐ	30g	Fructus Ligustri Lucidi
炒枣仁	chǎo zǎo rén	30g	Semen Ziziphi Spinosae (stir-fried)
龟甲	guī jiǎ	10g	Carapax et Plastrum Testudinis
炒麦芽	chǎo mài yá	15g	Fructus Hordei Germinatus (stir-fried)
何首乌	hé shǒu wū	15g	Radix Polygoni Multiflori

Modifications:

➤ With an aching lumbus, add *dù zhòng* (Cortex Eucommiae) 10 - 30g.

➤ With hair loss, increase the dosage of *hé shǒu wū* (Radix Polygoni Multiflori).

Chapter 7
Associated Disease Categories

(3) Non-interaction of Heart and Kidney

Signs and Symptoms: forgetfulness, fearful throbbing, deficiency vexation with sleeplessness, worry, low spirits, vexation and agitation, pessimism, heart palpitations, profuse dreaming, tidal fever, spontaneous sweating, aching limp lumbus and knees, tinnitus, dry mouth and tongue, dream emission, a red tongue with scant coating, and sunken fine pulses.

Other symptoms may include reduced eating, dizziness, a tendency to lie down, fatigue, despair, suicidal ideation, worry, and no strength to speak.

Treatment Principles: promote interaction of the heart and kidney, benefit the brain, calm the spirit.

Formula:

党参	dǎng shēn	15g	Radix Codonopsis
玄参	xuán shēn	30g	Radix Scrophulariae
丹参	dān shēn	30g	Radix et Rhizoma Salviae Miltiorrhizae
茯苓	fú líng	30g	Poria
远志	yuǎn zhì	10g	Radix Polygalae
当归	dāng guī	15g	Radix Angelicae Sinensis
五味子	wǔ wèi zǐ	10g	Fructus Schisandrae Chinensis
女贞子	nǚ zhēn zǐ	30g	Fructus Ligustri Lucidi
菟丝子	tù sī zǐ	30g	Semen Cuscutae
枸杞子	gǒu qǐ zǐ	15g	Fructus Lycii
炒枣仁	chǎo zǎo rén	30g	Semen Ziziphi Spinosae (stir-fried)
合欢皮	hé huān pí	30g	Cortex Albiziae
熟地黄	shú dì huáng	15g	Radix Rehmanniae Praeparata
生地	shēng dì	15g	Radix Rehmanniae

Modifications:

➤ With severe kidney depletion, add *hé shǒu wū* (Radix Polygoni Multiflori) 15g.

➤ With reduced food intake, add *jiāo mài yá* (Fructus Hordei Germinatus Ustus), *jiāo shān zhā* (Fructus Crataegi) and *jiāo shén qū* (Massa Medicata Fermentata Ustus) 30g each, or *shén qū* (Massa Medicata Fermentata) 15g.

➤ With qi stagnation, add *xiāng fù* (Rhizoma Cyperi) 10g and *yù jīn*

(Radix Curcumae) 15g.
➤ With persistent low spirits, add *chái hú* (Radix Bupleuri) 6g and *bái sháo* (Radix Paeoniae Alba) 30g.

(4) Phlegm Turbidity

Signs and Symptoms: forgetfulness, a tendency to lie down, low spirits, vexation and agitation, pessimism, despair, self-blame and self-reproach, regret, hypochondria with a suspicion of suffering from untreatable conditions, suicidal ideation, heaviness in the head, oppression, dizziness, thirst with no desire to drink, dry stool, red face and eyes, turbid thick phlegm, a red tongue with yellow slimy coating, and slippery rapid pulses

Other symptoms may include sense of impending doom, fidgetiness, fullness and oppression of the stomach duct and abdomen, a temptation to rage, a reluctance to leave the home, vexation, pacing, and agitation.

Treatment Principles: sweep phlegm, open orifices, awaken the brain, calm the spirit.

Formula:

陈皮	chén pí	10g	Pericarpium Citri Reticulatae
法半夏	fǎ bàn xià	10g	Rhizoma Pinelliae Praeparatum
茯苓	fú líng	30g	Poria
竹茹	zhú rú	6g	Caulis Bambusae in Taenia
礞石	méng shí	30g	Chlorite-schist (decocted first)
炒枳壳	chǎo zhǐ qiào	15g	Fructus Aurantii (stir-fried)
大黄	dà huáng	15g	Radix et Rhizoma Rhei (preserved in liquor)
莱菔子	lái fú zǐ	30g	Semen Raphani
炙甘草	zhì gān cǎo	6g	Radix et Rhizoma Glycyrrhizae Praeparata cum Melle

Modifications:
➤ With insomnia, add *chǎo suān zǎo rén* (Semen Ziziphi Spinosae, stir-fried) 30–60g.
➤ With thirst, add *shēng shí gāo* (Gypsum Fibrosum Cruda) (decocted first) 30–90g.

Chapter 7
Associated Disease Categories

Commentary

Depressive disorder with poor memory is commonly seen among middle-aged or elderly people. The poor mood is generally persistent, but these patients usually do not fully express their anger and frustration. Over a period of time, emotional repression damages the heart and spleen and qi and blood become depleted, thus reinforcing the condition. Liver qi stagnation can also result in this condition. Regarding the pathomechanism and outcome, in the initial stage, the liver fails to course and drain and the qi dynamic of the whole body is stagnated. Then heart-spleen dual deficiency or hyperactive heart fire patterns appear along with spleen-stomach disharmony and eventually kidney essence depletion. This condition is generally characterized by more deficiency than excess.

Treatment here should focus on supplementating the kidney and to a lesser extent the spleen. Nourishing essence, benefiting marrow, and fortifying the brain are also appropriate. That said, as most of these cases are chronic in nature, and many are triggered by patterns of stagnation and accumulation, moving qi and blood and coursing the liver are also useful adjunctive methods.

SORROW

The disease category of sorrow with depressive disorder is characterized by a tendency to weep or incessant sobbing, a sad facial expression, pessimism, and despair. The manifestations of depressive disorder are very complex, so in addition to low spirits there can also be worry, anxiety, insomnia, various physical pain symptoms, suspicion, or despair with suicidal ideation.

For sorrow with depressive disorder there are two typical etiologies. The first is a substantial emotional upset followed by intense, persistent negative emotions that manifest with weeping; the other is a pre-existing tendency to sorrow that is aggravated by upsetting incidents. The first is similar to reactive depression, while the second is similar to nervous depression.

Sorrow with depressive disorder is referred to as "tendency to sorrow" or "sorrow pattern" in Chinese medicine, and historically there is a unique approach to pattern differentiation and treatment.

This condition was first mentioned in the *The Yellow Emperor's Inner Classic* (*Huáng Dì Nèi Jīng*). The *Basic Questions – Treatise Explaining the Five Qi* (*Sù Wèn – Xuān Míng Wǔ Qì Piān*) states, "Essence-qi gathering in the lung causes sorrow."

The Basic Questions – Treatise on Wilting (*Sù Wèn – Wěi Lùn*) states, "Excessive sorrow causes expiry of the pericardium which leads to yang qi stirring internally. At the onset there will be collapse below the heart and one will frequently see blood in the urine."

The Spiritual Pivot – the Spirit (*Líng Shū – Běn Shén*) states, "When there is heart qi deficiency, there is sorrow", and "Sorrow of the liver affecting the center causes damage to the ethereal soul." Sorrow is the emotion associated with the lung, and excessive sorrow leads to dispersion of qi and therefore dysfunction of the internal organs.

Based on these ideas, later generations of physicians continued to discuss the tendency to sorrow and the associated manifestations. Jin Dynasty physician Liu Wan-su stated in the *Explanation of Mysterious Pathogeneses and Etiologies Based on the 'Basic Questions'* (*Sù Wèn Xuān Jí Yuán Bìng Shì*); "Fright, confusion, sorrow and laughing are all ascribed to heat." Also, "Sorrow is the mind associated with metal-lung. Metal's nature is dryness. The cause of dryness is fire. Heart fire is ascribed to heat, and often causes pain. Therefore, sorrow and agony are associated with dryness, heat, vexation and derangement of the heart-spirit, instead [of the usual metal function] of clearing and cleansing." Liu Wan-su considered sorrow to be a result of heat evil.

Etiology

Internal constraint of the seven emotions and damage due to excessive sadness are the primary causes of this disorder. These can damage the heart and lung causing qi and blood insufficiency as well as a depletion of visceral yin which allows the spirit to be disturbed. This leads to a susceptibility to excitement and sadness with a tendency towards sorrow-related patterns.

Pathomechanism

The primary location of this condition is the lung, but the heart

Chapter 7
Associated Disease Categories

and brain are affected as well. The key aspects of this dysfunction are associated with the corporeal soul of the lung and the brain-spirit. The nature of the condition is primarily qi and yin depletion. With lung qi deficiency, the corporeal soul fails to maintain its composure; this can result in shortness of breath, a desire to weep and profuse sweating with exertion. Over-thinking damaging the heart and spleen can also result in a tendency to sorrow.

Clinically, this is more frequently encountered as a deficiency pattern, so treatment here focuses on supplementation. Excessive sorrow itself will deplete qi and blood, and this can become the mechanism of a deeper imbalance of yin and yang over a period of time.

Pattern Differentiation and Treatment

(1) Heart and Lung Qi Dual Deficiency

Signs and Symptoms: heart palpitations, shortness of breath, a tendency to sorrow with a desire to weep, low spirits, insomnia or profuse dreaming, loose stools, a red tongue with a white coating, and sunken fine pulses.

Treatment Principles: supplement heart and lung.

Formula:

党参	dǎng shēn	20g	Radix Codonopsis
白术	bái zhú	15g	Rhizoma Atractylodis Macrocephalae
茯苓	fú líng	60g	Poria
当归	dāng guī	15g	Radix Angelicae Sinensis
炙甘草	zhì gān cǎo	15g	Radix et Rhizoma Glycyrrhizae Praeparata cum Melle
炒枣仁	chǎo zǎo rén	60g	Semen Ziziphi Spinosae (stir-fried)
紫菀	zǐ wǎn	10g	Radix et Rhizoma Asteris
款冬花	kuǎn dōng huā	10g	Flos Farfarae

Modifications:
- With kidney yang deficiency manifesting with aching lumbus and knees, add *bā jǐ tiān* (Radix Morindae Officinalis) 20g.
- With impotence and premature ejaculation, add *nǚ zhēn zǐ* (Fructus Ligustri Lucidi) 40g, *tù sī zǐ* (Semen Cuscutae) 80g, and *yín yáng*

huò (Herba Epimedii) 15g.
➤ With sweating with the slightest exertion, add *shēng huáng qí* (Radix Astragali raw) 30g.
➤ With insomnia, add *chǎo suān zǎo rén* (Semen Ziziphi Spinosae, stir-fried) 30g and *hé huān huā* (Flos Albiziae) 30g.

(2) VISCERAL AGITATION WITH A TENDENCY TO SORROW

Signs and Symptoms: sorrow with a desire to weep, crying without tears, a sense of relief after crying, heart vexation, sleeplessness, fidgeting, bound stool and constipation, a red tongue with a white coating or scant liquid, and fine sunken pulses.

Treatment Principles: nourish yin, moisten dryness.

Formula:

炙甘草	*zhì gān cǎo*	15g	Radix et Rhizoma Glycyrrhizae Praeparata cum Melle
小麦	*xiǎo mài*	30g	Fructus Tritici
大枣	*dà zǎo*	12g	Fructus Jujubae
炒枣仁	*chǎo zǎo rén*	60g	Semen Ziziphi Spinosae (stir-fried)
沙参	*shā shēn*	30g	Radix Adenophorae
生牡蛎	*shēng mǔ lì*	30g	Concha Ostreae Cruda (decocted first)
紫菀	*zǐ wǎn*	10g	Radix et Rhizoma Asteris

Modifications:
➤ With sleeplessness and frequent weeping, add *bǎi hé* (Bulbus Lilii) 40g and *mài mén dōng* (Ophiopogonis) 30g.
➤ With tidal fever and night sweats, add *dì gǔ pí* (Cortex Lycii) 30g.

Commentary

The pathomechanism here involves qi and yin depletion. When there is heart and lung qi deficiency, treatment should benefit qi and secure yin. If yin is insufficient, then it is difficult to store qi and this will aggravate the sorrow. Improper treatment with overly drying constraint-relieving medicinals can further destabilize yin and also result in greater qi deficiency. The outcomes of the different patterns are as follows:

(1) Heart and lung qi deficiency manifesting primarily with a tendency

Chapter 7
Associated Disease Categories

to sorrow can easily turn into qi deficiency with blood stasis, and blood stasis is in essence an excess of blood. *The Inner Classic (Nèi Jīng)* states, "Superabundant blood will cause anger", and in fact some patients may present with anger within the context of sorrow.

(2) Persistent untreated lung yin deficiency can lead to kidney yin depletion and irregularities of qi transformation. Meanwhile, there can be symptoms of fatigue and a lack of strength which indicate a decrease in the kidney-mind function. If there is no history of mental illness or other physical conditions, with proper treatment and medication, the prognosis is generally good.

FEAR

Fear with depressive disorder is a common clinical condition. This disease category refers to a mental disorder characterized by fear, uneasiness, and nervousness, along with subsequent low spirits, pessimism and suicidal ideation.

Etiology

1. Sudden exposure to a threat induces the descent of qi, dysfunction of the kidney's consolidation and storage function, and disorder of the brain-spirit. If the adverse stimulation is severe, or marked by an intense persistent physical reaction, then the liver and other organs may be affected as well. Liver qi stagnation with brain-spirit constraint may result.

2. Overindulgence in sexual activities with a constitutional insufficiency can lead to kidney essence depletion, insufficient engendering of marrow, and malnourishment of the brain-spirit. In other cases, severe or chronic physical conditions can also affect the kidney origin, leading to qi and blood depletion. This can affect the liver, gallbladder, heart, bones, and blood vessels and result in timidity, fear, uneasiness, and anxiety.

Pathomechanisms

1. The mind associated with the kidney is fear. Fear damaging the kidney can manifest with a tendency to fear, nervousness and timidity, possible incontinence, a greenish white facial complexion, profuse sweating, heart palpitations and, in severe cases, tremors of the body.

Since diseases of the mother affect the child, kidney damage leads to the liver failing to course and discharge effectively causing depression, low spirits, pessimism and despair. When kidney-water does not bear upward to the heart, the resulting pathogenic heart fire can cause fidgeting and a fearful paranoia.

2. Kidney deficiency leading to depleted essence that fails to engender marrow and nourish the brain-spirit results in decreased memory, distraction, slow thinking, a stiff facial expression, timidity, worry, and difficulty with social intercourse.

3. Non-interaction of heart and kidney and heart yang floating astray can manifest with insomnia, profuse dreaming, exhaustion, aching limp lumbus and knees, loss of ambition, a sense of time moving slowly and without purpose, and no faith in life.

Pattern Differentiation and Treatment

(1) Kidney-essence Insufficiency

Signs and Symptoms: constitutional weakness due to chronic diseases, susceptibility to fear, uneasiness, decreased memory, seminal emission at extreme fear, premature senility with white hair, aching limp lumbus and knees, and possible fecal and urinary incontinence; a feeling of mental oppression, depression, pessimism, despair, a loss of belief in one's health and future, and possible suicidal ideation; a pale tongue and fine sunken pulses.

Other symptoms may include insomnia, profuse dreaming, very light sleep, no desire to socialize, distancing self from family and acquaintances, torpid intake, and a sad facial expression.

Treatment Principles: secure the kidney, benefit essence, nourish the brain-spirit.

Formula:

熟地黄	shú dì huáng	15g	Radix Rehmanniae Praeparata
山药	shān yào	30g	Rhizoma Dioscoreae
山茱萸	shān zhū yú	15g	Fructus Corni
茯苓	fú líng	30g	Poria
泽泻	zé xiè	15g	Rhizoma Alismatis

Chapter 7
Associated Disease Categories

枸杞子	gǒu qǐ zǐ	15g	Fructus Lycii
牡丹皮	mǔ dān pí	10g	Cortex Moutan
菟丝子	tù sī zǐ	30g	Semen Cuscutae
何首乌	hé shǒu wū	30g	Radix Polygoni Multiflori
柴胡	chái hú	6g	Radix Bupleuri
白芍	bái sháo	30g	Radix Paeoniae Alba
当归	dāng guī	30g	Radix Angelicae Sinensis

Modifications:

➤ With insomnia, add *chǎo suān zǎo rén* (Semen Ziziphi Spinosae, stir-fried) 30g.

➤ With cold limbs, add *bā jǐ tiān* (Radix Morindae Officinalis) 15g and *Tiān Wáng Bǔ Xīn Dān* (Celestial Emperor Heart-Supplementing Elixir).

➤ With qi stagnation, add *xiāng fù* (Rhizoma Cyperi), *yù jīn* (Radix Curcumae) and *xiāng yuán* (Fructus Citri) 10g respectively.

(2) Liver-gallbladder Dual Deficiency

Signs and Symptoms: timidity, susceptibility to fear, indecisiveness, uneasiness, feeling unsettled all day, startling awake from sleep, fear and paranoia in severe cases, depression, a lack of interest and motivation, decreased memory, distraction, rib-side constraint, a pale red tongue, and wiry fine pulses.

Other symptoms may include decreased appetite, suspicion, insomnia, profuse dreaming, self-isolation, and fear of social contact.

Treatment Principles: supplement liver and gallbladder, nourish the brain-spirit.

Formula:

当归	dāng guī	15g	Radix Angelicae Sinensis
白芍	bái sháo	30g	Radix Paeoniae Alba
枸杞子	gǒu qǐ zǐ	25g	Fructus Lycii
茯神	fú shén	30g	Sclerotium Poriae Pararadicis
菟丝子	tù sī zǐ	30g	Semen Cuscutae
炒枣仁	chǎo zǎo rén	30g	Semen Ziziphi Spinosae (stir-fried)

太子参	tài zǐ shēn	30g	Radix Pseudostellariae
麦门冬	mài mén dōng	30g	Radix Ophiopogonis
柴胡	chái hú	6g	Radix Bupleuri
白术	bái zhú	15g	Rhizoma Atractylodis Macrocephalae
薄荷	bò he	6g	Herba Menthae

(3) Qi and Blood Depletion

Signs and Symptoms: typically associated with a constitutional insufficiency, persistent untreated diseases, or during recuperation from a major illness. Manifestations include palpitations, susceptibility to fear, depression, oppression, pessimism, despair, fatigue, no strength to speak, aching limpness all over the body, shortness of breath, spontaneous sweating, a pale tongue, and fine weak pulses.

Other symptoms may include reduced thirst, torpid intake, and no desire for human contact.

Treatment Principles: nourish qi, blood and the brain, calm the spirit.

Formula: Modified *Bā Zhēn Tāng* (Eight Gem Decoction)

生黄芪	shēng huáng qí	30g	Radix Astragali raw
党参	dǎng shēn	15g	Radix Codonopsis
白术	bái zhú	15g	Rhizoma Atractylodis Macrocephalae
大枣	dà zǎo	10g	Fructus Jujubae
太子参	tài zǐ shēn	30g	Radix Pseudostellariae
五味子	wǔ wèi zǐ	10g	Fructus Schisandrae Chinensis
当归	dāng guī	15g	Radix Angelicae Sinensis
川芎	chuān xiōng	20g	Rhizoma Chuanxiong
白芍	bái sháo	30g	Radix Paeoniae Alba
炒枣仁	chǎo zǎo rén	30g	Semen Ziziphi Spinosae (stir-fried)
炒麦芽	chǎo mài yá	30g	Fructus Hordei Germinatus

Modifications:

➢ With qi stagnation, add *chái hú* (Radix Bupleuri) 6g, *yù jīn* (Radix Curcumae) 10g, and *xiāng yuán* (Fructus Citri) 10g.

➢ With predominant kidney yang deficiency, add *ròu guì* (Cortex Cinnamomi) 10g and *xiān líng pí* (Herba Epimedii) 10g, or

Chapter 7
Associated Disease Categories

combined with *Jīn Guì Shèn Qì Wán* (Golden Cabinet Kidney Qi Pill).

Commentary

In this pattern, fear precedes the depressive symptoms with kidney or liver and kidney insufficiency as the most common cause. Fear patterns can develop after a chronic or severe disease, or manifest in patients with a constitutional weakness who receives a sudden fright. Over a long period of time, fear and timidity can also result in low spirits, pessimism, and despair.

There are two main groups of medicinals for clinical application:

1) *Shēng mǔ lì* (Concha Ostreae Cruda) (decocted first) 30g, *bǎi hé* (Bulbus Lilii) 30g, *chǎo zǎo rén* (Semen Ziziphi Spinosae, stir-fried) 30–60g, *mài mén dōng* (Ophiopogonis) 30g, *tài zǐ shēn* (Radix Pseudostellariae) 30g, *dāng guī* (Radix Angelicae Sinensis) 15g, and *bái sháo* (Radix Paeoniae Alba) 30g.

2) *Gǒu qǐ zǐ* (Fructus Lycii) 15g, *tù sī zǐ* (Semen Cuscutae) 30g, *shān zhū yú* (Fructus Corni) 10g, *hé shǒu wū* (Radix Polygoni Multiflori) 15g, *ròu cōng róng* (Herba Cistanches) 30g, *bǔ gǔ zhī* (Fructus Psoraleae) 15g, *yì zhì rén* (Fructus Alpiniae Oxyphyllae) 30g, and *chǎo zǎo rén* (Semen Ziziphi Spinosae, stir-fried) 30g.

BULIMIA

This disease category refers to bulimia nervosa accompanied by severe concurrent depressive symptoms. Bulimia nervosa is an eating disorder characterized by intermittent excessive eating and a fixation on controlling one's body weight. Although the manifestations are slightly different, most experts categorize this condition as the chronic stage of anorexia nervosa because the core symptom of both conditions is a fear of obesity. Bulimia nervosa patients tend to have more predominant emotional disorders than anorexia nervosa patients. The uncontrollable urge to eat makes them anxious, depressed and agitated; therefore, many researchers believe that bulimia has a stronger association with depressive conditions than does anorexia.

Etiology and Pathomechanism

This condition is most commonly seen in young females. With ungratified desires, liver qi becomes stagnated and the brain-spirit becomes inhibited. Alternately, constraint transforms into fire and disturbs the brain-spirit, but low spirits, pessimism, and despair can result in both cases. As the spleen and stomach are damaged by dietary irregularity, the qi dynamic in the middle is deranged, often leading to alternating bulimia and anorexia. Splenic failure of transportation and transformation leads to food damage and abdominal distention. With stomach qi failing to descend, there will be frequent vomiting after eating followed by a sense of relief. Persistent vomiting will cause great damage to the qi of the middle burner, and while the initial vomiting may be manually induced, as stomach qi becomes weaker, later vomiting may become spontaneous. The spleen will also fail to spread the essence of water and grain, causing emaciation. If the patient does not present with vomiting there will be stagnation in the middle burner, or phlegm-damp engendered internally due to failure of splenic transportation.

Clinical Guidelines

Bulimia is easily differentiated from swift digestion with rapid hungering as associated with stomach heat or dispersion-thirst. Bulimia nervosa can be difficult to treat because there can be simultaneous occurrences of qi constraint, deficiency, counterflow, and stagnation in a complex mingled excess and deficiency scenario. When treating depressive emotion, regulate the balance of qi and blood in the viscera and bowels while focusing treatment of the root pattern.

Psychological counseling and behavior modification are critical for all such patients. If the patient presents with severe malnourishment, amenorrhea, or other endocrine disturbances, one should definitely recommend additional medical support.

Diagnostic Criteria

Diagnostic criteria for bulimia nervosa

(1) Intermittent uncontrollable desire to eat, frequent binging (at least

Chapter 7
Associated Disease Categories

twice per week over a period of not less than three months).

(2) Morbid fear of obesity with frequent self-induced vomiting or diarrhea (usually through laxative abuse) or fasting.

(3) Other organic diseases or psychiatric disorder have been ruled out.

Pattern Differentiation and Treatment

(1) Liver-stomach Disharmony with Qi Counterflow, Brain-spirit Loss of Regularity

Signs and Symptoms: depression, pessimism, insomnia, fidgetiness, frequent laughing or crying, agitation, excessive eating followed by vomiting, fullness and oppression in the chest and rib-sides, distending pain in the stomach duct, frequent sighing, acid regurgitation, red margins on the tongue with a thin slimy coating, and wiry pulses.

Treatment Principles: course the liver, harmonize the stomach, downbear counterflow, calm the brain-spirit.

Formula: Modified *Sì Qì Tāng*（Four Qi Decoction）

法半夏	fǎ bàn xià	10g	Rhizoma Pinelliae Praeparatum
紫苏叶	zǐ sū yè	12g	Folium Perillae
厚朴	hòu pò	10g	Cortex Magnoliae Officinalis
生姜	shēng jiāng	6g	Rhizoma Zingiberis Recens
茯苓	fú líng	30g	Poria
香橼	xiāng yuán	10g	Fructus Citri
佛手	fó shǒu	10g	Fructus Citri Sarcodactylis
陈皮	chén pí	10g	Pericarpium Citri Reticulatae
竹茹	zhú rú	6g	Caulis Bambusae in Taenia
丹参	dān shēn	30g	Radix et Rhizoma Salviae Miltiorrhizae
川芎	chuān xiōng	20g	Rhizoma Chuanxiong
菊花	jú huā	10g	Flos Chrysanthemi
炒枣仁	chǎo zǎo rén	30g	Semen Ziziphi Spinosae (stir-fried)
远志	yuǎn zhì	6g	Radix Polygalae
郁金	yù jīn	30g	Radix Curcumae
天竺黄	tiān zhú huáng	15g	Concretio Silicea Bambusae

Modifications:
- With predominant food accumulation, add *shān zhā* (Fructus Crataegi) 10g and *shén qū* (Massa Medicata) 10g.
- With severe vomiting, add *dài zhě shí* (Haematitum) 30g.
- With predominant acid upflowing, add *hǎi piāo xiāo* (Endoconcha Sepiae) and *wǎ léng zǐ* (Concha Arcae) 30g each.
- With pain in the stomach duct, add *bái sháo* (Radix Paeoniae Alba) 30g, *suō luó zǐ* (Semen Aesculi) 30g, and *yuán hú* (Rhizoma Corydalis) 15g.
- With severe insomnia, add *chǎo zǎo rén* (Semen Ziziphi Spinosae, stir-fried) 30g, *yuǎn zhì* (Radix Polygalae) 6g and *hǔ pò miàn* (Succinum, powdered) 3g (infused).
- With slimy tongue fur, add *pèi lán* (Herba Eupatorii) 10g and *huáng lián* (Rhizoma Coptidis) 10g.
- With vexation, agitation and irascibility, add *shēng shí jué míng* (Concha Haliotidis Cruda) 30g, *cí shí* (Magnetitum) 30g, *shēng mǔ lì* (Concha Ostreae Cruda) (decocted first) 30g, and *shēng lóng chǐ* (Dens Draconis, raw) 30g.

(2) FOOD STAGNATION, SPLENIC TRANSPORTATION AND TRANSFORMATION FAILURE

Signs and Symptoms: vexation, agitation, depression, fidgetiness, excessive eating, vomiting of acid and putridity, belching, distending pain in the stomach duct, aggravation of the condition after eating, relief after vomiting, foul-smelling duck's slop stool or constipation, a thick slimy tongue coating, and rapid and excess pulses.

Treatment Principles: fortify the spleen, disperse food, harmonize the stomach, downbear counterflow, regulate qi, calm the spirit.

Formula: Modified *Bǎo Hé Wán* (Harmony-Preserving Pill)

山楂	shān zhā	10g	Fructus Crataegi
神曲	shén qū	10g	Massa Medicata Fermentata
莱菔子	lái fú zǐ	30g	Semen Raphani
陈皮	chén pí	10g	Pericarpium Citri Reticulatae
法半夏	fǎ bàn xià	10g	Rhizoma Pinelliae Praeparatum
茯苓	fú líng	30g	Poria

Chapter 7
Associated Disease Categories

连翘	lián qiào	10g	Fructus Forsythiae
竹茹	zhú rú	6g	Caulis Bambusae in Taenia
郁金	yù jīn	30g	Radix Curcumae
天竺黄	tiān zhú huáng	15g	Concretio Silicea Bambusae
旋覆花	xuán fù huā	10g	Flos Inulae
白术	bái zhú	15g	Rhizoma Atractylodis Macrocephalae
川芎	chuān xiōng	20g	Rhizoma Chuanxiong
丹参	dān shēn	30g	Radix et Rhizoma Salviae Miltiorrhizae
菊花	jú huā	15g	Flos Chrysanthemi
黄连	huáng lián	10g	Rhizoma Coptidis
栀子	zhī zǐ	10g	Fructus Gardeniae
火麻仁	huǒ má rén	30g	Fructus Cannabis
郁李仁	yù lǐ rén	30g	Semen Pruni

Modifications:

With poor sleep, add *chǎo zǎo rén* (Semen Ziziphi Spinosae, stir-fried) 30g, *hé huān pí* (Cortex Albiziae) 30g, *yuǎn zhì* (Radix Polygalae) 6g and *hǔ pò miàn* (Succinum, powdered) 3g (infused).

With agitation, add *lóng dǎn cǎo* (Radix et Rhizoma Gentianae) 10g and *bái sháo* (Radix Paeoniae Alba) 30g.

With predominant dry stools, add *jiǔ zhì dà huáng* (Radix et Rhizoma Rhei, preserved in liquor) (decocted later) 10g or *guā lóu rén* (Semen Trichosanthis) 30g.

With persistent slimy tongue fur, add *huò xiāng* (Herba Agastachis) 10g, and *pèi lán* (Herba Eupatorii) 10g.

(3) SPLENIC TRANSPORTATION AND TRANSFORMATION FAILURE, PHLEGM-RHEUM OBSTRUCTION, IMPAIRED MOVEMENT OF THE BRAIN-SPIRIT

Signs and Symptoms: low spirits, pessimism, despair, dizziness, weak extremities, fatigue, palpitations, flusteredness relieved by eating, rapacious appetite, occasional vomiting, chest oppression, a white slimy tongue coating, and slippery pulses.

Treatment Principles: fortify the spleen, resolve phlegm, downbear counterflow, disperse food, nourish the brain, calm the spirit.

Formula: *Xiǎo Bàn Xià Tāng*（Minor Pinellia Decoction） with *Líng*

Guì Zhú Gān Tāng (Poria, Cinnamon Twig, Atractylodes Macrocephala and Licorice Decoction)

法半夏	fǎ bàn xià	10g	Rhizoma Pinelliae Praeparatum
生姜	shēng jiāng	6g	Rhizoma Zingiberis Recens
茯苓	fú líng	30g	Poria
桂枝	guì zhī	10g	Ramulus Cinnamomi
白术	bái zhú	15g	Rhizoma Atractylodis Macrocephalae
党参	dǎng shēn	15g	Radix Codonopsis
扁豆	biǎn dòu	30g	Semen Lablab Album
薏苡仁	yì yǐ rén	30g	Semen Coicis
神曲	shén qū	15g	Massa Medicata Fermentata
香橼	xiāng yuán	15g	Fructus Citri
佛手	fó shǒu	10g	Fructus Citri Sarcodactylis
菊花	jú huā	15g	Flos Chrysanthemi
川芎	chuān xiōng	20g	Rhizoma Chuanxiong
丹参	dān shēn	30g	Radix et Rhizoma Salviae Miltiorrhizae
陈皮	chén pí	10g	Pericarpium Citri Reticulatae

Modifications:

➢ With severe palpitations and flusteredness, add *mài mén dōng* (Ophiopogonis) 30g, *tài zǐ shēn* (Radix Pseudostellariae) 30g and *wǔ wèi zǐ* (Fructus Schisandrae Chinensis) 10g.

➢ With insomnia, add *chǎo zǎo rén* (Semen Ziziphi Spinosae, stir-fried) 30g, *hé huān pí* (Cortex Albiziae) 30g and *yuǎn zhì* (Radix Polygalae) 6g.

➢ With food accumulation, add the *jiāo sān xiān* (Tres Immortales Usti) 30g each, or the *jiāo sì xiān* (Quattuor Immortales Usti) 40g each.

➢ With predominant qi and blood deficiency, add *rén shēn* (Radix et Rhizoma Ginseng) 6g, *dāng guī* (Radix Angelicae Sinensis) 15g, and *ē jiāo* (Colla Corii Asini) 10g.

➢ With yang deficiency, add *ròu guì* (Cortex Cinnamomi) 10g.

➢ With vomiting and counterflow, add *xuán fù huā* (Flos Inulae) 15g, *dài zhě shí* (Haematitum) 30g, and *zhú rú* (Caulis Bambusae in Taenia) 6g.

Chapter 7
Associated Disease Categories

➢ With food accumulation transforming into heat, add *huáng lián* (Rhizoma Coptidis) 10g and *zhī zǐ* (Fructus Gardeniae) 10g.

➢ With predominant damp, add *cǎo dòu kòu* (Semen Alpiniae Katsumadai) 10g, *huò xiāng* (Herba Agastachis) 10g, and *pèi lán* (Herba Eupatorii) 10g.

(4) Spleen and Stomach Deficiency, Failure to Nourish the Brain-spirit

Signs and Symptoms: low spirits, fatigue, lack of strength, pessimism, despair, rapacious appetite, intermittent vomiting after eating, lusterless facial complexion or emaciation, pain in the stomach duct and abdomen that is better with pressure, bright white facial complexion, cold in the extremities, no desire to drink or eat, thick liquid stool that feels cold and has no odor, a pale tongue with white coating, and sunken slow forceless pulses.

Treatment Principles: fortify the spleen, benefit qi, supplement deficiency, check counterflow, calm the brain-spirit.

Formula: *Bǔ Zhōng Yì Qì Tāng* (Center-Supplementing and Qi-Boosting Decoction) with *Xuán Fù Dài Zhě Tāng* (Inula and Hematite Decoction)

白术	bái zhú	15g	Rhizoma Atractylodis Macrocephalae
黄芪	huáng qí	30g	Radix Astragali
升麻	shēng má	10g	Rhizoma Cimicifugae
柴胡	chái hú	6g	Radix Bupleuri
人参	rén shēn	10g	Radix et Rhizoma Ginseng
炙甘草	zhì gān cǎo	10g	Radix et Rhizoma Glycyrrhizae Praeparata cum Melle
当归	dāng guī	15g	Radix Angelicae Sinensis
陈皮	chén pí	10g	Pericarpium Citri Reticulatae
竹茹	zhú rú	6g	Caulis Bambusae in Taenia
旋覆花	xuán fù huā	15g	Flos Inulae
代赭石	dài zhě shí	30g	Haematitum
菊花	jú huā	15g	Flos Chrysanthemi
川芎	chuān xiōng	20g	Rhizoma Chuanxiong
丹参	dān shēn	30g	Radix et Rhizoma Salviae Miltiorrhizae

郁金	*yù jīn*	30g	Radix Curcumae
天竺黄	*tiān zhú huáng*	15g	Concretio Silicea Bambusae

Modifications:

➢ With fatigue, lack of strength and low spirits, increase the dosage of *rén shēn* (Radix et Rhizoma Ginseng).

➢ With poor sleep, add *chǎo zǎo rén* (Semen Ziziphi Spinosae, stir-fried) 30g and *hé huān pí* (Cortex Albiziae) 30g.

➢ With headache, add *màn jīng zǐ* (Fructus Viticis) 15g; if the pain is severe, add *chuān xiōng* (Rhizoma Chuanxiong) 20g.

➢ With phlegm, add *bàn xià* (Rhizoma Pinelliae) 10g and *shēng jiāng* (Rhizoma Zingiberis Recens) 10g.

➢ With stomach cold and qi stagnation, add *mù xiāng* (Radix Aucklandiae) 10g, *yì zhì rén* (Fructus Alpiniae Oxyphyllae) 30g, *qīng pí* (Pericarpium Citri Reticulatae Viride) 10g, and *bái kòu rén* (Fructus Amomi Rotundus) 10g.

➢ With abdominal distention, add *zhǐ shí* (Fructus Aurantii Immaturus) 10g, *hòu pò* (Cortex Magnoliae Officinalis) 10g, *mù xiāng* (Radix Aucklandiae) 10g, and *shā rén* (Fructus Amomi) 10g.

➢ With abdominal pain, add *bái sháo* (Radix Paeoniae Alba) 30g and *gān cǎo* (Radix et Rhizoma Glycyrrhizae) 10g.

➢ With predominant cold, add *ròu guì* (Cortex Cinnamomi) 10g.

➢ With predominant dampness, add *cāng zhú* (Rhizoma Atractylodis) 15g.

➢ With yin deficiency, remove *shēng má* (Rhizoma Cimicifugae) and *chái hú* (Radix Bupleuri), and add *shú dì huáng* (Radix Rehmanniae Praeparata) 10g, *shān zhū yú* (Fructus Corni) 15g, and *shān yào* (Rhizoma Dioscoreae) 30g.

➢ With constipation, add *guā lóu rén* (Semen Trichosanthis) 30g and *huǒ má rén* (Fructus Cannabis) 30g, or *jiǔ zhì dà huáng* (Radix et Rhizoma Rhei, preserved in liquor) 10g.

➢ With diarrhea, remove *dāng guī* (Radix Angelicae Sinensis) and add *fú líng* (Poria) 30g, *cāng zhú* (Rhizoma Atractylodis) 15g, and *yì zhì rén* (Fructus Alpiniae Oxyphyllae) 30g.

➢ With food accumulation, add *shén qū* (Massa Medicata) 10g or *jiāo bīng láng* (Semen Arecae Ustum), *jiāo mài yá* (Fructus Hordei

Chapter 7
Associated Disease Categories

Germinatus Ustus), *jiāo shān zhā* (Fructus Crataegi Ustus) and *jiāo shén qū* (Massa Medicata Fermentata Ustus) 40g each.

(5) Stomach Yin Insufficiency, Counterflow Qi, Failure to Nourish the Brain-spirit

Signs and Symptoms: pessimism, despair, vexation, agitation, insomnia, fidgetiness, rapacious appetite, vomiting immediately after eating, dry mouth and throat, yellowish urine, dry stools, a red tongue with a scant coating, and fine rapid pulses.

Treatment Principles: benefit yin, harmonize the stomach, downbear counterflow, calm the spirit.

Formula: *Jú Pí Zhú Rú Tāng* (Tangerine Peel and Bamboo Shavings Decoction) with *Yì Wèi Tāng* (Stomach-Boosting Decoction)

法半夏	fǎ bàn xià	10g	Rhizoma Pinelliae Praeparatum
橘皮	jú pí	10g	Pericarpium Citri Reticulatae
枇杷叶	pí pá yè	10g	Folium Eriobotryae
麦门冬	mài mén dōng	30g	Radix Ophiopogonis
竹茹	zhú rú	6g	Caulis Bambusae in Taenia
赤茯苓	chì fú líng	30g	Poria Rubra
人参	rén shēn	10g	Radix et Rhizoma Ginseng
甘草	gān cǎo	10g	Radix et Rhizoma Glycyrrhizae
生地	shēng dì	30g	Radix Rehmanniae
玉竹	yù zhú	30g	Rhizoma Polygonati Odorati
沙参	shā shēn	30g	Radix Adenophorae
石斛	shí hú	30g	Caulis Dendrobii
天花粉	tiān huā fěn	30g	Radix Trichosanthis
菊花	jú huā	15g	Flos Chrysanthemi
川芎	chuān xiōng	20g	Rhizoma Chuanxiong
丹参	dān shēn	30g	Radix et Rhizoma Salviae Miltiorrhizae
郁金	yù jīn	30g	Radix Curcumae
天竺黄	tiān zhú huáng	15g	Concretio Silicea Bambusae

Modifications:
➤ With severe vomiting, add *pí pá yè* (Folium Eriobotryae) 10g.
➤ With liver stagnation, add *chái hú* (Radix Bupleuri) 6g, *bái sháo*

(Radix Paeoniae Alba) 30g, and *dāng guī* (Radix Angelicae Sinensis) 15g.
- With predominant qi stagnation, add *fó shǒu* (Fructus Citri Sarcodactylis) 10g and *xiāng yuán* (Fructus Citri) 15g.
- With predominant qi counterflow, add *xuán fù huā* (Flos Inulae) 15g and *dài zhě shí* (Haematitum) 30g.
- With poor sleep, add *chǎo zǎo rén* (Semen Ziziphi Spinosae, stir-fried) 30g and *hé huān pí* (Cortex Albiziae) 30g.
- With agitation, add *shēng shí jué míng* (Concha Haliotidis Cruda) 30g, *cí shí* (Magnetitum, decocted first) 30g, and *gōu téng* (Ramulus Uncariae Cum Uncis) 30g.
- With heart vexation and fidgeting, add *huáng lián* (Rhizoma Coptidis) 10g and *zhī zǐ* (Fructus Gardeniae) 10g.
- With dry stool, add *guā lóu rén* (Semen Trichosanthis) 30g and *huǒ má rén* (Fructus Cannabis) 30g.
- With food stagnation, add *shén qū* (Massa Medicata) 15g and *jiāo mài yá* (Fructus Hordei Germinatus Ustus), *jiāo shān zhā* (Fructus Crataegi Ustus) and *jiāo shén qū* (Massa Medicata Fermentata Ustus) 30g each.

Commentary

Bulimia nervosa can alternate with anorexia nervosa, since these two conditions share similar pathological and psychological mechanisms. Bulimia nervosa can be seen as an extension of anorexia nervosa, but with a later onset. Bulimia patients often worry about excessive eating, but will lose control at the sight sweet, fatty and greasy foods. The condition is also often related to a fear of obesity. After excessive eating, patients often induce vomiting, diarrhea or urination, or will fast intermittently; all of these abnormal dietary behaviors are often done secretly.

Nervous vomiting is also known as psychogenic bulimia nervosa, and this generally occurs when the patient is nervous or experiencing unpleasant emotions. The tendency to vomit after eating, or in other situations, may initially be through manual stimulation, however, later it may become reflexive. One aspect of this is that frequent vomiting weakens the stomach qi, leading to a situation where the stomach becomes overwhelmed in a normal digestive situation or is easily upset by

Chapter 7
Associated Disease Categories

emotions. In chronic cases, this aspect of the disorder must be addressed in order to restore the normal mechanical functioning of the spleen and stomach.

Pharmacological treatment of this condition focuses on anti-depressant and anti-anxiety medications. Antipsychotics are often applied as well, but these can only temporarily improve a patient's mood and compliance with treatment. There is no specifically effective medication for this condition, and the standard medical approach is to apply a combination of medication and psychotherapy.

The most effective applied psychotherapy is cognitive behavioral therapy, which can help to adjust the eating patterns and abnormal ideation. There is often a personality shift that appears before onset of the disorder; a tendency to codependent relationships, a choice of incompatible partners, fragile unstable moods, stubbornness, suspicion, lack of self confidence, and a tendency to become anxious, angry, and fearful. Patients often also have relationship or marriage problems. While addressing the behavior directly will help to resolve the condition, working with the psychological root of the issue with family or partners can also insure a better long term outcome.

Bulimia patients pay great attention to their appearance and also the impression of others; they may become obsessed with their attractiveness to the opposite gender. Psychological counseling is required in all cases. Once patients become engaged in the treatment process, they often become more interested in improving their low self-esteem and other malign psychological needs rather than controlling their weight.

GERIATRIC DEPRESSIVE DISORDER

In this discussion, the term geriatric refers anyone over the age of sixty. Geriatric depressive disorders include such disorders that occur for the first time at an advanced age, as well as to any depressive syndrome secondary to a physical condition related to aging and long term illness. This section focuses on pattern differentiation, treatment options, prevention, and follow-up.

Etiology

1. Ungratified emotions

A wide range of unique physical and psychological problems exist among the elderly; these problems can involve family, society, life, health, healthcare, and financial and emotional support in old age. As senior citizens gradually step out of the center of social living, they become more likely to feel conflicted regarding the realities of day to day life, furthermore, a strong sense of isolation commonly leads to increased frustration and despair.

Anger damages the liver, causing liver-wood to overwhelm and damage spleen-earth. Splenic failure of transformation function causes dampness to gather and engender phlegm. Phlegm obstructs the clear orifices, the brain spirit is disturbed and depression may result. In other cases, liver constraint transforms into fire; exuberant heart fire disturbs the brain-spirit to cause unstable emotions such as irascibility, vexation, agitation, frustration, and despair. If an elderly patient develops suicidal tendencies, they are usually severe.

2. Constitutional deficiency

The brain is the sea of marrow, the mansion of original spirit, and a function of the spirit mechanism. When people get to the age of sixty, viscera and bowel function naturally declines, the kidney origin fails, the dynamic between yin and yang becomes weaker, kidney essence stops engendering marrow and nourishing the brain, the sea of marrow becomes empty, the brain-spirit becomes weak, and the functions of recognition and acknowledgement are easily compromised. Once the spirit mechanism becomes weak and the brain-spirit is exhausted, then the brain-spirit can easily become constrained resulting in irregular emotional states. In other cases, when there is personal frustration, the brain-spirit can easily become constrained, resulting in depression. Financial difficulties and family disharmony can also easily aggravate the condition.

Chapter 7
Associated Disease Categories

3. Depletion due to enduring disease

In addition to physical debilitation, enduring diseases such as cardiovascular disease, malignant tumors, stroke, paralysis, and vision loss can all cause weakening of qi and blood, and impair function of the viscera and bowels. When the movement of qi and blood is inhibited, phlegm is generated internally which then obstructs the collaterals of the brain. This causes the brain-spirit to become constrained and induces depression. The elderly are commonly constitutionally deficient, with accompanying patterns of qi stagnation, blood stasis, phlegm obstruction, internal dampness, bowel qi stoppage, and spirit mechanism exhaustion; also, brain qi and visceral qi become less connected. Complex mixed cases of deficiency and excess also appear, and these depressive conditions tend to be more difficult.

Pathomechanism

When liver-kidney deficiency and spleen-kidney insufficiency impair proper nourishment of the brain, the mobility of the brain-spirit can be compromised, leading to depression. However, the pathomechanism usually involves ungratified emotions and unfulfilled desires. When intense, enduring and irresolvable mental stimulations are combined with patterns of liver-kidney deficiency, spleen-kidney insufficiency, brain marrow insufficiency, or phlegm stagnation attacking brain orifices; this also results in the exhaustion and disturbance of the brain-spirit. When patterns of deficiency, stasis, constraint, and phlegm combine, depression becomes more difficult to treat effectively. In addition, elderly patients usually present with a weak spleen and stomach and various physical conditions that cause an insufficiency in the source of engenderment and transformation; as qi and blood also fail to spread, the qi dynamic becomes congested and a variety of clinical manifestations will appear. In pattern differentiation, one must grasp the key mechanism of spleen-kidney dual deficiency and insufficiency of liver, kidney and brain marrow with impairment of the brain-spirit.

CM Diagnostic Criteria

(1) Age over sixty

(2) Low spirits that are hard to describe, or despair with a chief complaint of physical discomfort, generalized discomfort, hypochondria manifesting as a paranoia that they are suffering from a fatal disease, no pleasure in normally enjoyable activities, fatigue, lack of strength, frequently seeking medical care, a severe sense of isolation, self reproach, low self-esteem, and suicidal tendencies.

(3) The symptoms are comparatively light in the evening. The patient tends to wake up very early.

(4) Physical symptoms include low or absent appetite, weight loss, dry mouth, constipation, palpitations, flusteredness, and sweating that are marked by sudden onset. Also there may be a sense of dying, nausea, vomiting, dizziness, distention of the head, decreased memory, and feeble-minded behaviors.

(5) Symptoms remain unresolved for two weeks or longer.

(6) With or without other accompanying physical conditions.

(7) The possibility of senile dementia and drug effects are ruled out.

(8) A previous history of an unstable mood and suspicion, with the condition lasting for more than ten years.

If (1), (2), and (5) are present, a positive diagnosis can be made with reference to the other parameters.

Characteristics

(1) Low spirits, frustration, despair, a tendency to weep, misery that is hard to express, difficulty with relationships, a severe sense of rejection, and poor adaptability.

(2) Anxiety, nervousness, severe insomnia, constant nightmares, extreme fatigue upon waking, or chief a complaint of unresolved fatigue after sleeping.

(3) Sensitivity, suspicion, or paranoia towards acquaintances and family, typically marked by delusions of persecution and jealousy.

(4) Various primary complaints of physical discomfort such as hypochondria about fatal diseases, heart conditions, brain tumors, etc. Fear of death compounded with suicidal tendencies, an extremely poor appetite, emaciation, palpitations, and flusteredness that is triggered by the slightest incident. In severe cases, the patient will feel as if he is dying and will subsequently seek medical care in the emergency room.

Chapter 7
Associated Disease Categories

(5) People with a history of cancer surgeries can become insistent that they are not cured after the possibility of recurrence has been eliminated through multiple examinations. This is often accompanied by low self-esteem and severe sleep disorders.

(6) Timidity, poor social skills, or stubbornness.

Pattern Differentiation and Treatment

(1) INSUFFICIENCY OF THE SEA OF MARROW, BRAIN-SPIRIT IRREGULARITY

Signs and Symptoms: constitutional weakness, persistent low spirits, pessimistic attitude towards life, hypochondria about having a fatal disease, decreased interest in previously enjoyable activities, fatigue, lack of strength, slow thinking and movement, a severe sense of isolation, guilt, low self-esteem, suicidal tendencies or behavior; with improvement of symptoms in the evening, early waking, loose stools, frequent scanty urination, a pale tongue, and weak pulses.

Other symptoms may include poor appetite, weight loss, a dry mouth, constipation, palpitations, sweating, nausea, vomiting, dizziness, distention of the head, and mental symptoms of agitation, declining memory and comprehension, suspicion and sorrow, and a sense of dying during the onset of the depression.

Treatment Principles: supplement the kidney and marrow, nourish the brain, calm the spirit.

Formula:

熟地黄	*shú dì huáng*	30g	Radix Rehmanniae Praeparata
山药	*shān yào*	30g	Rhizoma Dioscoreae
龟甲	*guī jiǎ*	10g	Carapax et Plastrum Testudinis
当归	*dāng guī*	15g	Radix Angelicae Sinensis
生晒参	*shēng shài shēn*	3g	Radix et Rhizoma Ginseng Cruda
白术	*bái zhú*	10g	Rhizoma Atractylodis Macrocephalae
枸杞子	*gǒu qǐ zǐ*	15g	Fructus Lycii
女贞子	*nǚ zhēn zǐ*	20g	Fructus Ligustri Lucidi
何首乌	*hé shǒu wū*	30g	Radix Polygoni Multiflori

巴戟天	bā jǐ tiān	15g	Radix Morindae Officinalis
补骨脂	bǔ gǔ zhī	15g	Fructus Psoraleae
益智仁	yì zhì rén	30g	Fructus Alpiniae Oxyphyllae
仙灵脾	xiān líng pí	15g	Herba Epimedii

(2) Insufficiency of the Spleen and Kidney, Failure to Nourish the Brain

Signs and Symptoms: persistent low spirits, despair, loss of facial expression, a sallow complexion, emaciation, unwillingness to speak, decreased appetite, torpid intake, shortness of breath, cold limbs, declining memory, aching weak lumbus and knees, an enlarged tongue, and sunken fine and weak pulses.

Other symptoms may include palpable cold in the body and extremities, laziness, decreased self-care, increased isolation, and difficulty with human contact.

Treatment Principles: supplement spleen and kidney, nourish the brain, calm the spirit.

Formula:

熟地黄	shú dì huáng	30g	Radix Rehmanniae Praeparata
枸杞子	gǒu qǐ zǐ	15g	Fructus Lycii
肉苁蓉	ròu cōng róng	30g	Herba Cistanches
巴戟天	bā jǐ tiān	15g	Radix Morindae Officinalis
制首乌	zhì shǒu wū	30g	Radix Polygoni Multiflori Praeparata cum Succo Glycines Sotae
杜仲	dù zhòng	30g	Cortex Eucommiae
党参	dǎng shēn	15g	Radix Codonopsis
黄芪	huáng qí	30g	Radix Astragali
炒白术	chǎo bái zhú	15g	Rhizoma Atractylodis Macrocephalae (stir-fried)
茯苓	fú líng	30g	Poria
炒山药	chǎo shān yào	30g	Rhizoma Dioscoreae (mix-fried)
大枣	dà zǎo	10g	Fructus Jujubae
小茴香	xiǎo huí xiāng	10g	Fructus Foeniculi
神曲	shén qū	15g	Massa Medicata Fermentata

Chapter 7
Associated Disease Categories

(3) Qi Deficiency and Blood Stasis, Brain-spirit Irregularity

Signs and Symptoms: persistent low spirits, susceptibility to fright, forgetfulness, a tendency to sorrow, frequent weeping and sighing, a sad or blank facial expression, no sense of pleasure, shortness of breath, fatigue, lack of strength, unwillingness to speak, a tendency to lie down, profuse dreaming, decreased appetite, emaciation, scanty bowel movements, large volumes of clear urine, a dark purple tongue, and rough sunken fine pulses.

Other symptoms may include a lack of ease in mobility, a dry mouth with no desire to drink, self isolation and distancing from family and acquaintances, a lack of faith in life, and despair.

Treatment Principles: supplement qi, resolve stasis, awaken the brain, calm the spirit.

Formula:

黄芪	*huáng qí*	30g	Radix Astragali
当归	*dāng guī*	15g	Radix Angelicae Sinensis
枸杞子	*gǒu qǐ zǐ*	15g	Fructus Lycii
红花	*hóng huā*	10g	Flos Carthami
赤芍	*chì sháo*	20g	Radix Paeoniae Rubra
丹参	*dān shēn*	30g	Radix et Rhizoma Salviae Miltiorrhizae
川芎	*chuān xiōng*	15g	Rhizoma Chuanxiong
石菖蒲	*shí chāng pú*	6g	Rhizoma Acori Tatarinowii
远志	*yuǎn zhì*	10g	Radix Polygalae
益智仁	*yì zhì rén*	20g	Fructus Alpiniae Oxyphyllae
补骨脂	*bǔ gǔ zhī*	30g	Fructus Psoraleae
炒山药	*chǎo shān yào*	30g	Rhizoma Dioscoreae (mix-fried)

Empirical Insights

1. Some patients may have suffered from an unstable mood and a persistent sense of repression before entering old age. These patients may have had major persistent emotional stimulation in adolescence or middle age; they tend to be timid, and may have difficulties with relationships.

2. Some patients suffer from chronic diseases such as high blood

pressure, diabetes, coronary heart disease, or cerebral infarction, and have been on medications for a long time; some of these may be suffering from drug-induced disorders. These can lead to low spirits, a sense of pessimism, unstable mood, sleeplessness, decreased appetite and suspiciousness. Accompanying symptoms include personality changes and selfishness. When diagnosing, one should also differentiate depression from dementia.

These two conditions are the most commonly seen clinical presentations. When inquiring into the patient's history, the physician should pay attention to the cause and progression of the disease, and focus on enhancing communication with the patient. The key is to improve the patient's compliance and motivation. It is also recommended to begin treatment by focusing on the patient's sleep and appetite, gradually moving towards the goal of treating both root and branch.

Physical Conditions

While treating the elderly it is often the case that they will be suffering from concurrent chronic or acute physical ailments. Part of sound treatment involves making sure that the patient is managing these effectively, and, if treatment of these disorders is outside of the scope of Chinese medicine, they should be referred to appropriate clinicians.

Emphasis on Aftercare

Instruct the patient on how to maintain a healthy lifestyle; however, it is also important to not make sudden or drastic changes to their current way of life. Dietary therapies, simple physical exercise, social interaction, and entertainment can to help the patient become more optimistic about life.

Again, pay special attention to sleep patterns. The elderly tend to present with patterns of kidney deficiency, heart qi insufficiency, or non-interaction of the heart and kidney. They sleep lightly, and can wake up several times each night. Therefore, the elderly should follow a sleep schedule and when awake, they should remain as active as possible. Caffeine should be avoided, and less fluid should be taken in the evening to avoid nighttime urination. A healthy breakfast is important, and less should be eaten at dinner in order to facilitate proper digestion and better

Chapter 7
Associated Disease Categories

sleep. Moderate physical exercise should be performed; just enough to promote mild sweating.

Warming Yang and Opening Constraint

Constrained yang qi is one of the major causes of depression. The earliest liver-soothing and qi-regulating formula *Sì Nì Săn* (Frigid Extremities Powder) is indicated for inhibition of the qi dynamic, especially where *shaoyin* yang is constrained. For senile depression, warming yang is often the key to effective treatment. In the clinic, when treating depression among the elderly or those with weak constitutions, applying large doses of medicinals that warm kidney yang can greatly improve the outcome.

Our experience is that using a large quantity of *bā jǐ tiān* (Radix Morindae Officinalis), *xiān líng pí* (Herba Epimedii), and *ròu cōng róng* (Herba Cistanches), as well as moderate amount of *xiān máo* (Rhizoma Curculiginis) ensures the warming effect without excessively drying. Also, with prominent deficiency, use *shān zhū yú* (Fructus Corni) and *hé shǒu wū* (Radix Polygoni Multiflori) to nourish yin and blood. This treatment approach is an example of the axiom "seeking yang within yin".

To summarize, when treating geriatric disorders, one must understand the predominance of deficiency patterns, particularly of the spleen and kidney. Emphasize warming and supplementation of kidney qi and fortification of the spleen combined with heart-nourishing, liver-soothing, lung-securing and qi-benefiting methods of treatment. Once the brain-spirit becomes calm, depression will also be eliminated.

PEDIATRIC DEPRESSIVE DISORDER

Depressive disorders in children manifest similarly to those of adults, the primary difference being that due to children's young age, they may not be able to understand or describe the sorrow or depression that they feel. Some children or teenagers may express their emotions through acting out, self-isolation, or anger.

Etiology

The most common emotional etiologies for childhood depression are

ungratified emotional needs due to divorce or constant fighting between the parents, being treated poorly or excessively harshly by strict parents, being neglected, experiencing the death of family members, sudden changes in living environment, sexual abuse, abuse from parents, being bullied at school, punishment for being mischievous, failure to live up to the expectation of parents or teachers in examinations or competitions, or suffering caused by chronic health conditions.

Pathomechanism

While young patients are not always able to articulate their feelings effectively, there are predictable patterns of behavior to watch for; in some cases the patient may become inordinately meek or timid, manifesting with self isolation, timidity, suspicion, insecurity, pessimism, overly compliant, and with low self confidence. They will usually lose interest in previously enjoyable activities. Some patients will become more aggressive with unstable moods and irascibility, contempt for authority, a tendency to self-injury or inflicting harm on others, in extreme cases to the point of homicide.

In general, children with difficulty articulating feelings will somatacize their disorder, complaining of vague symptoms of physical discomfort including nausea, vomiting, anorexia, discomfort in the stomach duct or other vague presentations; medical examinations are usually without findings. Patience is required during the intake process to expose these manifestations and thus clarify diagnosis and treatment.

Pattern Differentiation and Treatment

(1) LIVER CONSTRAINT COMBINING WITH PHLEGM

Signs and Symptoms: unstable mood, irascibility, a tendency to hurt oneself or others, frequent worry, suspicion, self-isolation, dizziness, headaches, preferences for cold beverages, a red face and eyes, dry stools, yellowish turbid urine, a red tongue with a yellow coating, and wiry rapid pulses.

Other symptoms may include insomnia, profuse dreaming, stomach duct discomfort, and a lack of motivation.

Treatment Principles: rectify qi, sweep phlegm, awaken the brain,

Chapter 7
Associated Disease Categories

calm the spirit.

Formula:

菊花	jú huā	10g	Flos Chrysanthemi
川芎	chuān xiōng	10g	Rhizoma Chuanxiong
丹参	dān shēn	15g	Radix et Rhizoma Salviae Miltiorrhizae
白蒺藜	bái jí lí	30g	Fructus Tribuli
钩藤	gōu téng	30g	Ramulus Uncariae Cum Uncis
生石膏	shēng shí gāo	30g	Gypsum Fibrosum Cruda (decocted first)
珍珠母	zhēn zhū mǔ	30g	Concha Margaritiferae Usta
磁石	cí shí	60g	Magnetitum (decocted first)
黄连	huáng lián	15g	Rhizoma Coptidis
法半夏	fǎ bàn xià	10g	Rhizoma Pinelliae Praeparatum
栀子	zhī zǐ	10g	Fructus Gardeniae
大黄	dà huáng	10g	Radix et Rhizoma Rhei (preserved in liquor)
车前子	chē qián zǐ	30g	Semen Plantaginis
炒枣仁	chǎo zǎo rén	30–60g	Semen Ziziphi Spinosae (stir-fried)
石菖蒲	shí chāng pú	6g	Rhizoma Acori Tatarinowii
远志	yuǎn zhì	10g	Radix Polygalae
牛膝	niú xī	30g	Radix Achyranthis Bidentatae
天竺黄	tiān zhú huáng	10g	Concretio Silicea Bambusae
郁金	yù jīn	30g	Radix Curcumae

(2) Qi Stagnation and Blood Stasis

Signs and Symptoms: unstable mood, pessimism, vexation, agitation, no desire to see or talk to other people, a desire to die, a somber gray facial complexion, acne, dry stools, and a dark purple tongue.

Other symptoms may include decreased appetite and a tendency to frequently awaken.

Treatment Principles: rectify qi, resolve stasis, clear the brain, calm the spirit.

Formula:

柴胡	chái hú	6g	Radix Bupleuri

157

赤芍	chì sháo	30g	Radix Paeoniae Rubra
白芍	bái sháo	30g	Radix Paeoniae Alba
桃仁	táo rén	10g	Semen Persicae
红花	hóng huā	15g	Flos Carthami
牛膝	niú xī	15g	Radix Achyranthis Bidentatae
炒枣仁	chǎo zǎo rén	30g	Semen Ziziphi Spinosae (stir-fried)
天竺黄	tiān zhú huáng	15g	Concretio Silicea Bambusae
郁金	yù jīn	30g	Radix Curcumae
合欢皮	hé huān pí	30g	Cortex Albiziae

(3) Liver Constraint and Spleen Deficiency

Signs and Symptoms: a preference for laying down, no desire for company, no interest in school or previously enjoyable activities, a decline in focus and memory, emaciation, stomach duct discomfort, irregular bowel movements, long voidings of clear urine, a pale tongue with thin white coating, and sunken wiry fine pulses.

Other symptoms may include poor sleep, coldness towards family, no joy in life, a polarized preference for one parent while disliking the other, a reluctance to speak, repeated writings that indicate a negative or hostile attitude, and unconscious behaviors that show a negative attitude.

Treatment Principles: rectify qi, fortify spleen, nourish brain, quiet the spirit.

Formula:

柴胡	chái hú	6g	Radix Bupleuri
白芍	bái sháo	30g	Radix Paeoniae Alba
茯苓	fú líng	20g	Poria
当归	dāng guī	15g	Radix Angelicae Sinensis
陈皮	chén pí	15g	Pericarpium Citri Reticulatae
佛手	fó shǒu	15g	Fructus Citri Sarcodactylis
香橼	xiāng yuán	15g	Fructus Citri
炒枣仁	chǎo zǎo rén	30g	Semen Ziziphi Spinosae (stir-fried)
枸杞子	gǒu qǐ zǐ	15g	Fructus Lycii
菟丝子	tù sī zǐ	15g	Semen Cuscutae
甘草	gān cǎo	10g	Radix et Rhizoma Glycyrrhizae

Chapter 7
Associated Disease Categories

Empirical Insights

Children's depressive disorders have been increasing in recent years. Although is should be noted that many of these patients will present with premature physical development, the onset is most often related to dysfuntional relationships among family members. Figures from the educational environment can also cause problems; a lack of guidance and education around matters of sexuality may also be contributing factors. When clinical symptoms are discovered, it is best to start treatment as soon as possible.

From a Chinese medicine perspective, this condition is characterized by patterns of evil excess more often than those of upright qi deficiency. Common locations of the pathology include the heart, liver, and stomach, and the evils include fire, phlegm, and qi constraint. Treatment here should focus on dispelling the evils, emphasizing the clearing method. For patients older than thirteen, any frenetic movement of ministerial fire can manifest with frequent masturbation and dream emission; in such cases, the clearing and draining of internal fire should be emphasized.

Chapter 8
Treating Side Effects

The side-effects associated with many pharmaceutical medications can affect patient compliance, and in some cases cause severe toxic reactions. Drug-induced ailments can be very stubborn, lasting long after the medication has been discontinued. These include extracorticospinal tract reactions (specifically tardive dyskinesia), gastro-intestinal dysfunction, liver damage, sexual disorders, amenorrhea, cardiovascular changes, granulocytopenia, dermatitis, and abnormal weight gain.

SIDE-EFFECTS AND TOXICITY—THE CHINESE MEDICAL PERSPECTIVE

General speaking, antipsychotic and antidepressant medications often cause dryness and heat reactions within the body. They can lead to yin damage patterns, qi depletion, fluid damage, phlegm-heat ascending, stasis obstructing, and malnourishment of the sinews. Treatment is determined according to the relative severity of heat and deficiency, but usually focuses on clearing heat, nourishing yin, and moving blood.

1. Effects on the spleen and stomach

These classes of drugs first cause dryness and *yangming* heat manifesting with dry mouth, thirst with a desire to drink, drooling, change in appetite, and dry stools. Other symptoms include bad breath, yellowish urine, and, in severe cases, bowel obstruction and enteroparalysis. The tongue coating may appear yellow and dry, yellow and slimy, or even black.

Judging from those symptoms and the patient's constitution, the presenting patterns are mostly ascribed to fire, heat, phlegm-heat, or constrained heat. *Bái Hǔ Tāng* (White Tiger Decoction) and *Chéng Qì Tāng* (Qi-Coordinating Decoction) are indicated for *yangming* channel and *yangming* bowel excess patterns respectively, and are often applied with modifications to clear or purge internal heat.

2. Primary side-effects

Although psychiatric symptoms can be improved, extrapyramidal reactions may also occur. These include acute dystonia manifesting with sudden torticollis, tongue thrusting, mimetic convulsion, and opisthotonos.

Chapter 8
Treating Side Effects

Such reactions can be easily misdiagnosed as epilepsy, cephalitis or hysteria; laryngeal spasm can cause difficult breathing or apnea. The symptoms are generally ascribed to wind patterns; when combined with other yang-heat symptoms, the pattern can be differentiated as exuberant *yangming* heat engendering wind. This can be generally supported by the fact that those reactions occur mostly among young people and in males, with younger males being more constitutionally prone to *yangming* heat. Treatment methods that clear heat, nourish yin, and emolliate the sinews can be very effective.

The patient can also develop symptoms similar to Parkinson's syndrome such as akinesia, or slow movement, rigid spasms of the muscles, tremors of the tongue, lips and hands, a stiff facial expression, a bent body posture or festinating gait, and autonomic nerve dysfunction that manifests with drooling, profuse sweating, and seborrhea. These all reflect complex excess-deficiency patterns such as accumulated heat in the spleen combined with fluid depletion of the stomach and lung with liver yin damage. Treatments that clear heat and nourish yin-fluids can be effective.

Patients may also develop symptoms of flusteredness and anxiety which reflect heart and liver yin depletion with fire exuberance.

The most severe extra-pyramidal reaction is tardive dyskinesia, characterized by uncontrollable chewing, sucking and rolling of the tongue, twitching of the face, trunk or limbs, and eating disorders. From a Chinese medicine perspective, these symptoms are complex manifestations of heat exuberance and deficiency wind. In such cases, *shēng shí gāo* (Gypsum Crudum), *gé gēn* (Radix Puerariae Lobatae), *jī xuè téng* (Caulis Spatholobi), *shēng dì* (Radix Rehmanniae), *xuán shēn* (Radix Scrophulariae) and *mài mén dōng* (Radix Ophiopogonis) are effective for clearing heat, and nourishing yin and the sinews. Of course, for patterns of blood stasis obstructing the collaterals and vessels, corresponding treatment should be applied.

Even with no observable manifestations of wind, patients who have been taking these types of medications long term can still present with subjective discomfort involving sluggishness, muscular fatigue, and a tendency to lie down. Medicinals that nourish yin, clear heat, and nourish the sinews can improve these symptoms.

3. Severe side-effects

Reactions to medication primarily involve the spleen and stomach. When these organs are disrupted, splenic transportation of the essence of food is affected. In some cases, vigorous fire consumes qi and this also results in splenic insufficiency. When stomach fire is exuberant and the spleen is deficient, there will be an abnormal appetite. Sometimes the appetite remains normal, but since the spleen cannot uplift the clear and the stomach fails to downbear the turbid, the essence of food cannot be transported appropriately within the body, instead accumulating in the middle burner to form phlegm-dampness. This can manifest with deficiency obesity, lack of strength, sluggishness, fatigue, somnolence, a lusterless facial complexion, and lack of spirit in the eyes. Phlegm-turbidity obstructing the collaterals and vessels can result in blood stasis and other abnormal conditions. Evil heat can also bind with phlegm-damp to disturb the brain-spirit. Phlegm-heat can cause generalized discomfort, specifically of the head, also aggravating psychological symptoms.

With a concurrent constitutional deficiency, such insufficiency in the source of transformation can also lead to an accumulation of excess within the body. Along with weight gain and obesity among female patients, this will manifest with amenorrhea and frigidity; among men there will be sexual disorders such as impotence as the spleen and stomach fail to nourish kidney essence. Over a period of time, further insufficiencies of kidney essence, liver blood, brain marrow, and brain-spirit will manifest. Patients can also present with insufficiencies of the spirit, qi, and essence.

An insufficiency of heart qi or heart yin combined with phlegm-damp or phlegm-heat can manifest with pain in the anterior chest, palpitations, and flusteredness among younger patients. Some cases may appear as similar to chest impediment. *Shēng Mài Sǎn* (Pulse-Engendering Powder) should be applied with additional *guā lóu* (Fructus Trichosanthis) and *xiè bái* (Bulbus Allii Macrostemi).

After qi and yin are damaged, toxins and heat continue to affect the body. Malnourishment of the collaterals and vessels along with phlegm-turbidity can cause stasis and obstruction manifesting with amenorrhea or prolonged menstrual cycles, purple dark menses, ejaculatory incompetence, chest impediment, palpitations, liver dysfunction, and involuntary movement of the limbs. Pathological heat and toxins accumulating in the blood aspect can manifest with various types of dermatitis on the exterior; when these evils attack the organs, however, the situation can become life-threatening.

4. Nourishing yin and invigorating blood

Fire and heat patterns are commonly seen in brain-spirit related conditions, and evil heat is a predominant factor among the drug-induced ailments. Therefore, the treatment method of clearing heat is most commonly applied, especially from the *yangming* qi aspect. Relatively large dosages of *shēng shí gāo* (Gypsum Crudum) may be applied over a long period of time without side effects.

Most extra-pyramidal reactions are associated with yin damage and malnourishment of the sinews and vessels, therefore it is essential to nourish yin and emolliate the sinews. After taking these medications for a long time, yin depletion and fluid damage occurs. There is usually concurrent blood stasis and stagnation in the collaterals and vessels, so it is also important to invigorate blood as one aspect of treatment.

DRUG-INDUCED DIGESTIVE DYSFUNCTION

Drug related dysfunctions of the digestive system can manifest with a variety of symptoms: abnormal appetite, glomus and fullness in the stomach duct, clamoring stomach, nausea, vomiting, hiccoughing, dry mouth, thirst, bad breath, constipation, bowel obstruction, and even enteroparalysis where peristaltic function is compromised or absent. Some drug reactions are relatively minor and will become reduced or eliminated after taking the medication for a period of time, but other medications may cause severe reactions that require modification and Chinese medicinal support.

Etiology and Pathomechanism

When constrained emotions combine with heat exuberance, phlegm exuberance, or qi stagnation, these factors can become compounded by the internal heat caused by medications, and the spleen and stomach are usually affected. This can cause fluids to thicken and a greater accumulation of phlegm-damp manifesting with glomus and fullness, decreased appetite, acid vomiting, and clamoring stomach. In cases of stomach fire ascending, manifestations include hiccoughs, vomiting, bad breath, vexing thirst with a desire for cold drinks, bound stools or ungratifying diarrhea. Food accumulation manifests with distending fullness in the stomach duct and abdomen, abdominal pain aggravated by pressure, putrid belching and acid swallowing. Heat exuberance damaging stomach yin manifests with occasional retching or vomiting, a feeling of hunger with no desire to eat, and a dry mouth and throat. The roots of these manifestations all involve the presence stomach heat and fire.

Pattern Differentiation and Treatment

(1) INTESTINAL DRYNESS WITH BOWEL HEAT AND FLUID DAMAGE

Signs and Symptoms: dry bound stools, abdominal distention and pain, dry mouth, bad breath, a red face, heart vexation, short voidings of red urine, a red tounge with a dry yellow coating, and slippery and rapid pulses.

Treatment Principles: drain heat, abduct stagnation, moisten the intestines, free the stool.

Formula: Modified *Má Zǐ Rén Wán* (Cannabis Fruit Pill)

大黄	dà huáng	10g	Radix et Rhizoma Rhei (preserved in liquor)
枳实	zhǐ shí	10g	Fructus Aurantii Immaturus
厚朴	hòu pò	10g	Cortex Magnoliae Officinalis
火麻仁	huǒ má rén	30g	Fructus Cannabis
杏仁	xìng rén	10g	Semen Armeniacae Amarum
白芍	bái sháo	30g	Radix Paeoniae Alba
莱菔子	lái fú zǐ	30g	Semen Raphani
郁李仁	yù lǐ rén	30g	Semen Pruni

Modifications:
➢ With exuberant heat, add *shēng shí gāo* (Gypsum Crudum, decocted first) 80g and *zhī mǔ* (Rhizoma Anemarrhenae) 15g.
➢ With predominant fluid damage, add *Zēng Yè Tāng* (Humor-Increasing Decoction): *xuán shēn* (Radix Scrophulariae) 30g, *shēng dì* (Radix Rehmanniae) 30g and *mài mén dōng* (Radix

Chapter 8
Treating Side Effects

Ophiopogonis) 30g.

➢ With lung heat and qi ascending, add *guā lóu rén* (Semen Trichosanthis) 15g and *huáng qín* (Radix Scutellariae) 15g.
➢ With constrained anger damaging the liver and observable emotional symptoms, add *lú huì* (Aloe) and *zhū shā* (Cinnabaris).

(2) Stomach Heat Accumulation, Bowel-Qi Inhibition, Stomach Fire Rebelling Upwards

Signs and Symptoms: loud hiccoughs, bad breath, vexing thirst with a preference for cold drinks, fullness and oppression of the stomach duct and abdomen, bound stools, short voidings of red urine, a dry yellow tongue coating, and slippery rapid pulses.

Treatment Principles: clear stomach heat, drain heat, downbear counterflow.

Formula: Modified *Zhú Yè Shí Gāo Tāng* (Lophatherum and Gypsum Decoction)

竹叶	zhú yè	6g	Folium Phyllostachydis Henonis
生石膏	shēng shí gāo	60g	Gypsum Fibrosum Cruda (decocted first)
沙参	shā shēn	30g	Radix Adenophorae
麦门冬	mài mén dōng	30g	Radix Ophiopogonis
半夏	bàn xià	10g	Rhizoma Pinelliae
甘草	gān cǎo	10g	Radix et Rhizoma Glycyrrhizae
竹茹	zhú rú	6g	Caulis Bambusae in Taenia
柿蒂	shì dì	15g	Calyx Kaki

Modifications:

➢ With dry stools, add a proper amount of *Xiǎo Chéng Qì Tāng* (Minor Qi-Coordination Decoction), or *dà huáng* (Radix et Rhizoma Rhei) and *máng xiāo* (Natrii Sulfas).
➢ With vexing heat in the chest and diaphragm, use *Liáng Gé Sǎn* (Diaphragm-Cooling Powder).

(3) Phlegm-Food and Damp-Heat Brewing Internally with Inhibition of the Qi Mechanism

Signs and Symptoms: glomus and fullness in the stomach-duct and

abdomen, clamoring stomach, nausea, vomiting, dry mouth with no desire to drink, a bitter taste in the mouth, reduced food intake, a thick yellow slimy tongue coating, and slippery rapid pulses.

Treatment Principles: clear heat, resolve dampness, harmonize the stomach, disperse glomus.

Formula: *Xiè Xīn Tāng* (Heart-Draining Decoction) with *Lián Pò Yǐn* (Coptis and Officinal Magnolia Bark Beverage)

大黄	*dà huáng*	10g	Radix et Rhizoma Rhei
黄连	*huáng lián*	10g	Rhizoma Coptidis
黄芩	*huáng qín*	10g	Radix Scutellariae
厚朴	*hòu pò*	10g	Cortex Magnoliae Officinalis
石菖蒲	*shí chāng pú*	10g	Rhizoma Acori Tatarinowii
半夏	*bàn xià*	10g	Rhizoma Pinelliae
芦根	*lú gēn*	30g	Rhizoma Phragmitis
栀子	*zhī zǐ*	10g	Fructus Gardeniae
豆豉	*dòu chǐ*	10g	Semen Sojae
佩兰	*pèi lán*	15g	Herba Eupatorii

Modifications:

➤ With predominant nausea and vomiting, add *zhú rú* (Caulis Bambusae in Taenia) 6g, *shēng jiāng* (Rhizoma Zingiberis Recens) 6g, and *xuán fù huā* (Flos Inulae) 15g.

➤ With torpid intake and inability to eat, add *mài yá* (Fructus Hordei Germinatus) 15g, *jī nèi jīn* (Endothelium Corneum Gigeriae Galli) 10g, and *chǎo gǔ yá* (Fructus Setariae Germinatus, mix-fried) 15g.

➤ With clamoring stomach, add *Zuǒ Jīn Wán* (Left Metal Pill).

➤ With distention and fullness in the stomach duct and abdomen, putrid belching, acid swallowing, aversion to food, pain with a desire purge the bowels, or dry stools due to food stagnation, add *zhǐ shí* (Fructus Aurantii Immaturus) 10g, *dà huáng* (Radix et Rhizoma Rhei) 15g, *fú líng* (Poria) 30g, *bái zhú* (Rhizoma Atractylodis Macrocephalae) 15g, *zé xiè* (Rhizoma Alismatis) 30g, and *shén qū* (Massa Medicata Fermentata) 15g.

Chapter 8
Treating Side Effects

(4) Stomach Yin Insufficiency and Stomach Malnourishment

Signs and Symptoms: dull stomach pain, a feeling of hunger with no desire to eat, occasional retching, dry mouth and throat, vexing heat in the five hearts, thirst with desire to drink, dry bound stools resembling sheep's droppings, short intermittent hiccoughs, a red tongue with scanty fluid, and fine rapid pulses

Treatment Principles: nourish yin, benefit the stomach, regulate the middle.

Formula: Modified *Yì Wèi Tāng* (Yang-Raising Decoction)

生地	shēng dì	30g	Radix Rehmanniae
沙参	shā shēn	30g	Radix Adenophorae
麦门冬	mài mén dōng	30g	Radix Ophiopogonis
玉竹	yù zhú	30g	Rhizoma Polygonati Odorati
冰糖	bīng táng	30g	Saccharon Crystallinum

Modifications:
- With severe fluid damage, add *shí hú* (Caulis Dendrobii) 30g and *tiān huā fěn* (Radix Trichosanthis) 30g.
- With predominant abdominal distention, add *zhǐ qiào* (Fructus Aurantii) 15g, *fó shǒu* (Fructus Citri Sarcodactylis) 10g and *xiāng yuán* (Fructus Citri) 10g.
- With food stagnation, add *mài yá* (Fructus Hordei Germinatus) 10g and *gǔ yá* (Fructus Setariae Germinatus) 10g.
- With constipation, add *huǒ má rén* (Fructus Cannabis) 30g and *xuán shēn* (Radix Scrophulariae) 30g, or *guā lóu rén* (Semen Trichosanthis) 30g.
- With hiccoughing and vomiting, add *shēng jiāng* (Rhizoma Zingiberis Recens) 10g, *bàn xià* (Rhizoma Pinelliae) 10g, and *zhú rú* (Caulis Bambusae in Taenia) 6g.
- With qi depletion, add *xī yáng shēn* (Radix Panacis Quinquefolii) 15g.

DRUG-INDUCED WEIGHT GAIN

Abnormal weight gain as a side effect of medications will change after cessation or reduction of medication in most cases; however, in some cases it remains persistent. Obesity usually indicates a metabolic abnormality linked with many severe secondary cardiovascular or cerebrovascular diseases and diabetes, so iatrogenic obesity requires prompt management.

Etiology and Pathomechanism

Long term use of psychiatric medications can cause stomach fire effulgence that manifests with increased food intake and rapid digestion with consequential rapid hungering; on the other hand, toxic heat can cause a failure of splenic transportation and transformation resulting in digestive products that cannot spread to the lung and thus are transformed into phlegm-damp. With strong stomach function exaggerated by fire and a weak spleen failing to move and transform the exuberant dampness that obstructs the middle, phlegm-turbidity streams into the flesh, also resulting in obesity.

Another important cause of phlegm-damp gathering is the patients' tendency to lie down and the lack of energy caused by medication. With spleen deficiency, phlegm-damp will mostly accumulate in the abdomen to cause localized obesity.

In cases of chronic disease there will be eventual damage to the kidney; with kidney deficiency, turbidity is not discharged, the spleen and stomach are not supported by kidney yang and phlegm-damp forms easily. Phlegm-damp can also enter the collaterals and vessels resulting in patterns of phlegm binding with stasis.

Pattern Differentiation and Treatment

(1) Stomach Heat and Dampness Obstruction

Signs and Symptoms: obesity, excessive eating with frequent hungering, stagnation and oppression in the stomach-duct, a dry mouth

Chapter 8
Treating Side Effects

and tongue, bad breath, thirst with a desire to drink, bound stools, a red tongue with a yellow coating, and slippery rapid pulses.

Treatment Principles: drain heat, free the bowels, disinhibit dampness, resolve turbidity.

Formula: *Liáng Gé Sǎn* (Diaphragm-Cooling Powder) *with Sān Rén Tāng* (Three Kernels Decoction)

栀子	zhī zǐ	10g	Fructus Gardeniae
黄芩	huáng qín	10g	Radix Scutellariae
薄荷	bò he	6g	Herba Menthae (decocted later)
杏仁	xìng rén	10g	Semen Armeniacae Amarum
白蔻仁	bái kòu rén	10g	Fructus Amomi Rotundus
薏苡仁	yì yǐ rén	30g	Semen Coicis
厚朴	hòu pò	15g	Cortex Magnoliae Officinalis
白术	bái zhú	12g	Rhizoma Atractylodis Macrocephalae
滑石	huá shí	15g	Talcum
泽泻	zé xiè	30g	Rhizoma Alismatis
草决明	cǎo jué míng	12g	Semen Cassiae
大黄	dà huáng	15g	Radix et Rhizoma Rhei

(2) Internal Heat with Phlegm Obstruction

Signs and Symptoms: obesity, headache, dizziness, a distending sensation in the eyes, tinnitus, a drunken (bright red) facial complexion, numbness in the body and extremities, vexing heat in the five hearts, a red tongue tip with scant or thin coating on the tongue body, and fine wiry pulses.

Treatment Principles: resolve phlegm, downbear turbidity, dispel dampness, clear heat.

Formula: *Bàn Xià Bái Zhú Tiān Má Tāng* (Pinellia, Atractylodes Macrocephala and Gastrodia Decoction) with *Èr Chén Tāng* (Two Matured Substances Decoction)

半夏	bàn xià	10g	Rhizoma Pinelliae
白术	bái zhú	10g	Rhizoma Atractylodis Macrocephalae
天麻	tiān má	10g	Rhizoma Gastrodiae
羚羊角	líng yáng jiǎo	6g	Cornu Saigae Tataricae (infused)

紫苏叶	zǐ sū yè	10g	Folium Perillae
陈皮	chén pí	10g	Pericarpium Citri Reticulatae
夏枯草	xià kū cǎo	10g	Spica Prunellae
地龙	dì lóng	6g	Pheretima
白芥子	bái jiè zǐ	12g	Semen Sinapis
皂荚	zào jiá	6g	Fructus Gleditsiae
丹参	dān shēn	30g	Radix et Rhizoma Salviae Miltiorrhizae

Modifications:

➢ *Lóng dǎn cǎo* (Radix et Rhizoma Gentianae), *jīn qián cǎo* (Herba Lysimachiae), *yīn chén* (Herba Artemisiae Scopariae), *zhī zǐ* (Fructus Gardeniae), *cǎo jué míng* (Semen Cassiae), *zé xiè* (Rhizoma Alismatis), *yù jīn* (Radix Curcumae), and *hé yè* (Folium Nelumbinis) can also be used.

➢ With modifications, this formula can treat obesity patients with patterns of phlegm-damp transforming into heat with liver heat rushing upwards. It acts to clear the liver, disinhibit the gallbladder, and resolve turbidity.

(3) Spleen Deficiency with Dampness Obstruction

Signs and Symptoms: obesity, heavy and cumbersome limbs, fatigue, lack of strength, lassitude, somnolence, oppression in the chest, shortness of breath, distending fullness of the stomach-duct and abdomen, reduced food intake, loose stools, a pale tongue with a thin slimy coating, and moderate or soggy fine pulses.

Treatment Principles: fortify the spleen, benefit qi, resolve phlegm, eliminate dampness.

Formula: *Xiāng Shā Liù Jūn Zǐ Tāng* (Costusroot and Amomum Six Gentlemen Decoction) and *Píng Wèi Sǎn* (Stomach-Calming Powder) with *Wèi Líng Tāng* (Stomach-Calming Poria Decoction)

木香	mù xiāng	10g	Radix Aucklandiae
砂仁	shā rén	6g	Fructus Amomi
党参	dǎng shēn	15g	Radix Codonopsis
焦白术	jiāo bái zhú	12g	Rhizoma Atractylodis Macrocephalae (scorch-fried)

Chapter 8
Treating Side Effects

白茯苓	bái fú líng	30g	Poria Alba
川朴	chuān pò	10g	Cortex Magnoliae Officinalis
苍术	cāng zhú	12g	Rhizoma Atractylodis
陈皮	chén pí	10g	Pericarpium Citri Reticulatae
泽泻	zé xiè	30g	Rhizoma Alismatis
黄芪	huáng qí	30g	Radix Astragali
薏苡仁	yì yǐ rén	30g	Semen Coicis
竹茹	zhú rú	10g	Caulis Bambusae in Taenia
冬瓜皮	dōng guā pí	30g	Exocarpium Benincasae

(4) Spleen and Kidney Deficiency

Signs and Symptoms: obesity, fatigue, lack of strength, aching limp lumbus and back, dizziness, shortness of breath, aversion to cold, cold extremities, impotence, cold sensation in the genitals, deficiency puffy swelling, shortage of qi, no strength to speak, panting with exertion, dizziness, reduced food intake, cold pain in the lumbus and knees, loose stool or fifth-watch diarrhea, a pale tongue with a thin white coating, and sunken fine pulses.

Treatment Principles: benefit qi, fortify the spleen, warm yang, benefit the kidney.

Formula: *Sì Jūn Zǐ Tāng* (Four Gentlemen Decoction) with *Shèn Qì Wán* (Kidney Qi Pill)

党参	dǎng shēn	10g	Radix Codonopsis
白术	bái zhú	10g	Rhizoma Atractylodis Macrocephalae
茯苓	fú líng	12g	Poria
肉桂	ròu guì	5g	Cortex Cinnamomi
制附子	zhì fù zǐ	6g	Radix Aconiti Lateralis Praeparata
生地	shēng dì	15g	Radix Rehmanniae
泽泻	zé xiè	30g	Rhizoma Alismatis
牡丹皮	mǔ dān pí	10g	Cortex Moutan
淫羊藿	yín yáng huò	10g	Herba Epimedii
车前草	chē qián cǎo	10g	Herba Plantaginis
牛膝	niú xī	30g	Radix Achyranthis Bidentatae

Modifications:
- With predominant somnolence, add jasmine tea to the decoction.
- With scanty menstrual flow and profuse vaginal discharge, add *hóng huā* (Flos Carthami) 10g and *é zhú* (Rhizoma Curcumae) 10g.
- With predominant kidney deficiency, add *zhì shǒu wū* (Radix Polygoni Multiflori Praeparata cum Succo Glycines Sotae) 30g and *sāng jì shēng* (Herba Taxilli) 15g.
- Take 10 packets ground into fine powder; boil some powder each day to drink as a tea.

(5) Qi Stagnation and Blood Stasis

Signs and Symptoms: obesity, distending fullness of the rib-sides, glomus and fullness in the stomach duct, vexation, agitation, irascibility, a dry mouth and tongue, dizziness, blurred vision, insomnia, profuse dreaming, menstrual irregularities or amenorrhea, a dark tongue with stasis macules, and wiry rapid or fine wiry pulses.

Treatment Principles: move qi and blood, resolve constraint, eliminate blood stasis.

Formula: *Yuè Jú Wán* (Depression-Resolving Pill) with *Táo Hóng Sì Wù Tāng* (Peach Kernel and Carthamus Four Substances Decoction)

川芎	chuān xiōng	10g	Rhizoma Chuanxiong
苍术	cāng zhú	12g	Rhizoma Atractylodis
神曲	shén qū	15g	Massa Medicata Fermentata
焦栀子	jiāo zhī zǐ	10g	Fructus Gardeniae Praeparatus (scorched-fried)
柴胡	chái hú	10g	Radix Bupleuri
柿蒂	shì dì	6g	Calyx Kaki
法半夏	fǎ bàn xià	10g	Rhizoma Pinelliae Praeparatum
当归	dāng guī	12g	Radix Angelicae Sinensis
生地	shēng dì	30g	Radix Rehmanniae
赤芍	chì sháo	30g	Radix Paeoniae Rubra
红花	hóng huā	6g	Flos Carthami
泽兰	zé lán	30g	Herba Lycopi
泽泻	zé xiè	30g	Rhizoma Alismatis

Chapter 8
Treating Side Effects

| 荷叶 | *hé yè* | 30g | Folium Nelumbinis |
| 蒲黄 | *pú huáng* | 10g | Pollen Typhae |

Commentary

In Chinese medicine, obesity is considered as a condition of root deficiency and branch excess. Deficiency refers to insufficiencies either qi and yin, or qi and yang. Although there is potential for any of the viscera, and the gallbladder, to be involved, clinically, spleen-kidney qi deficiency patterns are most predominant. Failure of the liver to course and discharge is also a commonly seen pattern.

Branch excess refers to the accumulation of fat and phlegm-turbidity as well as the water-dampness, static blood, and qi stagnation that accompany these patterns.

The seven most commonly used Chinese medicinal approaches to weight loss are as follows:

(1) Fortify the spleen and resolve dampness: indicated for splenic transportation failure with gathering of internal dampness and obesity. Manifestations include abdominal fullness, a slimy tongue coating, and fine sunken pulses.

Representative formulas include *Zé Xiè Tāng* (Alisma Decoction), *Èr Zhú Fú Líng Tāng* (Two Atractylodes and Poria Decoction), and *Fáng Jǐ Huáng Qí Tāng* (Stephania Root and Astragalus Decoction).

With predominant deficiency, use *Shēn Líng Bái Zhú Sǎn* (Ginseng, Poria and Atractylodes Macrocephalae Powder), *Yì Gōng Sǎn* (Special Achievement Powder), *Zhǐ Zhú Wán* (Immature Bitter Orange and Atractylodes Macrocephala Pill) and *Wǔ Líng Sǎn* (Five Substances Powder with Poria).

(2) Dispel phlegm-turbidity: for manifestations of qi deficiency, chest oppression, somnolence, lassitude, a swollen tongue with a white slimy coating, and slippery pulses.

In moderate cases, use *Èr Chén Tāng* (Two Matured Substances Decoction), *Píng Chén Tāng* (Calming Matured Substances Decoction), or *Sān Zǐ Yǎng Qīn Tāng* (Three-Seed Filial Devotion Decoction).

In severe cases, use *Kòng Xián Dān* (Drool-Controlling Elixir) or *Dǎo Tán Tāng* (Phlegm-Expelling Decoction).

(3) Percolate water and disinhibit dampness: for manifestations of obesity, puffy water swelling, scanty urine, abdominal distention, a white tongue coating and fine sunken pulses.

Use *Wǔ Pí Yǐn* (Five-Peel Beverage), *Dǎo Shuǐ Fú Líng Tāng* (Poria Decoction), or *Xiǎo Fēn Qīng Yǐn* (Turbidity-Clearing Beverage).

(4) Free the bowels with mild purging: for those patients with a preference towards rich and sweet or fatty foods presenting with patterns of excess and accumulation. Manifestations include obesity, dry bound stools, difficulty moving, panting with exertion, a yellow thick tongue coating, and excess pulses.

Use *Dà Chéng Qì Tāng* (Major Purgative Decoction), *Xiǎo Chéng Qì Tāng* (Minor Purgative Decoction), *Tiáo Wèi Chéng Qì Tāng* (Stomach-Regulating and Purgative Decoction) or *dà huáng* (Radix et Rhizoma Rhei) alone; however, these medicinals should not be used over a long period of time.

(5) Resolve accumulation with dispersing and abducting: used for patterns manifesting with obesity, lassitude, abdominal fullness, food accumulation, and a white tongue coating.

Generally, to disperse meat accumulation, select *shān zhā* (Fructus Crataegi); to disperse accumulation of flour products, select *shén qū* (Massa Medicata Fermentata); to generally disperse food accumulation, select *mài yá* (Fructus Hordei Germinatus). These medicinals act specifically for obesity as associated with excessive nutrition.

(6) Course the liver and disinhibit the gallbladder: used for patterns manifesting with obesity, rib-side pain, agitation, dizziness, fatigue, abdominal distention, a red tongue with a yellow coating, and wiry pulses.

Formulas include *Wēn Dǎn Tāng* (Gallbladder-Warming Decoction), *Shū Gān Yǐn* (Liver-Coursing Beverage) consisting of *chái hú* (Radix Bupleuri), *bò he* (Herba Menthae), *jiāng huáng* (Rhizoma Curcumae

Longae), and *yù jīn* (Radix Curcumae)), *Xiāo Zhàng Săn* (Distention-Dispersing Powder) consisting of shā rén (Fructus Amomi) and *lái fú zǐ* (Semen Raphani), and *Xiāo Yáo Săn* (Free Wanderer Powder).

(7) Warm yang and disinhibit water: used for patterns manifesting with mental fatigue, aching limp lumbus and knees, lack of strength, deficiency obesity, puffy swelling, a greenish-white or dark somber facial complexion, physical cold, cold extremities, a pale tongue with a white coating, and fine weak forceless pulses.

Formulas include *Líng Guì Zhú Gān Tāng* (Poria, Cinnamon Twig, Atractylodes Macrocephala and Licorice Decoction) and *Bā Wèi Dì Huáng Wán* (Eight Ingredients Rehmannia Pill).

Dietary Management

With the patterns of spleen deficiency and dampness obstruction, advise the patient to consume white hyacinth bean (lablab), broad bean, peas, aduki bean, mung bean, carp, wax gourd (rind or flesh), celery cabbage, soybean sprout, mung bean sprout, corn, cucumber (or its skin), and watermelon (or its rind).

With spleen and kidney deficiency, select cowpeas, sword beans, lyceum berries, goat's milk, milk, lean mutton, sparrow meat, and walnuts.

With qi stagnation and blood stasis, select citron, oranges, tangerine (or its peel), buckwheat, sorghum, sword beans, radish, fennel, jasmine, hawthorn berries, eggplant, and vinegar.

With phlegm-heat obstructing internally, select snow fungus (tremella), wood ear, black beans, mulberry, lean pork, duck meat or eggs, sea cucumber, jelly fish, sesame, and pig kidney.

With stomach heat and damp obstruction, select celery cabbage, cabbage, celery, lettuce, bamboo shoots, water shield, lotus root, balsam pear, purslane, water chestnuts, and pears.

DRUG-INDUCED CHEST IMPEDIMENT

Drug-induced chest impediment refers to adverse cardiovascular system reactions with palpitations, flusteredness, and precordial region discomfort caused by antipsychotics and antidepressants. Many antipsychotics can cause tachycardia, orthostatic hypotension, arrhythmia, and electrocardiogram changes (extended or reversed T wave, extended Q-T or bundle branch block).

Etiology and Pathomechanism

Heat or toxins from medications affecting the middle burner can cause *yangming* heat exuberance that obstructs the qi dynamic. Phlegm-damp thus collects internally and transforms into fire. Fire disturbing the heart can manifest with palpitations, flusteredness, and tachycardia; phlegm-turbidity obstructing the qi dynamic in the upper burner can cause oppression of the chest, or chest pain and discomfort of the precordial region in severe cases; vigorous fire consuming qi can affect the transportation and transformation of the spleen and stomach, and the heart will be deprived of nourishment, resulting in heart palpitations and susceptibility to fright. In severe cases, yang deficiency leads to qi and blood inhibition, resulting in arrhythmia and bound intermittent pulses. If the toxins from medications affect the heart directly, these reactions can be acute and severe.

Pattern Differentiation and Treatment

(1) PHLEGM-FIRE DISTURBING THE HEART

Signs and Symptoms: palpitations, vexation, agitation, chest oppression, profuse phlegm, nausea, abdominal distention, a bitter taste in the mouth, and insomnia; the tongue appears red with a yellow slimy coating, and pulses are slippery and rapid or bound and intermittent.

Treatment Principles: clear heat, resolve phlegm, stabilize the mind, calm the spirit.

Formula: Modified *Huáng Lián Wēn Dǎn Tāng* (Coptis Gallbladder-Warming Decoction)

黄连	*huáng lián*	12g	Rhizoma Coptidis
黄芩	*huáng qín*	15g	Radix Scutellariae
半夏	*bàn xià*	10g	Rhizoma Pinelliae
陈皮	*chén pí*	15g	Pericarpium Citri Reticulatae

Chapter 8
Treating Side Effects

| 竹茹 | *zhú rú* | 6g | Caulis Bambusae in Taenia |
| 枳实 | *zhǐ shí* | 10g | Fructus Aurantii Immaturus |

Modifications:

➢ With predominant fire evil, add *zhī zǐ* (Fructus Gardeniae) 10g and *dǎn nán xīng* (Arisaema cum Bile) 10g.

➢ With oppression of the chest and profuse phlegm, add *guā lóu* (Fructus Trichosanthis) 30g and *bèi mǔ* (Bulbus Fritillaria) 10g.

➢ With predominant palpitations, add *shēng lóng gǔ* (Os Draconis Cruda, decocted first) 30g, *shēng mǔ lì* (Concha Ostreae Cruda, decocted first) 30g, *zhēn zhū mǔ* (Concha Margaritiferae Usta, decocted first) 30g, *yuǎn zhì* (Radix Polygalae) 10g, and *shí chāng pú* (Rhizoma Acori Tatarinowii) 6g.

➢ With fire damaging yin, add *shā shēn* (Radix Adenophorae) 30g and *mài mén dōng* (Radix Ophiopogonis) 30g.

➢ With a thick slimy tongue coating, add *pèi lán* (Herba Eupatorii) 10g.

(2) Qi Stagnation and Blood Stasis

Signs and Symptoms: palpitations, fearful throbbing, oppression, distention and pain in the anterior chest, irascibility, belching; the tongue appears dark purple or with stasis macules, and the pulses are rough or bound and intermittent.

Treatment Principles: rectify qi, move blood, free the vessels, settle fright.

Formula: *Chái Hú Shū Gān Sǎn*（Bupleurum Liver-Soothing Powder）combined with *Xuè Fǔ Zhú Yū Tāng*（Blood Stasis Expelling Decoction）

赤芍	*chì sháo*	30g	Radix Paeoniae Rubra
桃仁	*táo rén*	15g	Semen Persicae
红花	*hóng huā*	15g	Flos Carthami
丹参	*dān shēn*	30g	Radix et Rhizoma Salviae Miltiorrhizae
川芎	*chuān xiōng*	20g	Rhizoma Chuanxiong
三七粉	*sān qī fěn*	3g	Radix et Rhizoma Notoginseng (powdered and infused)

郁金	yù jīn	30g	Radix Curcumae
延胡索	yán hú suǒ	15g	Rhizoma Corydalis
降香	jiàng xiāng	10g	Lignum Dalbergiae Odoriferae
香附	xiāng fù	10g	Rhizoma Cyperi
琥珀面	hǔ pò miàn	3g	Succinum (powdered and infused)

Modifications:

➢ With qi deficiency likely to result in stasis, add *dǎng shēn* (Radix Codonopsis) 15g and *huáng qí* (Radix Astragali) 30g.

➢ With blood deficiency, add *hé shǒu wū* (Radix Polygoni Multiflori) 30g, *shú dì huáng* (Radix Rehmanniae Praeparata) 15g, and *gǒu qǐ zǐ* (Fructus Lycii) 30g.

➢ With phlegm-turbidity, add *guā lóu* (Fructus Trichosanthis) 30g, *xiè bái* (Bulbus Allii Macrostemi) 15g, and *bàn xià* (Rhizoma Pinelliae) 15g.

(3) HEART QI INSUFFICIENCY WITH HEART MALNOURISHMENT

Signs and Symptoms: palpitations, fearful throbbing, susceptibility to fright, chest oppression, shortness of breath, fatigue, lack of strength, spontaneous sweating, no strength to speak, dizziness, a pale tongue with a white coating, and fine weak or slow moderate pulses.

Treatment Principles: nourish the heart, benefit qi, quiet the spirit, settle fright.

Formula: Supplemented *Sì Jūn Zǐ Tāng* (Four Gentlemen Decoction)

人参	rén shēn	10g	Radix et Rhizoma Ginseng
茯苓	fú líng	30g	Poria
白术	bái zhú	15g	Rhizoma Atractylodis Macrocephalae
黄芪	huáng qí	30g	Radix Astragali
甘草	gān cǎo	10g	Radix et Rhizoma Glycyrrhizae
丹参	dān shēn	30g	Radix et Rhizoma Salviae Miltiorrhizae
红花	hóng huā	10g	Flos Carthami
山药	shān yào	30g	Rhizoma Dioscoreae

Modifications:

➢ With heart blood deficiency, add *shú dì huáng* (Radix Rehmanniae

Chapter 8
Treating Side Effects

Praeparata) 15g, and *ē jiāo* (Colla Corii Asini) 10g.

➤ With heart qi constraint, palpitations, vexation, oppression, and low spirits, add *chái hú* (Radix Bupleuri) 10g, *yù jīn* (Radix Curcumae) 30g and *hé huān pí* (Cortex Albiziae) 30g.

(4) Heart Blood Insufficiency

Signs and Symptoms: palpitations, dizziness, lusterless facial complexion, fatigue, lack of strength, sleeplessness, profuse dreaming, a pale red tongue with a thin white coating, and fine sunken or bound intermittent pulses.

Treatment Principles: supplement qi and blood, quiet the spirit.

Formula: Modified *Guī Pí Tāng* (Spleen-Restoring Decoction)

当归	*dāng guī*	15g	Radix Angelicae Sinensis
白芍	*bái sháo*	30g	Radix Paeoniae Alba
阿胶	*ē jiāo*	10g	Colla Corii Asini
龙眼肉	*lóng yǎn ròu*	15g	Arillus Longan
黄芪	*huáng qí*	40g	Radix Astragali
白术	*bái zhú*	15g	Rhizoma Atractylodis Macrocephalae
人参	*rén shēn*	10g	Radix et Rhizoma Ginseng
茯苓	*fú líng*	30g	Poria
甘草	*gān cǎo*	10g	Radix et Rhizoma Glycyrrhizae
远志	*yuǎn zhì*	10g	Radix Polygalae
酸枣仁	*suān zǎo rén*	30g	Semen Ziziphi Spinosae
木香	*mù xiāng*	10g	Radix Aucklandiae

Modifications:

➤ With heart vexation, insomnia, spontaneous sweating, night sweats, a pale red tongue with scanty fluid and fine rapid pulses, add *xuán shēn* (Radix Scrophulariae) 30g, *shēng dì* (Radix Rehmanniae) 30g and *mài mén dōng* (Radix Ophiopogonis) 30g.

➤ With insomnia and profuse dreaming, add *hé huān pí* (Cortex Albiziae) 30g, *bǎi zǐ rén* (Semen Platycladi) 30g and *yè jiāo téng* (Caulis Polygoni Multiflori) 30g.

➤ With torpid intake and abdominal distention, add *jī nèi jīn* (Endothelium Corneum Gigeriae Galli) 15g, *chén pí* (Pericarpium

Citri Reticulatae) 10g, *shā rén* (Fructus Amomi) 10g, *mài yá* (Fructus Hordei Germinatus) 15g and *gǔ yá* (Fructus Setariae Germinatus) 15g.

➢ With phlegm-damp, add *bàn xià* (Rhizoma Pinelliae) 15g and *cāng zhú* (Rhizoma Atractylodis) 15g.

➢ With blood stasis, add *chuān xiōng* (Rhizoma Chuanxiong) 20g, and *dān shēn* (Radix et Rhizoma Salviae Miltiorrhizae) 30g.

➢ With blood deficiency and heat, add *huáng lián* (Rhizoma Coptidis) 10g and *huáng bǎi* (Cortex Phellodendri Chinensis) 10g.

(5) HEART YIN DEPLETION

Signs and Symptoms: palpitations, susceptibility to fright, vexing heat in the five hearts, dry mouth, thirst, a red tongue with scanty coating, and fine or fine and rapid pulses.

Treatment Principles: enrich yin, downbear fire, quiet the heart and spirit.

Formula: *Tiān Wáng Bǔ Xīn Dān* (Celestial Emperor Heart-Supplementing Elixir) or modified *Zhū Shā Ān Shén Wán* (Cinnabar Spirit-Calming Pill) with predominant yin deficiency, use *Tiān Wáng Bǔ Xīn Dān*:

天门冬	tiān mén dōng	30g	Radix Asparagi
麦门冬	mài mén dōng	30g	Radix Ophiopogonis
生地	shēng dì	30g	Radix Rehmanniae
玄参	xuán shēn	30g	Radix Scrophulariae
当归	dāng guī	15g	Radix Angelicae Sinensis
丹参	dān shēn	30g	Radix et Rhizoma Salviae Miltiorrhizae
人参	rén shēn	10g	Radix et Rhizoma Ginseng
茯苓	fú líng	30g	Poria
五味子	wǔ wèi zǐ	15g	Fructus Schisandrae Chinensis
朱砂	zhū shā	1g	Cinnabaris
远志	yuǎn zhì	10g	Radix Polygalae
柏子仁	bǎi zǐ rén	30g	Semen Platycladi

With yin deficiency and effulgent fire, use modified *Zhū Shā Ān Shén Wán*:

Chapter 8
Treating Side Effects

朱砂	zhū shā	1g	Cinnabaris
珍珠母	zhēn zhū mǔ	30g	Concha Margaritiferae Usta
当归	dāng guī	15g	Radix Angelicae Sinensis
生地	shēng dì	30g	Radix Rehmanniae
黄连	huáng lián	10g	Rhizoma Coptidis
栀子	zhī zǐ	10g	Fructus Gardeniae
莲子	lián zǐ	10g	Semen Nelumbinis

Modifications:

➢ With vexing heat of the five hearts, tinnitus, and aching lumbus associated with kidney yin depletion and frenetic stirring of heart fire, add *huáng lián* (Rhizoma Coptidis) 10g, *ē jiāo* (Colla Corii Asini) 15g, *bái sháo* (Radix Paeoniae Alba) 30g, and a piece of egg yolk.

➢ With stasis, add *chì sháo* (Radix Paeoniae Rubra) 30g and *dān shēn* (Radix et Rhizoma Salviae Miltiorrhizae) 30g.

➢ With predominant palpitations, add *Shēng Mài Yǐn* (Pulse-Engendering Beverage) consisting of *rén shēn* (Radix et Rhizoma Ginseng) 10g, *wǔ wèi zǐ* (Fructus Schisandrae Chinensis) 15g and *mài mén dōng* (Radix Ophiopogonis) 30g.

(6) Devitalized Heart Yang

Signs and Symptoms: palpitations, chest oppression, shortness of breath, chest pain, a bright white facial complexion, physical cold and cold limbs, a pale tongue with thin white coating, and slow sunken or bound intermittent pulses.

Treatment Principles: warm and supplement heart yang, quiet the spirit, settle fright.

Formula: Modified *Guì Zhī Gān Cǎo Lóng Gǔ Mǔ Lì Tāng* (Cinnamon Twig, Licorice, Dragon Bones and Oyster Shell Decoction)

桂枝	guì zhī	12g	Ramulus Cinnamomi
甘草	gān cǎo	10g	Radix et Rhizoma Glycyrrhizae
人参	rén shēn	10g	Radix et Rhizoma Ginseng
黄芪	huáng qí	30g	Radix Astragali

| 生龙骨 | *shēng lóng gǔ* | 30g | Os Draconis (decocted first) |
| 生牡蛎 | *shēng mǔ lì* | 30g | Concha Ostreae Cruda (decocted first) |

DRUG-INDUCED URINARY BLOCK

Drug-induced urinary block is characterized by difficult or scanty urination with dribbling, hypertonicity of the lower abdomen, or inability to urinate. This is a commonly seen side-effect that occurs more frequently in the elderly, especially those with prostate disorders.

Etiology and Pathomechanism

There are a variety of mechanisms for this pathology, most if which evolve from the hot and acrid nature of the pharmaceuticals used in the treatment of psychiatric disorders: If the pharmaceuticals are of a warm and drying nature the heat they induce in the body can congest the body fluids in the three burners, and the qi dynamic and waterway become inhibited. When heat obstructs the lung qi and it fails to effuse in the upper burner, this can result in the lung failing to regulate the waterways, consequentially leading to inhibited urination. If the spleen qi in the middle burner fails to raise the clear yang effectively then the turbid yin cannot be downborn, and this can also result in difficult urination. Kidney origin deficiency in the lower burner can lead to failure of storage or insufficient bladder qi; this can lead to inhibited urination, and urinary block, enuresis, or even urinary incontinence. If damp heat moves downwards and affects qi transformation in the lower burner, there will be dribbling urinary stoppage that leads to urinary blockage. Pre-existing liver qi constraint or liver qi constraint that is exacerbated by sluggish fluid metabolism combined with the toxin from medications can also affect the coursing and draining function of the liver and its channel resulting in inhibited urination.

Pattern Differentiation and Treatment

(1) **D**AMP-HEAT IN THE **B**LADDER

Signs and Symptoms: dribbling urinary stoppage, short voidings of scanty red urine with a burning sensation, a bitter taste and stickiness in the mouth, thirst with no desire to drink, a red tongue with yellow slimy coating, and sunken, rapid pulses.

Treatment Principles: clear heat, disinhibit the damp-heat, disinhibit urine.

Formula: Modified *Bā Zhèng Sǎn* (Eight Corrections Powder)

车前子	*chē qián zǐ*	10g	Semen Plantaginis
瞿麦	*qú mài*	15g	Herba Dianthi
滑石	*huá shí*	30g	Talcum
大黄	*dà huáng*	15g	Radix et Rhizoma Rhei (preserved in liquor)
栀子	*zhī zǐ*	15g	Fructus Gardeniae
萹蓄	*biǎn xù*	10g	Herba Polygoni Avicularis
木通	*mù tōng*	10g	Caulis Akebiae
甘草	*gān cǎo*	10g	Radix et Rhizoma Glycyrrhizae

Modifications:
- With a thick slimy tongue coating, add *cāng zhú* (Rhizoma Atractylodis) 15g, and *huáng bǎi* (Cortex Phellodendri Chinensis) 15g.
- With heart vexation and sores on the mouth and tongue, add *Dǎo Chì Sǎn* (Red Guiding Powder).
- With damp-heat in the lower burner scorching kidney yin manifesting with dry mouth and tongue, heat in the palms and soles, tidal fever and spontaneous sweating, add *shēng dì* (Radix Rehmanniae) 30g, *chē qián zǐ* (Semen Plantaginis) 10g, *niú xī* (Radix Achyranthis Bidentatae) 30g, and *dì gǔ pí* (Cortex Lycii) 15g.
- With damp-heat brewing and binding in the three burners affecting qi transformation manifesting with scanty urine or urinary block, dark facial complexion, chest oppression, vexation, agitation, nausea, and vomiting, use *Huáng Lián Wēn Dǎn Tāng* (Coptis Gallbladder-Warming Decoction) with added *chē qián zǐ* (Semen Plantaginis) 10g, *dà huáng* (Radix et Rhizoma Rhei) 10g, and *tōng cǎo* (Medulla Tetrapanacis) 10g.

(2) Lung Heat Exuberance

Signs and Symptoms: ungratifying urination or dribbling urinary stoppage, dry throat, vexing thirst with desire to drink, rapid breathing, cough, a thin yellow tongue coating, and rapid pulses.

Treatment Principles: clear lung heat, disinhibit the waterways.

Formula: Modified *Qīng Fèi Yǐn* (Lung-Clearing Beverage)

黄芩	huáng qín	15g	Radix Scutellariae
桑白皮	sāng bái pí	15g	Cortex Mori
鱼腥草	yú xīng cǎo	30g	Herba Houttuyniae
麦门冬	mài mén dōng	30g	Radix Ophiopogonis
芦根	lú gēn	30g	Rhizoma Phragmitis
天花粉	tiān huā fěn	30g	Radix Trichosanthis
地骨皮	dì gǔ pí	15g	Cortex Lycii
车前子	chē qián zǐ	10g	Semen Plantaginis
茯苓	fú líng	30g	Poria
猪苓	zhū líng	15g	Polyporus
泽泻	zé xiè	30g	Rhizoma Alismatis

Modifications:

➢ With constipation, add *dà huáng* (Radix et Rhizoma Rhei) 10g, and *xìng rén* (Amarum) 15g.

➢ With red urine and a burning sensation during urination, add *Bā Zhèng Sǎn* (Eight Corrections Powder).

(3) Liver Qi Constraint

Signs and Symptoms: blocked or ungratifying urination, distending fullness of the lower abdomen, vexation, and irascibility; the tongue appears red and the pulses are wiry.

Treatment Principles: course and disinhibit the qi dynamic, disinhibit urine.

Formula: Modified *Chén Xiāng Sǎn* (Aquilaria Powder)

沉香	chén xiāng	6g	Lignum Aquilariae Resinatum
橘皮	jú pí	15g	Pericarpium Citri Reticulatae

Chapter 8
Treating Side Effects

柴胡	*chái hú*	10g	Radix Bupleuri
青皮	*qīng pí*	10g	Pericarpium Citri Reticulatae Viride
乌药	*wū yào*	10g	Radix Linderae
当归	*dāng guī*	10g	Radix Angelicae Sinensis
郁金	*yù jīn*	30g	Radix Curcumae
王不留行	*wáng bù liú xíng*	10g	Semen Vaccariae
石韦	*shí wéi*	10g	Folium Pyrrosiae
车前子	*chē qián zǐ*	10g	Semen Plantaginis
冬葵子	*dōng kuí zǐ*	30g	Fructus Malvae
茯苓	*fú líng*	30g	Poria

Modifications:
➤ With severe liver qi stagnation, add *mù xiāng* (Radix Aucklandiae) 10g, *zhǐ shí* (Fructus Aurantii Immaturus) 10g, *bīng láng* (Semen Arecae) 10g, and *dà huáng* (Radix et Rhizoma Rhei) 10g.

(4) Spleen Qi Failing to Ascend

Signs and Symptoms: frequent urgency with inability to urinate, scant ungratifying urination, sagging distention of the lower abdomen, shortness of breath, a low faint voice, fatigue, decreased appetite, a pale tongue, and weak pulses.

Treatment Principles: upbear the clear, downbear the turbid, transform qi, disinhibit water.

Formula: *Bǔ Zhōng Yì Qì Tāng* (Center-Supplementing and Qi-Boosting Decoction) combined with *Chūn Zé Tāng* (Spring Pond Decoction)

人参	*rén shēn*	10g	Radix et Rhizoma Ginseng
党参	*dǎng shēn*	10g	Radix Codonopsis
黄芪	*huáng qí*	30g	Radix Astragali
白术	*bái zhú*	15g	Rhizoma Atractylodis Macrocephalae
桂枝	*guì zhī*	10g	Ramulus Cinnamomi
肉桂	*ròu guì*	10g	Cortex Cinnamomi
升麻	*shēng má*	10g	Rhizoma Cimicifugae
柴胡	*chái hú*	10g	Radix Bupleuri
茯苓	*fú líng*	30g	Poria

猪苓	zhū líng	15g	Polyporus
泽泻	zé xiè	30g	Rhizoma Alismatis
车前子	chē qián zǐ	10g	Semen Plantaginis

Modifications:
➢ With kidney qi insufficiency, add *Jì Shēng Shèn Qì Wán* (Life-Saving Kidney Qi Pill).

(5) Kidney Yang Debilitation

Signs and Symptoms: blocked or dribbling ungratifying urination, white facial complexion, timidity, cold limp lumbus and knees, a pale enlarged tongue with sunken, fine pulses weak in the cubit positions.

Treatment Principles: warm yang, benefit qi, supplement kidney, disinhibit urine.

Formula: Modified *Jì Shēng Shèn Qì Wán* (Life-Saving Kidney Qi Pill)

附子	fù zǐ	6g	Radix Aconiti Lateralis Praeparata
肉桂	ròu guì	10g	Cortex Cinnamomi
桂枝	guì zhī	10g	Ramulus Cinnamomi
熟地黄	shú dì huáng	15g	Radix Rehmanniae Praeparata
山药	shān yào	30g	Rhizoma Dioscoreae
山茱萸	shān zhū yú	20g	Fructus Corni
车前子	chē qián zǐ	10g	Semen Plantaginis
茯苓	fú líng	30g	Poria
泽泻	zé xiè	30g	Rhizoma Alismatis

TARDIVE DYSKINESIA

Tardive dyskinesia is a persistent motion disorder caused by long term use of antipsychotics. It commonly occurs among those who have been on antipsychotics for more than one year, also tending to occur after medication is reduced or discontinued. The condition is characterized by involuntary stiff rhythmic movements that do not occur during sleep, and are aggravated by nervousness and excitement; there is also muscular hypotonia with poorly

Chapter 8
Treating Side Effects

coordinated movement. Currently, there is no specific Western medical treatment for this condition; however, Chinese medicine has been shown to be effective in relieving the symptoms in some cases.

Etiology and Pathomechanism

The pharmaceutical toxins brew and bind internally and eventually transform into heat. As heat and toxin gathers in the *yangming*, stomach yin becomes depleting and the spleen is malnourished. When heat flares upward, fluids fail to nourish the upper body and the sinews become dry and prone to spastic movement, manifesting with involuntary movements of the mouth, tongue and cheek. Toxic heat can also affect liver blood more globally to cause general malnourishment of the sinews leading to liver wind, causing involuntary and rhythmic tremors of the extremities, commonly accompanied by a red tongue with yellow coating and wiry rapid pulses. When internal heat is constrained for too long, yin and blood are deeply affected; manifestations include a red tongue with a scanty coating, or a pale red tongue with no coating, and fine rapid pulses. Some patients may also present with a stiff or tilted neck because as the *yangming* channel becomes depleted, muscular contractions will occur the along its running course on the sides of the neck.

Pattern Differentiation and Treatment

(1) Yangming Heat Exuberance with Yin Humor insufficiency

Signs and Symptoms: involuntary and rhythmic movements of the mouth, tongue and lips, tilted neck, difficulty eating, dry throat and tongue, thirst with a desire for cold drinks, vexation, agitation, dry bound stools, and in severe cases delirious speech, a red tongue with a dry yellow coating, and wiry rapid forceful pulses.

Treatment Principles: flush *yangming*, clear heat, enrich yin.
Formula:

生石膏	*shēng shí gāo*	80 – 400g	Gypsum Fibrosum Cruda (decocted first)
石斛	*shí hú*	30g	Caulis Dendrobii
麦门冬	*mài mén dōng*	30g	Radix Ophiopogonis

生地	shēng dì	30g	Radix Rehmanniae
天花粉	tiān huā fěn	30g	Radix Trichosanthis
瓜蒌	guā lóu	30g	Fructus Trichosanthis
黄连	huáng lián	10g	Rhizoma Coptidis
大黄	dà huáng	10g	Radix et Rhizoma Rhei (preserved in liquor and decocted later)

Modifications:
➢ With severe vexation and thirst, add *zhī mǔ* (Rhizoma Anemarrhenae) 10g and *zhī zǐ* (Fructus Gardeniae) 10g.

(2) Liver Yin Insufficiency with Malnourishment of the Sinews

Signs and Symptoms: involuntary and rhythmic movements of the extremities accompanied by tongue thrusting and clenching of the jaw, a lusterless facial complexion, dizziness, blurred vision, disturbing dreams, tinnitus, dry and rough feeling eyes, scant menses or amenorrhea, a red tongue with a scanty coating, and wiry fine pulses.

Treatment Principles: nourish liver yin, moisten the sinews.

Formula:

生地	shēng dì	30g	Radix Rehmanniae
熟地黄	shú dì huáng	30g	Radix Rehmanniae Praeparata
女贞子	nǚ zhēn zǐ	30g	Fructus Ligustri Lucidi
白芍	bái sháo	30g	Radix Paeoniae Alba
当归	dāng guī	20g	Radix Angelicae Sinensis
鸡血藤	jī xuè téng	30g	Caulis Spatholobi
牛膝	niú xī	30g	Radix Achyranthis Bidentatae

Modifications:
➢ With insomnia, add *yè jiāo téng* (Caulis Polygoni Multiflori) 30g and *chǎo zǎo rén* (Semen Ziziphi Spinosae, stir-fried) 30g.

(3) Spleen and Kidney Deficiency with Middle Burner Qi Insufficiency

Signs and Symptoms: involuntary lip-licking, sucking, and movement of the tongue, difficulty swallowing, and constant movement of the

Chapter 8
Treating Side Effects

extremities. A tendency to lie down, no strength to move or speak, fatigue, palpitations, forgetfulness, reduced sleeping with profuse dreaming, abdominal distention, torpid intake, emaciation, a withered-yellow facial complexion, a pale tender tongue with a thin white coating or a smooth mirror-like tongue surface. Pulses are sunken, fine and weak.

Treatment Principles: nourish the heart, fortify the spleen, benefit qi, foster yin.

Formula:

党参	dǎng shēn	15g	Radix Codonopsis
白术	bái zhú	10g	Rhizoma Atractylodis Macrocephalae
茯苓	fú líng	30g	Poria
生地	shēng dì	30g	Radix Rehmanniae
麦门冬	mài mén dōng	30g	Radix Ophiopogonis
夜交藤	yè jiāo téng	30g	Caulis Polygoni Multiflori
枸杞子	gǒu qǐ zǐ	15g	Fructus Lycii
女贞子	nǚ zhēn zǐ	30g	Fructus Ligustri Lucidi
炒枣仁	chǎo zǎo rén	60g	Semen Ziziphi Spinosae (stir-fried)
焦麦芽	jiāo mài yá	30g	Fructus Hordei Germinatus Ustus
焦山楂	jiāo shān zhā	30g	Fructus Crataegi
焦神曲	jiāo shén qū	30g	Massa Medicata Fermentata Ustus

(4) Liver Qi Stagnation with Blood stasis

Signs and Symptoms: involuntary movements of the extremities, involuntary chewing and movements of the tongue, low spirits, vexation, agitation, irascibility, distending pain of the rib-sides, menstrual irregularities, a dark purple tongue with static macula, and sunken, wiry, rough pulses.

Treatment Principles: course the liver, rectify qi, invigorate blood, resolve stasis.

Formula:

柴胡	chái hú	6g	Radix Bupleuri
陈皮	chén pí	10g	Pericarpium Citri Reticulatae
木香	mù xiāng	10g	Radix Aucklandiae

香附	xiāng fù	10g	Rhizoma Cyperi
桃仁	táo rén	15g	Semen Persicae
红花	hóng huā	10g	Flos Carthami
赤芍	chì sháo	30g	Radix Paeoniae Rubra
当归	dāng guī	15g	Radix Angelicae Sinensis
鸡血藤	jī xuè téng	30g	Caulis Spatholobi
牛膝	niú xī	30g	Radix Achyranthis Bidentatae

Modifications:

➢ An oral liquid form of *Xuè Fǔ Zhú Yū Tāng* (Blood Stasis Expelling Decoction) can be applied as an alternative, twice daily, one tube each time.

(5) Stomach Yin Insufficiency with Contraction of the Neck Muscles

Signs and Symptoms: dry mouth and tongue, twirling and rolling movements of the tongue, lip licking, pouting movements, rigidity, tilting and pain of the neck and back, involuntary extension of the neck, backward bending of the neck and upper extremities, hypertonicity and pain in the lumbus and lower limbs when walking or when nervous, profuse sweating, a red tongue with thin yellow coating or no coating, and wiry fine pulses.

Treatment Principles: nourish yin, resolve the flesh.

Formula:

生石膏	shēng shí gāo	80-550g	Gypsum Fibrosum Cruda (decocted first)
玄参	xuán shēn	30g	Radix Scrophulariae
麦门冬	mài mén dōng	30g	Radix Ophiopogonis
生地	shēng dì	30g	Radix Rehmanniae
鸡血藤	jī xuè téng	30g	Caulis Spatholobi
葛根	gé gēn	30 – 80g	Radix Puerariae Lobatae
炒麦芽	chǎo mài yá	30g	Fructus Hordei Germinatus (stir-fried)

One decoction daily, divided in two portions. 30 – 60 packets constitute one course of treatment.

Chapter 8
Treating Side Effects

Representative Cases

A 33-year-old female with schizophrenia became an inpatient on January 6th, 1988. She was treated with Fluphenazine for 73 days and her mental status had become stabilized. The patient was discharged and the medication was discontinued, however, the condition then relapsed and became aggravated. In May, 1988, she was prescribed Perphenazine, 20mg daily. She started to present with a tilted neck, and eventually the neck and nape became rigid and extremely painful after the family took her home and discontinued the medication. In June, 1993, she was admitted to the Chinese medicine department. Her diagnosis at intake was schizophrenia with tardive dyskinesia. The principal manifestations included tilted neck with involuntary and rhythmic tremors, and leaning backward and to the right.

More than 70 packets of yin-nourishing and flesh-resolving medicinals were applied, leading to slight improvement of the condition. The dosage of *shēng shí gāo* (Gypsum Fibrosum Cruda) was increased to 420g, and *gé gēn* (Radix Puerariae Lobatae) 60g. After another 50 packets all of the symptoms were substantially relieved. The formula was continued with modifications. By July 1994, the neck symptoms were basically resolved. One packet was taken every two days for another three months. The patient was considered as clinically cured, and follow-up visits showed no abnormality.

A 15-year-old boy with mental disorders was prescribed Haloperidol, 8mg daily. The psychiatric condition stabilized, however, after the dosage was decreased, he developed a tilted neck, inability to walk straight, a stiff tongue and intermittent rhythmic tremor of the extremities. After taking Diazepam and artane, his symptoms were slightly improved, but relapsed after two days. He was then diagnosed with tardive dyskinesia. Other manifestations included dry stools, a red tongue with a yellow coating, and wiry slippery pulses.

Pattern differentiation: *yangming* heat exuberance.

Treatment Principles: open and discharge *yangming*, enrich yin, clear heat.

14 packets of *shēng shí gāo* (Gypsum Fibrosum Cruda), *gé gēn* (Radix

Puerariae Lobatae), *jī xuè téng* (Caulis Spatholobi), *xuán shēn* (Radix Scrophulariae), *mài mén dōng* (Radix Ophiopogonis) and *chǎo mài yá* (Fructus Hordei Germinatus, stir-fried) were applied. The symptoms were substantially relieved. After another 14 packets, all symptoms were completely resolved.

Commentary

For best results, it is important to receive Chinese medicinal treatment within one year of the onset of this condition because the functioning of the viscera and bowels will not have become severely damaged. If a tilted neck is the only symptom, then surgical treatment or nerve blocking therapies can only temporarily resolve the symptoms of the local musculature; this cannot permanently resolve the condition. In our clinic, there was one patient who had recieved surgical intervention and was subsequently treated with Chinese medicine for two years with no resolution of the symptoms.

If the condition is chronic or the patient is elderly, symptoms will be characterized by involuntary movements of the mouth and tongue, involuntary flexion and extension of the tips of the four extremities, an inability to sit still, and temporary symptomatic relief during sleep. These cases are difficult to treat. For elderly patients, the key treatment principle is to secure the root. In order to avoid damaging yin, acrid and drying medicinals are prohibited or should be used with caution.

When treating recalcitrant disorders with obvious physical manifestations of channel damage, dosages for some medicinals can be quite high. For example: when *shēng shí gāo* (Gypsum Fibrosum Cruda) is used as the chief medicinal, the common dosage is 80–380g; when *gé gēn* (Radix Puerariae Lobatae) is the primary selection for treating rigid or tilted neck, the common dosage is 30–80g. *Gé gēn* (Radix Puerariae Lobatae) can resolve the flesh, eliminate vexation, and nourish fluids. Once the *yangming* channel is moistened, the condition will resolve.

DRUG-INDUCED SEXUAL DISORDERS

These conditions are more commonly seen in males of 20–50 years of age. Clinical manifestations include low libido, impotence, spermatorrhea

Chapter 8
Treating Side Effects

and premature ejaculation; there are also cases of abnormal erection. Among women there can be low libido or vaginal dryness with severe pain during sexual intercourse; there are also cases of hyperactive sexual function. Chinese medicine has been proven effective in managing these conditions.

Etiology and Pathomechanism

The spleen and stomach are the sea of water and grain. The spleen transforms and transports the essence of water and grain, and this essence goes on to nourish and restore the kidney essence, so the supply of the kidney yang and kidney qi relies on this mechanism. Long-term application of antipsychotic drugs can affect the function of the spleen, stomach and kidney. Common manifestations include dry mouth and tongue, ungratifying defecation, and stiffness of the body. Eventually both kidney yin and kidney yang will become depleted, and sexual disorders appear. There are also relatively rare cases of yang hyperactivity causing sexual dysfunction.

Pattern Differentiation and Treatment

(1) KIDNEY YANG INSUFFICIENCY

Signs and Symptoms: low libido, impotence, seminal emission, premature ejaculation, a somber dark or white bright facial complexion, dizziness, blurred vision, aching limp lumbus and knees, a pale red tongue with thin white coating, and sunken fine pulses.

Treatment Principles: supplement the kidney, invigorate yang.

Formula:

女贞子	nǚ zhēn zǐ	30g	Fructus Ligustri Lucidi
菟丝子	tù sī zǐ	60g	Semen Cuscutae
仙灵脾	xiān líng pí	10g	Herba Epimedii
仙茅	xiān máo	10g	Rhizoma Curculiginis
补骨脂	bǔ gǔ zhī	10g	Fructus Psoraleae
肉桂	ròu guì	5g	Cortex Cinnamomi
五味子	wǔ wèi zǐ	15g	Fructus Schisandrae Chinensis
金樱子	jīn yīng zǐ	15g	Fructus Rosae Laevigatae
海螵蛸	hǎi piāo xiāo	10g	Endoconcha Sepiae

(2) KIDNEY YIN INSUFFICIENCY

Signs and Symptoms: impotence, dream emission, disturbed sleep, dizziness, fatigue, lack of strength, tinnitus, spontaneous sweating at night, occasional short voidings of red urine with a burning sensation, a red tongue with no coating, and sunken fine rapid pulses.

Treatment Principles: enrich yin, clear heat.

Formula:

盐知母	yán zhī mǔ	10g	Rhizoma Anemarrhenae (mix-fried with brine)
盐黄柏	yán huáng bǎi	15g	Cortex Phellodendri Chinensis (mix-fried with brine)
女贞子	nǚ zhēn zǐ	30g	Fructus Ligustri Lucidi
菟丝子	tù sī zǐ	30g	Semen Cuscutae
地骨皮	dì gǔ pí	30g	Cortex Lycii
生地	shēng dì	20g	Radix Rehmanniae
夜交藤	yè jiāo téng	30g	Caulis Polygoni Multiflori
柏子仁	bǎi zǐ rén	30g	Semen Platycladi
远志	yuǎn zhì	10g	Radix Polygalae
琥珀面	hǔ pò miàn	3g	Succinum (powdered and infused)

(3) YIN AND YANG DUAL DEFICIENCY

Signs and Symptoms: low libido, impotence, seminal emission, somber lusterless facial complexion, fatigue, lack of strength, loose stool, long voidings of clear urine, aching limp lumbus and knees, decreased memory, tendency to lay down, no strength to move, a red tongue with no coating, and sunken, fine weak pulses.

Treatment Principles: supplement yin and yang.

Formula:

何首乌	hé shǒu wū	30g	Radix Polygoni Multiflori
女贞子	nǚ zhēn zǐ	30g	Fructus Ligustri Lucidi
枸杞子	gǒu qǐ zǐ	15g	Fructus Lycii
菟丝子	tù sī zǐ	60g	Semen Cuscutae

Chapter 8
Treating Side Effects

仙茅	*xiān máo*	10g	Rhizoma Curculiginis
仙灵脾	*xiān líng pí*	10g	Herba Epimedii
补骨脂	*bǔ gǔ zhī*	10g	Fructus Psoraleae
山茱萸	*shān zhū yú*	15g	Fructus Corni
山药	*shān yào*	30g	Rhizoma Dioscoreae
玄参	*xuán shēn*	30g	Radix Scrophulariae
杜仲	*dù zhòng*	30g	Cortex Eucommiae

(4) BLOOD STASIS WITH HYPERSEXUALITY

Signs and Symptoms: insomnia, vexation, agitation, hypersexuality, frequent and excessively long sexual intercourse or frequent masturbation, a dark tongue with purple spots or with stasis maculae and white coating, and wiry rough pulses.

Treatment Principles: resolve stasis, clear heat.

Formula:

桃仁	*táo rén*	15g	Semen Persicae
红花	*hóng huā*	10g	Flos Carthami
益母草	*yì mǔ cǎo*	30g	Herba Leonuri
丹参	*dān shēn*	30g	Radix et Rhizoma Salviae Miltiorrhizae
知母	*zhī mǔ*	10g	Rhizoma Anemarrhenae
黄芩	*huáng qín*	10g	Radix Scutellariae
黄柏	*huáng bǎi*	10g	Cortex Phellodendri Chinensis
牛膝	*niú xī*	30g	Radix Achyranthis Bidentatae

One decoction daily, divided in two portions taken morning and night.

Representative Case

A 25-year-old female had suffered from insomnia, dull affect, excessive suspicion, and isolation for more than one year. In 1991, she was treated for her psychiatric condition with Sulpiride and the symptoms subsided; meanwhile, amenorrhea and galactorrhea both occurred. After cessation of the treatment, her menstruation remained irregular with an interval period of two weeks and dark purple menses. After getting married in December, 1994, she suffered from low libido, vaginal dryness and severe pain during sexual intercourse.

At the initial visit to our clinic, the patient presented with emaciation, a bright white facial complexion, aching limp lumbus and knees, a pale red tongue with thin white coating, and sunken fine pulses.

Pattern differentiation: yin and yang dual deficiency.

The Western prescription medication remained unchanged. The following Chinese medicinals were prescribed:

Nǚ zhēn zǐ (Fructus Ligustri Lucidi) 40g, *tù sī zǐ* (Semen Cuscutae) 60g, *gǒu qǐ zǐ* (Fructus Lycii) 15g, *hé shǒu wū* (Radix Polygoni Multiflori) 30g, *shān zhū yú* (Fructus Corni) 20g, *xiān líng pí* (Herba Epimedii) 12g, *shā shēn* (Radix Adenophorae) 30g, *mài mén dōng* (Radix Ophiopogonis) 30g, *bǎi hé* (Bulbus Lilii) 40g, *dān shēn* (Radix et Rhizoma Salviae Miltiorrhizae) 30g, and *chǎo mài yá* (Fructus Hordei Germinatus, stir-fried) 30g.

With modifications over the course of time, 105 packets were taken. The patient's libido and sexual function both improved, and there was no longer dryness or pain during sexual intercourse. Formulas that nourish blood, emolliate the liver, and supplement the spleen and kidney were applied for the next three months, and menstruation was restored to normal. After that, medicinals that nourish the liver, spleen and kidney were given at one packet every two days, and the patient's condition stabilized. In May, 1996, she became pregnant. *Shā rén* (Fructus Amomi) and *huáng qín* (Radix Scutellariae) were applied to calm and stabilize the fetus; meanwhile, the prescription for Sulpiride was changed to 0.3g daily. In January 1997, she delivered a healthy male infant.

Commentary

This condition is commonly neglected because these patients feel reluctant to report their symptoms proactively when they initially occur. As these side effects are very common with many classes of psychiatric medications, and are predictable aspects of the patterns that cause psychiatric complaints, making inquiry into the sexual function and history of patients can be a useful gauge for both diagnosis and the effectiveness of treatment.

Chapter 8
Treating Side Effects

DRUG-INDUCED AMENORRHEA

Psychiatric medications such as Chlorpromazine, Perphenazine, Fluphenazine, Sulpiride, Penfluridol, and Risperidone can all cause menstrual irregularities. If menstruation has been absent for more than three months since the patient began taking antipsychotic or antidepressant medications and all other possible causes for amenorrhea have been eliminated, this can be diagnosed as drug-induced amenorrhea. The condition is most commonly seen among young unmarried women, and less frequently in middle-aged women.

Etiology and Pathomechanism

Prolonged application of antipsychotics can damage the spleen and stomach which causes insufficiency of the transforming source, meaning that the essence of water and grain fails to nourish kidney essence and blood; this leads to malnourishment of the penetrating and conception vessels. Since there is no accumulation of blood to discharge, amenorrhea occurs. The nature of this type is predominantly deficiency, although *yangming* heat is a typical side effect of antipsychotic medications which can also damage blood in the penetrating and conception vessels, also leading to menstrual irregularity or amenorrhea due to a relative deficiency of blood.

The toxin from medications can also affect the liver's function of blood storage and regulation of the menses. The qi dynamic becomes inhibited, therefore amenorrhea occurs. This is mostly an excess presentation.

Both deficiency and excess conditions are commonly seen in the in clinical settings, and, as these cases are frequently long standing, complex mixed patterns may also be seen.

Pattern Differentiation and Treatment

(1) Qi Stagnation and Blood Stasis

Signs and Symptoms: unstable mood, vexation, agitation, irascibility, poor food intake, restless sleep, amenorrhea for months or years, scurrying distention of the rib-sides, frequent galactorrhea, a dark purple tongue

with a thin white coating, and wiry rough pulses. There is usually no discomfort in the lower abdomen.

Treatment Principles: rectify qi, resolve stasis.

Formula:

柴胡	chái hú	10g	Radix Bupleuri
香附	xiāng fù	10g	Rhizoma Cyperi
郁金	yù jīn	20g	Radix Curcumae
桃仁	táo rén	15g	Semen Persicae
红花	hóng huā	10g	Flos Carthami
赤芍	chì sháo	30g	Radix Paeoniae Rubra
莪术	é zhú	10g	Rhizoma Curcumae
川芎	chuān xiōng	20g	Rhizoma Chuanxiong

(2) Qi Deficiency and Blood Stasis

Signs and Symptoms: heart palpitations, fearful throbbing, shortness of breath, no strength to speak, fatigue, limp extremities, vexing heat in the five hearts, tidal fever with sweating, amenorrhea for years, a red tongue with thin white coating, and sunken, wiry, fine pulses.

Treatment Principles: benefit qi, invigorate blood.

Formula:

生黄芪	shēng huáng qí	20g	Radix Astragali raw
党参	dǎng shēn	15g	Radix Codonopsis
太子参	tài zǐ shēn	30g	Radix Pseudostellariae
丹参	dān shēn	30g	Radix et Rhizoma Salviae Miltiorrhizae
桃仁	táo rén	15g	Semen Persicae
红花	hóng huā	10g	Flos Carthami
益母草	yì mǔ cǎo	30g	Herba Leonuri
香附	xiāng fù	10g	Rhizoma Cyperi
牛膝	niú xī	30g	Radix Achyranthis Bidentatae

(3) Spleen-kidney Deficiency

Signs and Symptoms: torpid food intake, emaciation, fatigue, lack of strength, shortness of breath, no strength to speak, amenorrhea for years, a bright white facial complexion, a pale red tongue with no coating, and sunken fine weak pulses.

Treatment Principles: supplement spleen and kidney.

Formula:

党参	dǎng shēn	15g	Radix Codonopsis
炒白术	chǎo bái zhú	10g	Rhizoma Atractylodis Macrocephalae (stir-fried)
丹参	dān shēn	30g	Radix et Rhizoma Salviae Miltiorrhizae
益母草	yì mǔ cǎo	30g	Herba Leonuri
当归	dāng guī	15g	Radix Angelicae Sinensis
白芍	bái sháo	30g	Radix Paeoniae Alba
熟地黄	shú dì huáng	30g	Radix Rehmanniae Praeparata
大枣	dà zǎo	10g	Fructus Jujubae
炒麦芽	chǎo mài yá	30g	Fructus Hordei Germinatus

(4) Effulgent Yin Deficiency Fire

Signs and Symptoms: heart vexation, agitation, bitter taste in the mouth, dry throat, mouth and tongue sores, yellowish red urine, dry stool, and amenorrhea for months. The tongue appears red and the pulses are wiry and rapid. This pattern is commonly accompanied by psychiatric symptoms.

Treatment Principles: enrich yin, clear heat, nourish blood, free the menses.

Formula:

生石膏	shēng shí gāo	60-300g	Gypsum Fibrosum Cruda (decocted first)
知母	zhī mǔ	10g	Rhizoma Anemarrhenae
生地	shēng dì	30g	Radix Rehmanniae
玄参	xuán shēn	30g	Radix Scrophulariae
栀子	zhī zǐ	10g	Fructus Gardeniae
益母草	yì mǔ cǎo	30g	Herba Leonuri
大黄	dà huáng	10g	Radix et Rhizoma Rhei (preserved in liquor and decocted later)

(5) Spleen Deficiency with Damp Exuberance

Signs and Symptoms: depression, occasional vexation and agitation, fatigue, no strength to speak, somnolence, torpid intake, nausea, distending fullness of the chest and abdomen, obesity, amenorrhea for months or years, coughing with phlegm, a pale tongue with thin or slimy coating and tooth marks, and sunken slippery pulses.

Treatment principle: fortify the spleen, dispel dampness.
Formula:

茯苓	fú líng	30g	Poria
山药	shān yào	30g	Rhizoma Dioscoreae
陈皮	chén pí	15g	Pericarpium Citri Reticulatae
半夏	bàn xià	10g	Rhizoma Pinelliae
礞石	méng shí	60g	Chlorite-schist (decocted first)
胆南星	dǎn nán xīng	10g	Arisaema cum Bile
竹茹	zhú rú	6g	Caulis Bambusae in Taenia
砂仁	shā rén	10g	Fructus Amomi

One decoction daily, divided in two portions taken morning and night.

(6) Blood Deficiency with Stasis

Signs and Symptoms: decreased menstrual flow with blood clots or spotting, dizziness, blurred vision, heart palpitations, fearful throbbing, empty sagging or distending pains of the lower abdomen, a normal or dark purple tongue with static maculae, and fine rough or wiry rough pulses.

Treatment Principles: supplement and invigorate blood, free the menses.

Formula: Modified *Táo Hóng Sì Wù Tāng* (Peach Kernel and Carthamus Four Substances Decoction)

桃仁	táo rén	15g	Semen Persicae
红花	hóng huā	10g	Flos Carthami
川芎	chuān xiōng	20g	Rhizoma Chuanxiong
当归	dāng guī	15g	Radix Angelicae Sinensis
白芍	bái sháo	30g	Radix Paeoniae Alba
赤芍	chì sháo	30g	Radix Paeoniae Rubra
熟地黄	shú dì huáng	15g	Radix Rehmanniae Praeparata
何首乌	hé shǒu wū	30g	Radix Polygoni Multiflori

Chapter 8
Treating Side Effects

三棱	sān léng	15g	Rhizoma Sparganii
莪术	é zhú	15g	Rhizoma Curcumae
水蛭	shuǐ zhì	10g	Hirudo
虻虫	méng chóng	10g	Tabanus

Representative Case

A 36-year-old female was diagnosed with schizophrenia in 1989. After systematic treatment, the patient was discharged. Sulpiride was continued at 0.4g daily. The patient's condition was stable and she was able to maintain a functional job and family; however, her menstrual flow progressively decreased and became almost absent over time. In February, 1997, she paid her first visit to our department after suffering from amenorrhea for five months. The patient presented with dizziness, generalized discomfort, slow speech, timidity, a dark purple tongue, and wiry rough pulses.

Diagnosis:

(1) Schizophrenia

(2) Drug-induced amenorrhea

Pattern differentiation:

Liver constraint with blood stasis, loss of regulation of the penetrating and conception vessel

Formula:

Fó shǒu (Fructus Citri Sarcodactylis) 10g, *xiāng fù* (Rhizoma Cyperi) 10g, *chén pí* (Pericarpium Citri Reticulatae) 15g, *dān shēn* (Radix et Rhizoma Salviae Miltiorrhizae) 30g, *yì mǔ cǎo* (Herba Leonuri) 30g, *táo rén* (Semen Persicae) 20g, *hóng huā* (Flos Carthami) 15g, *chuān xiōng* (Rhizoma Chuanxiong) 12g, *chì sháo* (Radix Paeoniae Rubra) 30g, *nǚ zhēn zǐ* (Fructus Ligustri Lucidi) 30g, *jī xuè téng* (Caulis Spatholobi) 40g, and *chǎo zǎo rén* (Semen Ziziphi Spinosae, stir-fried) 60g.

After seven packets, the patient reported a lower abdominal sensation as if menstruation was soon to arrive, but it did not. After another three packets, a five-day menstrual period occurred with medium flow. The menses were initially dark, becoming normal after the third day. Her tongue became pale red with a thin white coating, and pulses were wiry and fine. There was no complaint of physical discomfort.

Blood-nourishing and liver-emolliating medicinals were continued at one packet every two days along with the Sulpiride. Follow-up over the next three menstrual periods showed no abnormality. Chinese medicinal treatment was was then stopped.

Commentary

Amenorrhea is defined as absent menstruation for three months or more. During this time the patient can easily develop unstable moods with anger, vexation, irascibility, and an increased appetite. When drug-induced amenorrhea occurs among women who are not sexually active, occasionally there appear itching sensations in the nipples, galactorrhea, increased appetite, and weight gain. Some patients may present with distending fullness of the rib-sides, irascibility, and flusteredness for a certain period of days every month that would roughly correspond with their pre- or peri- menstrual time periods, and this generally resolves spontaneously. Conversely, patients that have had no such "false premenstrual" conditions who start experiencing them after treatment can regard this as a positive sign, as the movement, while not sufficient to bring on a cycle, has stirred the normal mechanisms and caused these symptoms.

Sulpiride can increase prolactin levels, so the amenorrhea caused by this drug is most difficult to treat and is also commonly accompanied by weight gain.

In order to treat this condition most effectively, it is important to initiate treatment as soon as possible, within the first three to four months after the onset. When treating female patients taking psychiatric medications long term, be sure to regularly inquire into their menstrual history and also attempt to manage their menstruation cycles before clinical amenorrhea occurs.

Chapter 9
Recovery and Recurrence

There are many different possible outcomes for those patients with depressive disorders. In theory, depression/depressive disorders would be associated a favorable prognosis and the recovering patient would feel no different than from before the onset of the condition. Although most patients will recover with treatment, many will relapse, and others will not respond favorably even with extended treatment. On the other hand, some individuals will recover spontaneously without any treatment.

Recurrence is a typical characteristic of depressive disorder, and many patients will suffer with repeated episodes. Recurrence also causes changes in personality and social skills, work ability, and/or may cause other mental disabilities. Therefore, rehabilitation is a critical scenario for patients recovering from depressive disorder. Rehabilitation and recovery from depressive disorders can include multiple issues such as preventive therapies, reducing disability, restoring and enhancing social abilities, improving quality of life, and reducing the cost of continuing health care. This chapter focuses on recovery, rehabilitation, and prevention, particularly as associated with the application of Chinese medicine.

Factors in the Recurrence of Depressive Disorders

Preventing recurrence is a critical issue in recovery. Research and studies show a recurrence rate of 50% among depression patients with a single episode, 75% for those with two episodes, and a rate as high as 90% for patients with three or more episodes. Generally speaking, people with the following characteristics are more vulnerable to recurrence:

1) Those not fully recovered or significantly improved who withdraw from treatment.
2) Those with persistent negative thinking even after proper treatment.
3) Those with a history of repeated relapses.
4) Those who continue to live in a stressful state or environment.
5) Those who feel continually dissatisfied with their social and living status who cannot adapt to their objective situation.
6) Those with other concurrent physiological or somatic diseases.

From the Chinese medical point of view, the recurrence of depression is closely associated to mental and emotional issues associated with one's environment and lifestyle. It is also clear that patients who have recently recovered should be careful to avoid mental and emotional upsets. Measures should be taken to ensure the stability of their living and working status, and to help avoid conflicts with other people.

However, relapse is also closely associated with the individual constitution. Those patients with constitutional tendencies toward liver constraint, liver and spleen deficiency, spleen and kidney deficiency, and those with yin deficiency of both liver and kidney are more likely to relapse into depression.

Seasonal changes are also an important factor in recurrence. Depression tends to recur in the autumn and winter, especially with abnormal or suddenly changing weather at the turn of the seasons. The Chinese folk term, "autumn sadness" also reflects traditional Chinese ideas regarding the downward-moving character of autumn-metal, and how this phase influences the emotions. Modern medicine also shows that mood can be seriously affected by a lack of sunlight.

Preventing Recurrence

Each subsequent episode of depressive disorder makes the condition more difficult to cure, so preventive measures and maintenance therapy should be continued after recovery. Patients should be encouraged to remain compliant throughout the course of treatment because after a certain period of time many patients tend to stop taking their prescribed medications. Poor compliance is associated with several factors, including the side effects of medication, a lack of education, or even the simple inconvenience and cost of travelling to the clinic.

Ideally, depressive disorder patients should receive regular outpatient reviews and continue with all therapies, including psychological counseling. Scheduled review and consultation should be used to counsel patients on the importance of compliance, and also to assess the presence of possible drug side effects. Chinese medicine therapies based on syndrome differentiation are effective for resolving the side effects of antidepressants.

For a patient's first episode of depression, recovery should be maintained with Western medications or Chinese medicinals for 6-9 months. For a second episode, maintenance therapy should continue for at least 5 years. Those with three episodes may need to take antidepressants indefinitely. Patients with a family history of depressive disorder or bipolar affective disorder, or with onset at a young age (< 20 years old), and those who have a history of suicide-attempts should also remain medicated for an extended period. The maintenance dosage for Western drugs is usually 1/3 of the normal therapeutic dosage. Such medications must never be withdrawn suddenly, and their dosages should be reduced very gradually. Chinese medicinal formulas can be reduced to one daily portion, then to a half portion each day or one portion every two days, and then to one portion every other day and finally 2 portions weekly.

The key to preventing recurrence is early detection and early treatment, and therefore it is also important to pay close attention for any signs of recurrence at to provide treatment at the earliest possible stage. Recurrence generally includes the following signs and symptoms:

Changes in sleep—symptoms include insomnia, difficulty sleeping or waking up, or other unusual changes in the normal sleep pattern.

Poor concentration—signs may include difficulty in classes or at work, memory lapses, neglecting to greet others, or sitting silently as if lost.

Less energy—signs may include excessive lying in bed or sitting alone, a feeling of fatigue which cannot be relieved by sleep, decreased work efficiency, and poor personal hygiene.

Frustration and irritation—anger without reason, quarrelling, an inability to control emotion, impatience, impulsiveness, frequent conflicts with family or colleagues, and breaking things.

Loss of interest—no pleasure in previously enjoyed activities, also accompanied by low spirits, boredom, or even a tendency to give away previously valued objects.

Decline in libido—may also include a lack of interest in one's self-image or appearance, little interest in one's spouse, not wanting to talk to friends, and/or frigidity and impotence.

Depression is an emotion common to all human beings. Chinese medical theory describes the seven affects, all of which are normal emotions. Depressed emotion will appear when facing stress, frustration, painful situations, or aging and sickness. However, depressive disorder is a pathological psychological condition that requires intervention. Normally depressed emotions should be differentiated from those of pathological depression through following the following signs:

① "Normal" depressive emotions are based on an objective

Chapter 9
Recovery and Recurrence

background, that is, they are caused by "good reasons". Pathological depressive disorders often come about with no obvious reason or external stimulus. There may be negative influences involved, but reactions and behaviors associated with them are generally exaggerated.

2) Normal emotional changes are usually temporary in nature, with normal psychological defenses used to restore mental balance. For pathological depression, the symptoms will remain persistent without treatment, or they may even become more severe. According to psychological medical criteria, normal depression should not persist for over 2 weeks.

3) Typical depressive disorders have a rhythmic or cyclic characteristic, often with severe symptoms in the morning and milder symptoms in the evening. Many patients will report extremely painful bad moods in the early morning; in fact, this time period is when many patients will attempt suicide. Such patients will usually feel better after 3-4 pm with no problems in the evening.

4) Persistent insomnia, impaired mental function, weight loss, loss of appetite and libido, and vague discomfort throughout the entire body even though physical examination is normal.

Dietary Guidelines for Recovery and Rehabilitation

Chinese and Western medical systems both consider the daily diet as an important factor in the successful treatment of depressive disorder. One recent report states that fish, eggs, and other foods rich in omega-3 fatty acids can improve a person's mental health. Research has shown that omega-3 fatty acids can not only prevent the onset of depressive disorder, but also help to improve learning ability. A study involving over fourteen-thousand pregnant women showed that those who ate more fish during pregnancy were less prone to depressive disorder, in fact, their children also showed reduced behavioral problems and learning disabilities. Also, children with low omega-3 levels are more likely to suffer from mood disorders in adulthood. Seafoods are not only rich in minerals and vitamins, but also serve as main source of omega-3 fatty acids.

Autumn is the season associated with the highest incidence and recurrence of depression, so recovering patients should be sure to maintain a nutritious diet during this season. Depressed patients often have autonomic nervous system disorders and poor digestion, so consuming foods that are relatively easy to digest are recommended.

Recent research shows that neurasthenia is associated with a lack of the trace elements zinc and copper. (Ed. Note: Although the term neurasthenia is seen largely as antiquated in the West, it is commonly accepted diagnosis in Asian psychology, perhaps because it incorporates CM and cultural concepts of body-mind.). Zinc deficiency also has a negative impact on energy metabolism and oxidation-reduction of the brain nerve cells. Copper deficiency leads to disorders of the internal inhibition process of nerve cells, causing over-excitement of the endocrine system and insomnia; neurasthenia may also develop over time. Oyster and herring are very rich in zinc, but high levels also exist in lean meats, liver and kidney, diary products, apples, and walnuts. Foods with high levels of copper include squid, razor clam, blood clam, escargot, shrimp, loach, lamb, mushroom, and corn.

In general, depressive disorder patients should consider the following dietary guidelines:

1) A high-fiber diet with foods that moisten the intestines can prevent constipation.

2) Sufficient water is required to maintain the basic function of the internal organs and also to promote the elimination of harmful substances.

3) Those with insomnia should avoid spicy, pickled, smoked and other overly stimulating foods.

In Chinese medicine, dietary therapy is applied according to the physical constitution and also syndrome differentiation. The goal of food therapy is to improve the individual constitution of the patient, cultivate healthy qi, balance the qi and blood of the viscera and bowels, and to eliminate any remaining internal causes. Because the onset of depressive disorder is closely associated with the physical constitution, food therapy can address the core of the disease to a certain extent. However, internal pathogenic factors of cold, heat, phlegm, fire, constraint, and deficiency can all result from an improper diet.

The Song Dynasty text, *Formulas from Benevolent Sages Compiled during the Taiping Era* (Tài Píng Shèng Huì Fāng) states, "Intake of food can eliminate pathogenesis and settle the viscera and bowels, clear the mind and refresh emotions, and also nourish qi and blood. One who is

Chapter 9
Recovery and Recurrence

able to use food as a treatment for calming the emotions and eliminating disease is a superior practitioner". This passage shows that certain foods can eliminate pathogens and resolve toxins while also regulating organ function. However, in all cases, food therapy should be applied only after assessing the individual constitution and presenting patterns.

The following is a list of food-based remedies that are useful for addressing the accompanying symptoms of depressive disorder.

1. Poor Sleep

1) Sugar water: Sugar water taken at bedtime makes it easier to fall asleep by inhibiting the activities of cerebral cortex.

2) Milk: Milk contains tryptophan, an essential amino acid that promotes sleep by raising serotonin levels in the brain.

3) Fruit: For those who cannot sleep due to overwork, fruits such as apples and banana can be helpful for relieving muscle fatigue. Some also recommend placing oranges or orange peel near the pillow because its aroma is said to promote relaxation.

4) Bread: a small amount of bread taken at bedtime can also promote sleep.

5) Millet: millet is a grain rich in tryptophan. In Chinese medicine, millet acts to nourish the spleen and harmonize the stomach. Millet congee can be taken for dinner or before bedtime.

2. Palpitations

1) *Gān Mài Dà Zǎo Tāng* (Licorice, Wheat and Jujube Decoction): Contains *xiǎo mài* (Fructus Tritici) 30g, *dà zǎo* (Fructus Jujubae) 10g, and *gān cǎo* (Radix et Rhizoma Glycyrrhizae) 6g. Boil with water, remove the dregs and drink.

2) Jujube soup: Stew *dà zǎo* (Fructus Jujubae) in water on medium heat until boiling, cook until well-done. Add brown sugar and take as soup.

3) Longan, date seed, and euryale seed soup: Contains *lóng yǎn ròu* (Arillus Longan) 10g, *chǎo zǎo rén* (Semen Ziziphi Spinosae) 10g, and *qiàn shí* (Semen Euryales) 12g. Prepare as a soup and drink before bedtime.

4) Lotus seed congee: Contains *lián zǐ* (Semen Nelumbinis) 50g, *lóng yǎn ròu* (Arillus Longan) 30g, and crystal sugar. Peel off the *lián zǐ* (Semen Nelumbinis) skin and let the plumule remain, grind to powder, add some

water and make a paste. Put the paste into boiling water with the *lóng yǎn ròu* (Arillus Longan) and crystal sugar to make a congee.

3. Dizziness

1) *Qīng Luò Yǐn* (Channel-Clearing Beverage): Contains fresh lotus leaf edges 6g, fresh honeysuckle flower 6g, watermelon skin 6g, one fresh lentil flower, skin of the fruit of a towel gourd 6g, and fresh lophatherum 6g. Add to 2 glasses of water, boil until one glass remains. Take twice a day.

2) Chrysanthemum and longjing tea: Contains chrysanthemum 10g and longjing tea 10g. Add boiling water and take as tea. Also effective for dizziness and blurry vision.

3) Black fungus soup: Contains black *hēi mù ěr* (Auricularia) 30g, and *dà zǎo* (Fructus Jujubae) 30pcs. Boil with water and take warm.

4) Finger citron and ginger soup: Contains *fó shǒu* (Fructus Citri Sarcodactylis) 10g and fresh *shēng jiāng* (Rhizoma Zingiberis Recens) 6g. Boil in water, remove the dregs. Add sugar and drink while warm.

5) Chinese hawthorn and lotus leaf tea: Contains *shān zhā* (Fructus Crataegi) 30g and *hé yè* (Folium Nelumbinis) 12g. Boil in two bowls of water until one bowl remains, remove the dregs and drink as tea.

4. Constipation

1) Carrot juice 100g, three times a day.

2) For chronic constipation, hypertension: Put fresh spinach into boiling water for 3 minutes, remove and add sesame oil. Eat three times a day.

3) For constipation, gastric and duodenal ulcer, chronic cholecystitis: Potato juice, 1/2 glass on empty stomach both morning and night, continue for 10–20 days.

4) Sesame oil, take 70ml daily as one daily dose.

Chapter 10
Case Studies

1. Liver Constraint with Phlegm Binding

Mr. Zhang, married, age 34.

The patient reported feelings of deep desperation and paranoia after encountering an unpleasant series of situations in his work life. He was previously diagnosed with depression, and had been on medication for three months at the time of the initial interview. His mood had been fluctuating severely, and he was unable to fully recover. At the initial visit, signs and symptoms included dry stools, abnormally yellow urine, a red tongue with a thick yellow slimy coating, and wiry rapid pulses.

Diagnosis: Moderate depressive disorder.

Pattern Differentiation: Liver constraint with phlegm binding and disturbing the brain-spirit.

Treatment Principles: Clear the liver, resolve phlegm, clear the brain, calm the spirit.

Prescription: *chái hú* (Radix Bupleuri) 6g, *jú huā* (Flos Chrysanthemi) 15g, *dān shēn* (Radix et Rhizoma Salviae Miltiorrhizae) 20g, *bái jí lí* (Fructus Tribuli) 30g, *shēng shí gāo* (Gypsum Fibrosum Cruda, decocted first) 80g, *huáng lián* (Rhizoma Coptidis) 10g, *chén pí* (Pericarpium Citri Reticulatae) 15g, *tiān zhú huáng* (Concretio Silicea Bambusae) 15g, *yù jīn* (Radix Curcumae) 30g, *chǎo zǎo rén* (Semen Ziziphi Spinosae, stir-fried) 60g, *shén qū* (Massa Medicata Fermentata) 15g, and *fǎ bàn xià* (Rhizoma Pinelliae Praeparatum) 10g.

7 packets were initially prescribed, one decocted and taken morning and night as one divided dose.

Second Visit:

After taking 7 packets, the patient felt clear-headed and slightly calmer. His appetite was improved, defecation was once again gratifying, and his paranoia was diminished, however, the bad mood and low libido remained. Other signs included a yellowish white facial complexion with somber gray areas beneath the eyes, and a red tongue with a white slimy coating.

Fú líng (Poria) 30g, *zhēn zhū mǔ* (Concha Margaritiferae Usta, decocted first) 60g and *tù sī zǐ* (Semen Cuscutae) 10g were added to the previous formula. 14 more packets were prescribed.

Third Visit:

Appetite, sleep and mood were greatly improved, and the patient was willing leave his home for the first time in a long while. However, he continued to report a sense of frustration.

Prescription: *chuān xiōng* (Rhizoma Chuanxiong) 15g, *jú huā* (Flos Chrysanthemi) 15g, *dān shēn* (Radix et Rhizoma Salviae Miltiorrhizae) 20g, *chén pí* (Pericarpium Citri Reticulatae) 15g, *huáng lián* (Rhizoma Coptidis) 10g, *yù jīn* (Radix Curcumae) 30g, *tiān zhú huáng* (Concretio Silicea Bambusae) 15g, *chǎo zǎo rén* (Semen Ziziphi Spinosae, stir-fried) 60g, *pèi lán* (Herba Eupatorii) 10g, *ròu cōng róng* (Herba Cistanches) 30g and *jī xuè téng* (Caulis Spatholobi) 40g.

7 additional packets were prescribed.

Fourth Visit:

The patient's mood had returned to normal, and he considered himself to be fully recovered. However, his libido was still slightly low. To reinforce the effect of the previous treatments, the following medicinals were prescribed:

Jú huā (Flos Chrysanthemi) 10g, *dān shēn* (Radix et Rhizoma Salviae Miltiorrhizae) 30g, *chuān xiōng* (Rhizoma Chuanxiong) 12g, *tiān zhú huáng* (Concretio Silicea Bambusae) 10g, *yù jīn* (Radix Curcumae) 30g, *gǒu qǐ zǐ* (Fructus Lycii) 15g, *tù sī zǐ* (Semen Cuscutae) 60g, *ròu cōng róng* (Herba Cistanches) 30g, *xiān líng pí* (Herba Epimedii) 15g, *shēng shí gāo* (Gypsum Fibrosum Cruda, decocted first) 80g, *zhēn zhū mǔ* (Concha Margaritiferae Usta, decocted first) 60g, and *chǎo zǎo rén* (Semen Ziziphi Spinosae, stir-fried) 60g.

After 15 packets, his libido was greatly improved and sleep returned to normal. To reinforce the treatment effect, the patient was instructed to continue with one packet every two days.

Commentary:

Before the condition arose, the patient's personality was somewhat timid. His initial encounter with unpleasant circumstances at work first caused a pattern of liver constraint and qi stagnation. This caused the liver to fail to course effectively, also affecting the spleen. When spleen-earth fails to course, phlegm-damp brews internally; enduring liver qi constraint transformed into fire to disturb the brain-spirit, manifesting as an emotional condition. With liver conditions, "the child steals the mother's qi" and kidney damage results, manifesting in low libido. The kidney failed to engender marrow, and the sea of marrow in the brain became deficient, so the pattern developed into an excess-deficiency complex with qi constraint and phlegm-heat. With kidney deficiency also present from the onset, the patient manifested frustration, timidity, and lack of a strong will.

Treatment primarily focused on soothing the liver, resolving phlegm, and clearing heat. By the fourth visit, the excess evil was almost completely resolved and therefore signs of deficiency became more pronounced. At that time, the focus of treatment was changed to primarily supplementing the kidney and securing the root. By invigorating kidney essence and strengthening the brain-spirit, the effect of treatment became long lasting because the patient's constitution had improved, with no recurrence of symptoms when encountering other negative situations.

During the treatment, the patient was also prescribed one tablet of Deanxit (Flupentixol) in the morning and one with lunch, and 0.8mg of Alprazolam in the evening.

2. Spleen and Kidney Dual Deficiency

Mr. Pan, married, age 48.

The patient had been suffering from neurasthenia for 20 years. During the past two months he had also developed feelings of deep anxiety and sleeplessness. He was diagnosed with "depressive disorder with psycholepsy" by another hospital, and unsuccessfully treated with Fluoxetine for one month.

The primary manifestations included abdominal pain with an urge to defecate at dawn, loose stools with a sense of relief immediately after defecation, no pleasure in eating, stomach duct discomfort, vexation and agitation, fidgeting, frequent urination at night, a lack of strength and fatigue of the four limbs, emaciation, lower back pain and limp knees, and sleeplessness that was gradually aggravated despite taking 4mg of Clonazepam daily; there was also tiredness in the morning, dizziness, suicidal ideation, palpitations at the slightest exertion, indecisiveness, and a slight cough. His facial complexion was bright white, with a pale tongue and sunken fine pulses.

Diagnosis: Moderate depressive disorder.

Pattern Differentiation: Spleen-kidney dual deficiency and malnourishment of the brain.

Treatment Principles: Supplement the spleen, kidney and brain, calm the spirit.

Prescription: *shēng huáng qí* (Radix Astragali raw) 30g, *chǎo bái zhú* (Rhizoma Atractylodis Macrocephalae, stir-fried) 10g, *fú líng* (Poria) 30g, *chǎo suān zǎo rén* (Semen Ziziphi Spinosae, stir-fried) 60g, *hé huān pí* (Cortex Albiziae) 30g, *bǔ gǔ zhī* (Fructus Psoraleae) 30g, *huái shān yào* (Rhizoma Dioscoreae) 30g, *tù sī zǐ* (Semen Cuscutae) 60g, *xiān líng pí* (Herba Epimedii) 10g, *shén qū* (Massa Medicata Fermentata) 10g, *yì zhì rén* (Fructus Alpiniae Oxyphyllae) 15g, *zhì gān cǎo* (Radix et Rhizoma Glycyrrhizae Praeparata cum Melle) 10g, and *dà zǎo* (Fructus Jujubae) 10g.

7 packets were prescribed, decocted.

Second Visit:

His loose stools, lack of strength, and appetite were all improved. The patient also developed a strong desire and will to recover. His mood was improved, but some anxiety remained persistent. *Hé shǒu wū* (Radix Polygoni Multiflori) 20g and 3 slices of *shēng jiāng* (Rhizoma Zingiberis Recens) were added to the previous formula. Another 15 packets were prescribed.

Third Visit:

Loose stools were reduced to an occasional occurrence. Appetite, strength, and mood were observably improved. His suicidal tendencies were decreased, but the patient still felt pessimistic. Since the previous formula had been effective, another 20 packets were prescribed with the addition of *shēng shài shēn* (Radix et Rhizoma Ginseng Cruda) 1g. The depression was greatly relieved, and his stools became firm with no urgency. To reinforce the effect of treatment, the patient continued with one packet of this formula every three days.

Commentary:

This patient had a weak constitution and a history of intractable disease. Long term sleeplessness and weakness of the spleen, stomach, and kidney also caused a deficiency of upright qi. When the brain-spirit is already weak, emotional stimulation can disrupt qi and blood and constrain the qi dynamic. Deficiency patterns and constraint will often occur together with deficiency as the root pattern and constraint as the branch manifestation. In this pattern, spleen and kidney dual deficiency and insufficiency of kidney origin [primordial energy of the kidney] was predominant. This leads to qi not being invigorated and clear yang not being uplifted, also resulting in malnourishment of the brain-spirit. Therefore, treatment here primarily focused on securing the root and supplementing the kidney. During treatment, the antidepressant medication was continued at the same dosage, and no side effects were reported.

3. Depression due to Dual Depletion of Qi and Blood

Ms Chen, age 38.

For six months the patient had been suffering from dizziness, headache, a lack of strength, fatigue in the extremities, decreased appetite, emaciation, low spirits, and pessimism. Previous treatments showed no observable effect. After a consultation with psychiatrists, she was diagnosed with "psycholepsy" and treated with 20mg of Fluoxetine daily for two months. Once again there was no obvious effect.

The patient presented with a somber green-blue and yellowish complexion with a dark blue-green caste of the eye sockets, no pleasure in eating, depression, generalized discomfort, fatigue, worry, sleeplessness, a sense of tightness in the head, a pale tongue with a thin white coat, and fine weak sunken pulses.

Diagnosis: Moderate depressive disorder.

Pattern Differentiation: Qi and blood insufficiency, malnourishment of the brain.

Treatment Principles: Supplement qi, blood, and kidney yang.

Prescription: *jú huā* (Flos Chrysanthemi) 10g, *dān shēn* (Radix et Rhizoma Salviae Miltiorrhizae) 20g, *chuān xiōng* (Rhizoma Chuanxiong) 15g, *gŏu qĭ zĭ* (Fructus Lycii) 15g, *shān yào* (Rhizoma Dioscoreae) 30g, *shān*

Chapter 10
Case Studies

zhū yú (Fructus Corni) 15g, *tù sī zǐ* (Semen Cuscutae) 30g, *xiān líng pí* (Herba Epimedii) 15g, *ròu cōng róng* (Herba Cistanches) 30g, and *chǎo suān zǎo rén* (Semen Ziziphi Spinosae, stir-fried) 60g.

7 packets were prescribed, decocted. Taken as two divided portions, once each morning and night.

Second Visit:

The patient did not react to the initial treatment. *Dāng guī* (Radix Angelicae Sinensis) 10g and *bái sháo* (Radix Paeoniae Alba) 30g were added to the previous formula, and the dosage of *chǎo zǎo rén* (Semen Ziziphi Spinosae, stir-fried) was increased to 70g.

Third Visit:

There was no observable effect or improvement in mood, and the possibility of a physical condition was ruled out. Detailed inquiry revealed that the patient had received six abortions, and that her husband required her to participate in sexual activity almost daily. Since multiple pregnancies had taxed his wife so severely, the husband was also counseled regarding proper birth control, and on the importance of regulating their sexual activities. Another 20 packets of the previous formula were prescribed.

Fourth Visit:

The patient continued with the previous formula while also regulating their sexual activity. Her mental status, physical constitution, and appetite were all greatly improved. However, her facial complexion was still somber, and she reported fatigue in the daytime as well as some head discomfort. Lab exams showed a relatively low volume of hemoglobin (100g/L). Her tongue still appeared pale with thin white coating. Treatment continued to primarily supplement qi and blood and nourish the brain while also calming the spirit, invigorating yang, and opening constraint.

Prescription: *shú dì huáng* (Radix Rehmanniae Praeparata) 15g, *gǒu qǐ zǐ* (Fructus Lycii) 15g, *shān yào* (Rhizoma Dioscoreae) 15g, *shān zhū yú* (Fructus Corni) 30g, *tù sī zǐ* (Semen Cuscutae) 60g, *bǔ gǔ zhī* (Fructus Psoraleae) 30g, *xiān líng pí* (Herba Epimedii) 15g, *dāng guī* (Radix Angelicae Sinensis) 15g, *shēng huáng qí* (Radix Astragali raw) 60g, and *hé shǒu wū* (Radix Polygoni Multiflori) 30g.

7 packets were prescribed. She was also instructed to take three packets of *Shēng Mài Yǐn* (Pulse-Engendering Beverage) daily.

Fifth Visit:

All of the symptoms were greatly relieved; the patient appeared to be both calm and optimistic. In order to reinforce the treatment effect, she continued taking Chinese medicinals along with Western medicines.

Commentary:

Due to excessive sexual activity and multiple abortions, qi and blood were both depleted, which also weakened the viscera and bowels. This pattern aggravated the already malnourished condition of the brain-spirit, resulting in depressive disorder. The patient was diagnosed with depression at the initial visit, with the pattern being spleen and kidney insufficiency, qi and blood dual deficiency, and malnourishment of the brain-spirit. While the diagnosis, pattern differentiation, and resulting prescription were all correct, there was no reaction to the initial treatment. This indicated that the root cause had not been addressed.

The heart stores the spirit and governs blood; the spleen is the abode of intention and governs blood; the liver is the abode of the ethereal soul and stores blood; the kidney stores essence, maintains composure of the mind, governs the bones and also the engendering of marrow. These qualities are all closely related to the function of the brain-spirit. Excessive blood loss due to multiple abortions and essence loss due to frequent pregnancies and sexual activities will always lead to qi and blood deficiency with essence depletion; the main manifestations include fatigue, lack of strength, and ungratifying emotions.

In this case, the patient was middle-aged, so her viscera and bowel function was easily restored. Once the root cause was eliminated, this allowed for successful supplementation of qi, blood, and kidney yang as well as for proper nourishing of the brain-spirit.

The key to this case lies in her compliance with the physician's suggestion to reduce her sexual activity. Detailed inquiry into the patient's lifestyle can often be an important factor in determining proper diagnosis

Chapter 10
Case Studies

and treatment. Obstetric and gynecological history, sexual psychology, sexual function and sexual activity are often neglected during intake, especially among unmarried young women. In addition, the symptoms in this case also suggest that her depression was related to kidney deficiency.

For depression due to kidney deficiency or mild internal heat, large dosages of yang-invigorating medicinals such as *bā jǐ tiān* (Radix Morindae Officinalis), *guī bǎn* (Plastrum Testudinis), *shān zhū yú* (Fructus Corni) and *xiān líng pí* (Herba Epimedii) can be applied. Once kidney qi becomes invigorated, liver qi can assert orderly reaching and coursing again, and then there can be emotional relief. The treatment method of invigorating yang and opening constraint can be surprisingly effective when used appropriately.

4. Liver and Stomach Disharmony

Mr. Yang, married, age 40.

In December of 2003 the patient reported awakening in the night with a sense of tightness and oppression on both sides of his head, and he was unable to remain lying down comfortably. He also had a dry mouth, dimmed vision, trembling hands, and severe emotional tension such that he was unable to go back to sleep. At six o' clock the next morning he experienced a stroke-like sensation with trembling hands, shaking of the body, fear, anxiety and inability to speak clearly. He immediately sought medical help from a local hospital where the physician was unable to reach a clear diagnosis from CT scans. A cerebral infarction was suspected, so a transfusion of *Nao Sai Tong*, *Nao Xue Tong* and salvia injections were applied immediately. This resulted in profuse sweating and seminal emission. A second CT scan of the brain showed no abnormality.

The next day the patient reported feeling electrified all over his body, discomfort in the stomach duct and abdomen, constipation, belching, nausea, and vomiting of sour water. An ultrasound examination in another hospital showed no abnormality in the liver, gallbladder, pancreas, or spleen. Meanwhile, patient also had a sense of heat effusion with blurred vision, blank staring, a desire to weep, and a miserable facial expression. The physician considered his condition to be a relapsing of a recent common cold; however, treatment based on this diagnosis did not have any effect.

Following exams in three other hospitals, no organic disease was found. One hospital prescribed Bacillus kicheniformis capsules which resulted in five to six daily bowel movements, aggravated tremors, a sense of being on verge of collapse, and profuse sweating. The patient voluntarily discontinued this treatment.

After going to a psychiatric hospital the patient was diagnosed with depression. Deanxit was prescribed, one tablet in the morning and one at noon, as well as 0.8mg of Alprazolam in the evening, and all symptoms were improved. At this point it was decided that the patient required integrative treatment with Chinese and Western medicine.

Detailed inquiry revealed the patient had been through a series of personal frustrations in the previous two months, and also that he had been drinking a half liter of white liquor each day for many years. Before the onset of this condition, the patient had suffered with a bad cold with intermittent relapses. Other complaints included distention and fullness of the stomach duct, stifling oppression in the chest, hiccoughing, belching, acid reflux, depression, sleeplessness, generalized aching, anxiety, and suicidal thoughts. At the initial visit, his tongue appeared red with a thick yellow slimy coating, his stool was dry, and the pulses were wiry slippery and rapid.

Diagnosis: Moderate depressive disorder.

Pattern Differentiation: Liver and stomach disharmony with irregularity of the brain-spirit.

Prescription: *jú huā* (Flos Chrysanthemi) 10g, *chuān xiōng* (Rhizoma Chuanxiong) 10g, *dān shēn* (Radix et Rhizoma Salviae Miltiorrhizae) 30g, *yún líng* (Poria) 30g, *fó shǒu* (Fructus Citri Sarcodactylis) 12g, *xiāng yuán* (Fructus Citri) 15g, *shā rén* (Fructus Amomi) 6g, *mù guā* (Fructus Chaenomelis) 30g, *Chái hú* (Radix Bupleuri) 6g, *bái sháo* (Radix Paeoniae Alba) 30g, *shén qū* (Massa Medicata Fermentata) 15g, *cǎo dòu kòu* (Semen Alpiniae Katsumadai) 10g, *suō luó zǐ* (Semen Aesculi) 30g, *gān cǎo* (Radix et Rhizoma Glycyrrhizae) 3g, *chǎo zǎo rén* (Semen Ziziphi Spinosae, stir-fried) 60g, *zhēn zhū mǔ* (Concha Margaritiferae Usta, decocted first) 60g, *wǎ léng zǐ* Concha Arcae) 20g.

7 packets were prescribed, one daily decoction divided into two portions, taken morning and night. Western medication was continued as prescribed by the specialists.

Second Visit:

After taking the medicinals for three days, the stomach discomfort began to resolve, his appetite improved, and he smiled for the first time. However, he also reported a lack of strength, poor sleep, a fluctuating mood, regular defecation, and long voiding of clear urine. His tongue was red with yellow thick slimy coating, and pulses were wiry and fine.

Huáng lián (Rhizoma Coptidis) 10g, *pèi lán* (Herba Eupatorii) 10g and *shān zhū yú* (Fructus Corni) 15g were added to the previous formula, and 14 more packets were prescribed.

Third Visit:

The patient's condition continued to improve, with his mood normal and the stomach duct discomfort eliminated. He was prescribed with 20 more packets of the formula and discharged from the hospital.

Fourth Visit:

The patient was clear-headed, but he reported occasional stomach duct discomfort, dull pain in the lower abdomen, poor sleep, and a sense of uneasiness when thinking about family issues. The patient was instructed to care for his mental health and to continue taking his Chinese medicinals and Western medicine while gradually decreasing the dosage.

Commentary:

This case is characterized by complicated symptoms and strong subjective signs with no positive examination results. The main signs involved the gastrointestinal system and his emotional state. Treatment was therefore focused on soothing the liver and harmonizing the stomach. In a few days, most of the gastrointestinal symptoms were relieved, and this increased the patient's compliance and confidence in the treatment plan.

5. Liver Constraint Transforming into Fire, Static Blood Obstruction

Ms. Li, age 22.

The patient had a one year history of mental illness; she presented with depression, a flat affect, reluctance to speak, poor social skills, poor memory, and distraction. She was emaciated and also reported low self-esteem regarding her physical appearance and relationships. There was also vexation, agitation, frequent outbursts of anger, irregular menstruation, and suicidal thoughts. Her tongue was red with a white coating, and pulses were slippery and rapid.

Diagnosis: Moderate depressive disorder

Pattern Differentiation: Liver Constraint transforming into fire harassing upwards, blood stasis obstruction.

Treatment Principles: course the liver, drain fire, resolve stasis, calm the spirit.

Prescription: *jú huā* (Flos Chrysanthemi) 15g, *chuān xiōng* (Rhizoma Chuanxiong) 15g, *dān shēn* (Radix et Rhizoma Salviae Miltiorrhizae) 20g, *bái jí lí* (Fructus Tribuli) 30g, *gōu téng* (Ramulus Uncariae Cum Uncis) 30g, *huáng lián* (Rhizoma Coptidis) 10g, *zhī zǐ* (Fructus Gardeniae) 15g, *tiān zhú huáng* (Concretio Silicea Bambusae) 15g, *yù jīn* (Radix Curcumae) 30g, *shén qū* (Massa Medicata Fermentata) 10g, *chǎo zǎo rén* (Semen Ziziphi Spinosae, stir-fried) 60g, *lái fú zǐ* (Semen Raphani) 30g, *chē qián zǐ* (Semen Plantaginis) 10g, *shēng shí gāo* (Gypsum Fibrosum Cruda, decocted first) 120g, *cí shí* (Magnetitum, decocted first) 60g, and *zhēn zhū mǔ* (Concha Margaritiferae Usta, decocted first) 60g.

14 packets were prescribed, one decocted daily and taken in two portions, morning and night. Antidepressant and anti-anxiety medications included Amitriptyline 50mg and Alprazolam 0.8mg in the evening.

Second Visit:

There was a slight improvement in her mood, her appetite was slightly better, and she was now able watch television undistracted for short periods of time. However, the patient continued to express frustration and pessimism, and she refused to leave the house. Her angry outbursts had decreased in frequency, bowel movements were once every two days, and the tongue appeared red with a white coating. The previous formula had obviously taken effect, so *zhī mǔ* (Rhizoma Anemarrhenae) 12g was added, and the dosage of *shēng shí gāo* (Gypsum Fibrosum Cruda) was increased to 160g. Another 14 packets were prescribed.

Amitriptyline was increased to 25mg in the morning and at noon, and 50mg in the evening.

Chapter 10
Case Studies

Third Visit:

Her condition had significantly improved. The patient was more active, willing to communicate with her parents, and she agreed to further treatment.

Prescription: *jú huā* (Flos Chrysanthemi) 15g, *chuān xiōng* (Rhizoma Chuanxiong) 15g, *dān shēn* (Radix et Rhizoma Salviae Miltiorrhizae) 30g, *yún líng* (Poria) 30g, *tiān zhú huáng* (Concretio Silicea Bambusae) 15g, *zhī mǔ* (Rhizoma Anemarrhenae) 15g, *huáng bǎi* (Cortex Phellodendri Chinensis) 6g, *yù jīn* (Radix Curcumae) 30g, *huáng lián* (Rhizoma Coptidis) 10g, *mài mén dōng* (Ophiopogonis) 30g, *chǎo zǎo rén* (Semen Ziziphi Spinosae, stir-fried) 70g, *lái fú zǐ* (Semen Raphani) 30g, *xuán shēn* (Radix Scrophulariae) 30g, *shēng dì* (Radix Rehmanniae) 30g, and *shēng shí gāo* (Gypsum Fibrosum Cruda, decocted first) 120g.

14 packets were prescribed.

After taking this formula, the patient's mental status gradually returned to normal, and she showed a willingness to go back to school. The dosage of the Western medication was gradually decreased, and there were no further office visits. A two year follow-up showed no abnormality or relapse.

6. Liver Constraint and Blood Stasis

Mr. Zhao, age 56.

In the fall of 2001 the patient had suffered a deep personal setback and frustration, and his emotional condition began to deteriorate. Manifestations included a flat facial affect, extreme frustration, slow movements, tremors in the extremities, a lack of confidence, a pessimistic attitude, difficulty walking and a fear of falling down, a desire to lay down, forgetfulness, and distraction. Also, his irregular diet caused a functional gastrointestinal disorder; during the previous five years he only had one bowel movement every seven to ten days.

Other symptoms included emaciation, stiffness in the extremities, and poor sleep. Neurological examinations showed no abnormalities, and Parkinson's disease was ruled out. The psychiatry department diagnosed him with depression, but Fluoxetine and Lorazepam had no observable effect. The patient was then willing to receive integrative medical treatments.

In addition to the above-mentioned symptoms, the patient also presented with a reluctance to speak, an extremely low libido, vexation and agitation, dry stools, a dark red tongue with stasis spots and scant fluids, a white tongue coating, and wiry pulses.

Diagnosis: Major depressive disorder.

Pattern Differentiation: Liver constraint and blood stasis disturbing the brain-spirit.

Treatment Principles: Course the liver, resolve stasis, awaken the brain, calm the spirit.

Prescription: *chái hú* (Radix Bupleuri) 6g, *fó shǒu* (Fructus Citri Sarcodactylis) 10g, *bái sháo* (Radix Paeoniae Alba) 30g, *xiāng yuán* (Fructus Citri) 15g, *yún líng* (Poria) 30g, *tiān zhú huáng* (Concretio Silicea Bambusae) 15g, *yù jīn* (Radix Curcumae) 30g, *chǎo zǎo rén* (Semen Ziziphi Spinosae, stir-fried) 60g, *ròu cōng róng* (Herba Cistanches) 30g, *táo rén* (Semen Persicae) 10g, *hóng huā* (Flos Carthami) 15g, *chì sháo* (Radix Paeoniae Rubra) 30g, *shān zhū yú* (Fructus Corni) 15g, and *shén qū* (Massa Medicata Fermentata) 15g. Seven packets of herbs were prescribed, taken as divided packets once each morning and night.

Fluoxetine was continued at 20mg daily.

Second Visit:

His appetite had improved and his bowel movements had come more frequently. There were purple spots on the tongue with white coating.

Xiān líng pí (Herba Epimedii) 15g and *gǒu qǐ zǐ* (Fructus Lycii) 15g were added to the previous formula. 14 additional packets were prescribed. Western medication was also continued.

Third Visit:

Patient started to display a more pleasant affect, and he was now able to take walks and perform household chores. The stiffness of his limbs was greatly relieved, and he was also able to talk to his family. His tongue appeared pale red with white coating, and pulses were wiry and slippery.

Prescription: *jú huā* (Flos Chrysanthemi) 15g, *chuān xiōng* (Rhizoma Chuanxiong) 20g, *dān shēn* (Radix et Rhizoma Salviae Miltiorrhizae) 20g, *tiān zhú huáng* (Concretio Silicea Bambusae) 15g, *yù jīn* (Radix Curcumae) 30g, *chén pí* (Pericarpium Citri Reticulatae) 15g, *ròu cōng róng* (Herba

Cistanches) 30g, *gŏu qĭ zĭ* (Fructus Lycii) 15g, *xiān líng pí* (Herba Epimedii) 15g, *chì sháo* (Radix Paeoniae Rubra) 30g, *bái sháo* (Radix Paeoniae Alba) 30g, *chăo zăo rén* (Semen Ziziphi Spinosae, stir-fried) 70g, *mài mén dōng* (Ophiopogonis) 30g, *jī xuè téng* (Caulis Spatholobi) 40g, *shēng dì* (Radix Rehmanniae) 30g, *shēng shí gāo* (Gypsum Fibrosum Cruda, decocted first) 80g, and *băi hé* (Bulbus Lilii) 30g. Another fourteen packets.

Fourth Visit:

The patient's condition was stabilized and most symptoms were eliminated. He was instructed to continue taking Chinese medicine once every other day; Western medications was also continued.

Commentary:

In this case, enduring liver constraint caused qi stagnation that transformed into heat. Over a period of time, blood stasis resulted, causing a major case of depression. There are three key points regarding the pathological process:

1) He had suffered from constrained emotions for a long time, and there was liver qi stagnation.

2) Enduring qi stagnation inhibited the movement of blood, causing stasis.

3) Enduring liver constraint caused damage to the liver. "The child steals the mother's qi" is applicable here because liver damage had led to kidney damage, and signs of kidney yang depletion had appeared. With kidney damage, kidney-zhi was also affected.

The treatment principles were to course the liver, move blood, and supplement kidney yang. When coursing the liver, large dosages of *chái hú* (Radix Bupleuri) should not be used long term because this medicinal can attack and dry the liver instead of helping it. Applying a large dosage of *bái sháo* (Radix Paeoniae Alba) can supplement liver yin while astringing; this prevents excessive opening with an inability to close that can be caused by qi-moving medicinals such as *fó shŏu* (Fructus Citri Sarcodactylis) and *xiāng yuán* (Fructus Citri).

When treating depression, only by using a combination of opening and closing, and upbearing and downbearing methods can organ function be restored. Enduring disease can also affect the brain-spirit and kidney-

zhi, therefore large dosages of *tù sī zǐ* (Semen Cuscutae), *xiān líng pí* (Herba Epimedii) and *ròu cōng róng* (Herba Cistanches) were applied to invigorate qi and blood. Once the kidney source was fulfilled, all the viscera became once again harmonious. *Yún líng* (Poria) and *shén qū* (Massa Medicata Fermentata) were added in order to prevent the qi-moving and kidney-supplementing medicinals from damaging the spleen and stomach.

7. Qi Stagnation and Blood Stasis

Ms. Wang, age 19.

The patient had grown up in a strict, conservative and controlling family. When she was 19, she rejected the marriage that her family arranged for her, and was thus confined to the house. The patient subsequently started to despair and weep, and she was unwilling to see people. She also developed auditory hallucinations of her teachers and classmates calling her back to school. As her psychotic condition progressed, she started exhibiting delirious speech, sleeplessness, an inability to eat, and she became emaciated. The family considered this to be a sign of spirit possession and a shaman was sent for. During the treatment process, the skin on the patient's the abdomen was burned. In her despair, she then drove a nail into her head with a hammer. Her skull was penetrated, but her brain was undamaged.

The Western medicine department diagnosed her with depression and prescribed Amitriptyline 50mg and 0.8mg Alprazolam in the evenings. After a week, her condition had not improved. Her suicidal tendencies, frustration, and fatigue remained even though the family had promised not to interfere with her marriage. The family then requested integrative medical treatment.

At the initial visit the patient entered the clinic with the assistance of her parents. Her head was bandaged, and she presented with emaciation, frustration, a flat facial affect, an unwillingness to interact, extreme passivity, no will to live or desire to be cured, despair, episodes of auditory hallucinations, sleeplessness with nightmares occurring immediately after closing her eyes, reduced intake of food, turbid yellow urine, absent urination for six or seven days, burnt skin on the abdomen with pain resulting in limited movement, dry stools, a dark red tongue with purple spots on the edge, a yellow slimy tongue coating, and wiry rapid pulses.

Chapter 10
Case Studies

Diagnosis: Major depressive disorder.

Pattern Differentiation: Qi stagnation with blood stasis and dampness obstructing the middle burner.

Treatment Principles: Rectify qi, resolve constraint and dampness, awaken the spirit.

Prescription:

Chái hú (Radix Bupleuri) 6g, *bái sháo* (Radix Paeoniae Alba) 30g, *chì sháo* (Radix Paeoniae Rubra) 30g, *xiāng fù* (Rhizoma Cyperi) 15g, *chǎo zhǐ qiào* (Fructus Aurantii, stir-fried) 10g, *tiān zhú huáng* (Concretio Silicea Bambusae) 15g, *yù jīn* (Radix Curcumae) 30g, *hóng huā* (Flos Carthami) 9g, *niú xī* (Radix Achyranthis Bidentatae) 30g, *huáng lián* (Rhizoma Coptidis) 10g, *pèi lán* (Herba Eupatorii) 10g, *lái fú zǐ* (Semen Raphani) 30g, *jiǔ zhì dà huáng* (Radix et Rhizoma Rhei, preserved in liquor) 15g, *chǎo suān zǎo rén* (Semen Ziziphi Spinosae, stir-fried) 60g, *jī xuè téng* (Caulis Spatholobi) 40g, *jīn yín huā* (Flos Lonicerae Japonicae) 20g, *shēng shí gāo* (Gypsum Fibrosum Cruda, decocted first) 160g, and *zhēn zhū mǔ* (Concha Margaritiferae Usta, decocted first) 60g.

Amitriptyline was also prescribed, 50mg each evening.

> **Second Visit:**

The patient's mood appeared to be improved, as were her sleep and appetite. Her entire body had relaxed somewhat, and bowel movements occurred smoothly once a day. The auditory hallucinations had disappeared, but she still had pessimistic attitude towards life. There was still pronounced yellow urine, a dark tongue with purple spots, and a thin white slimy tongue coating. Her pulses were wiry and fine.

Prescription:

1) Amitriptyline

2) Acupuncture on the head and back once every two days

3) Chinese Medicinals: *Jú huā* (Flos Chrysanthemi) 15g, *chuān xiōng* (Rhizoma Chuanxiong) 20g, *dān shēn* (Radix et Rhizoma Salviae Miltiorrhizae) 20g, *tiān zhú huáng* (Concretio Silicea Bambusae) 15g, *yù jīn* (Radix Curcumae) 30g, *huáng lián* (Rhizoma Coptidis) 10g, *pèi lán* (Herba Eupatorii) 10g, *chǎo zǎo rén* (Semen Ziziphi Spinosae, stir-fried) 60g, *fó shǒu* (Fructus Citri Sarcodactylis) 10g, *chén pí* (Pericarpium Citri Reticulatae) 15g, *fǎ bàn xià* (Rhizoma Pinelliae Praeparatum) 15g, *shí chāng pú* (Rhizoma

Acori Tatarinowii) 6g, *jiǔ zhì dà huáng* (Radix et Rhizoma Rhei, preserved in liquor) 15g, *lái fú zǐ* (Semen Raphani) 30g, *niú xī* (Radix Achyranthis Bidentatae) 30g, *shēng shí gāo* (Gypsum Fibrosum Cruda, decocted first) 160g, *cí shí* (Magnetitum, decocted first) 30g, *zhēn zhū mǔ* (Concha Margaritiferae Usta, decocted first) 60g, and *jīn yín huā* (Flos Lonicerae Japonicae) 20g.

14 packets were prescribed.

Third Visit:

The patient's mood was significantly improved. She was willing to talk openly, receive further treatment, and her facial expression had become pleasant. The abdominal burn had healed, and her headaches from the injury were substantially improved. The patient could walk without the assistance of others, and she displayed a positive attitude towards life. Her appetite was relatively normal, and bowel movements occurred daily with loose stools. The tongue appeared dark with no spots and a thin slimy coating. Her pulses were wiry and slippery.

Prescription:

1) Amitriptyline

2) Chinese Medicinals: *jú huā* (Flos Chrysanthemi) 15g, *chuān xiōng* (Rhizoma Chuanxiong) 20g, *dān shēn* (Radix et Rhizoma Salviae Miltiorrhizae) 20g, *chén pí* (Pericarpium Citri Reticulatae) 15g, *tiān zhú huáng* (Concretio Silicea Bambusae) 15g, *yù jīn* (Radix Curcumae) 30g, *huáng lián* (Rhizoma Coptidis) 10g, *pèi lán* (Herba Eupatorii) 10g, *jiǔ zhì dà huáng* (Radix et Rhizoma Rhei, preserved in liquor) 15g, *lái fú zǐ* (Semen Raphani) 30g, *niú xī* (Radix Achyranthis Bidentatae) 30g, *jī xuè téng* (Caulis Spatholobi) 30g, *xuán shēn* (Radix Scrophulariae) 30g, *mài mén dōng* (Ophiopogonis) 30g, *shēng shí gāo* (Gypsum Fibrosum Cruda, decocted first) 120g, and *zhēn zhū mǔ* (Concha Margaritiferae Usta) (decocted first) 60g.

14 packets were prescribed.

Fourth Visit:

The patient's mood had returned to normal, she showed regret for her previous suicidal behavior, and she was positive about her schoolwork and relationships in the future. Her appetite, urine and stool were regular.

Chapter 10
Case Studies

To reinforce the treatment, the previous formula was continued at one packet every two days, and Amitriptyline was continued for half a year at 25mg daily. After several more visits, her condition was completely resolved and the patient was able to enter college and develop a stable relationship.

Commentary:

The onset, course and clinical manifestations of this case were considered to be a manifestation of enduring qi constraint transforming into heat and blood stasis. With the addition of the mental provocation, the spirit was affected and she became very deranged and with self-damaging behavior. This was an acute and major condition that definitely required treatment with integrative medicine. Acupuncture treatments were used to promote the downward movement of heat evil, move blood, and free the vessels. Acupuncture is most effective for treating this kind of acute major depressive disorder when accompanied by suicidal tendencies; according to clinical studies, a series of twenty-four treatments can bring significant changes.

In this case, the key to Chinese medicinal treatment is to course the liver without damaging liver yin, so qi-moving medicinals should not be used excessively. One should be especially cautious when using *Chái hú* (Radix Bupleuri) so as to not damage liver yin and blood. *bái sháo* (Radix Paeoniae Alba) or *chì sháo* (Radix Paeoniae Rubra) are usually combined with *chái hú* (Radix Bupleuri) to nourish blood and emolliate the liver.

When dampness gathers in the middle burner, it should be resolved before it accumulates and transforms into phlegm. Therefore, *huáng lián* (Rhizoma Coptidis) and *pèi lán* (Herba Eupatorii) were added Because *huáng lián* (Rhizoma Coptidis) acts to clear heat and dry dampness and *pèi lán* (Herba Eupatorii) aromatically transforms dampness.

Turbid evils usually exit through the lower orifices. To free the six bowels and dispel evils through the proper outlet, *jiǔ zhì dà huáng* (Radix et Rhizoma Rhei, preserved in liquor), *lái fú zǐ* (Semen Raphani), and *niú xī* (Radix Achyranthis Bidentatae) were added.

To avoid the typical side effects of Amitriptyline such as dry mouth and tongue, *jī xuè téng* (Caulis Spatholobi) and a large dosage of *shēng shí gāo* (Gypsum Fibrosum Cruda) were added. These medicinals act to clear heat and engender fluids.

Adding medicinals such as *xuán shēn* (Radix Scrophulariae) 30g, *mài mén dōng* (Ophiopogonis) 30g and *shēng dì* (Radix Rehmanniae) can also prevent generalized discomfort caused by antidepressant medications.

8. Bulimic Depressive Disorder

Ms. Bai, unmarried, age 20.

Initial Visit: August 10th, 2004

The patient had a history of being excessively competitive and self-centered, her mood fluctuating with the slightest frustration. When she was in college she started to control her diet in order to stay fit, she later began to induce vomiting immediately after eating. Over a period of time, the amount of food she ate increased substantially. At first, she manually induced vomiting with her fingers; but eventually this developed into spontaneous vomiting that gave her some temporary psychological relief. Two hours after eating she would become agitated and hungry again.

The patient suffered weight loss, low spirits, and depression. This gradually led to emaciation, a somber facial complexion, menstrual block, and edema of the lower extremities. She had visited many Western internal medicine departments, and the usual diagnosis was "dystrophia".

Primary complaints included depression, emaciation, low self-esteem, feelings of resentment toward others, overeating, amenorrhea for four months, poor sleep, a lack of strength, an inability to walk steadily or for long periods of time, and a denial of the existence of the condition. Her tongue was pale with thin white coating, and pulses were wiry and fine.

She was 165cm (5'4") tall and weighed 37.5kg (82.7 lbs); BP 90/70mmHg. Western medical diagnostics showed no abnormalities of the heart, lung, liver and spleen, nor any condition affecting the nervous system.

WM Diagnosis: bulimia nervosa with dystrophia.

CM Diagnosis: bulimia with depression.

Pattern Differentiation: heart-spleen dual deficiency, malnourishment of the brain-spirit.

Chapter 10
Case Studies

Treatment Principles: secure the heart, benefit the spleen, nourish the brain, calm the spirit.

Prescription:

1) Psychological counseling
2) Fluoxetine (Prozac)
3) Chinese Medicinals: *Jú huā* (Flos Chrysanthemi) 15g, *chuān xiōng* (Rhizoma Chuanxiong) 20g, *dān shēn* (Radix et Rhizoma Salviae Miltiorrhizae) 30g, *fú líng* (Poria) 30g, *dǎng shēn* (Radix Codonopsis) 15g, *chǎo bái zhú* (Rhizoma Atractylodis Macrocephalae, stir-fried) 10g, *shān yào* (Rhizoma Dioscoreae) 30g, *dà zǎo* (Fructus Jujubae) 10g, *fó shǒu* (Fructus Citri Sarcodactylis) 10g, *xiāng yuán* (Fructus Citri) 15g, *ròu cōng róng* (Herba Cistanches) 30g, *chǎo zǎo rén* (Semen Ziziphi Spinosae, stir-fried) 60g, *bǎi hé* (Bulbus Lilii) 30g, *dāng guī* (Radix Angelicae Sinensis) 15g, and *huǒ má rén* (Fructus Cannabis) 30g.

5 packets were prescribed, decocted once daily and taken as two portions, once each morning and night.

Second Visit: August 16th

While the overeating remained persistent, and there was no observable effect on her mood, the patient was now able to acknowledge her illness and therefore showed some willingness to control her diet. She still presented with a strong urge to overeat.

Another 7 packets of the formula were prescribed along with prepared *Tiān Wáng Bǔ Xīn Dān* (Celestial Emperor Heart-Supplementing Elixir), 1 pill twice daily. Psychological counseling and Western medication were also continued.

Third Visit: August 23rd

The general status of the patient was improved as her facial expressions were more animated, and the frequency of overeating was reduced with less urge to overeat. After eating, however, there was still a desire to vomit.

Xuán fù huā (Flos Inulae) 10g and *dài zhě shí* (Haematitum) 30g were added to the previous formula. 7 packets were prescribed, and Western medication was continued.

Fourth Visit: August 30th

The patient's condition was greatly improved with a better mood and less desire to overeat. The patient's physical strength had also increased. The amount of food taken each day became manageable, but there was still some discomfort with a persistent desire to vomit after eating. There was an occasional dry mouth with thirst.

Xuán shēn (Radix Scrophulariae), mài mén dōng (Ophiopogonis), shēng dì (Radix Rehmanniae), jiāo mài yá (Fructus Hordei Germinatus Ustus), jiāo shān zhā (Fructus Crataegi) and jiāo shén qū (Massa Medicata Fermentata Ustus) 30g each were added to the formula, and 6 more packets were prescribed. Psychological counseling was continued, and the patient was advised to go back to school.

Fifth Visit: September 5th

The patient was managing her diet effectively, presented with vivid facial expressions, and was able to go back to school. She still reported profuse dreaming. Her menstrual period had lasted for only one day with scant pale menses and clotting.

Yù jīn (Radix Curcumae) 15g and xiāng fù (Rhizoma Cyperi) were added to the previous formula, and an additional 10 packets were prescribed.

On September 15th, the patient's mother reported that she had stopped overeating completely. Her mood was animated, but there were dry stools on some occasions.

Commentary:

Bulimia is commonly accompanied by depression. In Western medicine, antidepressant medications are often used as the primary medicine in conjunction with small doses of antipsychotics. These patients can manifest signs of qi deficiency, yin deficiency, blood deficiency, damp-heat, or even yin-yang dual deficiency. Western pharmaceuticals can partially relieve the psychological symptoms, but not the physical conditions. Furthermore, there may be intolerable side effects. When differentiating this disorder according to Chinese medicine, the physician should also pay attention to the patient's psychological health and recommend appropriate counseling as needed.

Chapter 11
Applications of Chinese Medicine in Psychiatry

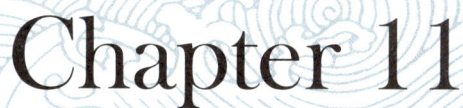

The Chinese medical perspective is that permutations of the human mind and emotions are associated with the functions and mutual interactions of qi, blood, body fluids, and the viscera and bowels. To treat the various types of depression and other psychiatric disorders, medicinals should be applied in correspondence with changes in these functions; thus, in Chinese medicine there is no "separate" treatment of mental and emotional conditions.

Qi

Regarding qi, exposure to intense or persistent irregular emotional extremes can affect the qi dynamic of the viscera and bowels, causing both physical and psychological symptoms.

Commonly selected medicinals include the following:

For liver constraint with qi stagnation, use *chái hú* (Radix Bupleuri) 6g, *bái sháo* (Radix Paeoniae Alba) 30g, *xiāng fù* (Rhizoma Cyperi) 10g, *fó shǒu* (Fructus Citri Sarcodactylis) 10g, and *dāng guī* (Radix Angelicae Sinensis) 10g.

The maximum dose for *chái hú* (Radix Bupleuri) is 10g, with prolonged usage it may cause excessive stimulation. *Bái sháo* (Radix Paeoniae Alba) 30g can be added to emolliate the liver and prevent the drying nature of *chái hú* (Radix Bupleuri) from damaging liver yin and blood.

For heart qi insufficiency, which is commonly seen in people with chronic conditions, use *shēng huáng qí* (Radix Astragali, raw) 30–60g, *tài zǐ shēn* (Radix Pseudostellariae) 30g and *mài mén dōng* (Ophiopogonis) 30g.

For qi stagnation of the stomach and intestines, use *lái fú zǐ* (Semen Raphani) 15g, *chǎo zhǐ qiào* (Fructus Aurantii, stir-fried) 15g and *jiǔ zhì dà huáng* (Radix et Rhizoma Rhei, preserved in liquor, added later to the decoction) 10 – 15g.

With qi counterflow, modified *Xuán Fù Dài Zhě Tāng* (Inula and Hematite Decoction) can be added. Profuse flatus after administration indicates a good outcome.

Blood

Disorders of blood include blood deficiency, blood heat, and irregular movement of blood; all of these patterns can cause mental disorders. In mild cases there will be symptoms of neurosis such as neurasthenia,

Chapter 11
Applications of Chinese Medicine in Psychiatry

forgetfulness, insomnia, profuse dreaming, and vexation and agitation; in severe cases there will be fright and fear, speaking or laughing to oneself, and self-isolation.

Use *dāng guī* (Radix Angelicae Sinensis) 10–30g, *bái sháo* (Radix Paeoniae Alba) 30g, *mài mén dōng* (Ophiopogonis) 30g, *wŭ wèi zĭ* (Fructus Schisandrae Chinensis) 15g, *ē jiāo* (Colla Corii Asini) 15g, and *nǚ zhēn zĭ* (Fructus Ligustri Lucidi) 30g.

Blood Stasis

Clinical observation demonstrates that premenstrual emotional instability is commonly caused by blood stasis; stasis can also be linked to sudden surges of anger and rage among men.

In the *Introduction to Medicine* (*Yī Xué Rù Mén*), Li Yan innovated the concept of "blood confounding the orifices of the heart" and a corresponding treatment using *táo rén* (Semen Persicae), *hóng huā* (Flos Carthami), and *sū mù* (Lignum Sappan). Also, in the *Correction of Errors in Medical Works* (*Yī Lín Găi Cuò*), Wang Qing-ren created *Diān Kuáng Mèng Xĭng Tāng* (Mania and Withdrawal Dream-Awakening Decoction) for the treatment of psychiatric disorders related to blood stasis.

Commonly used medicinals include *táo rén* (Semen Persicae) 15g, *hóng huā* (Flos Carthami) 15g, *chuān xiōng* (Rhizoma Chuanxiong) 15g, *chì sháo* (Radix Paeoniae Rubra) 30g, *dì lóng* (Pheretima) 10g, *zé lán* (Herba Lycopi) 10g, *xiāng fù* (Rhizoma Cyperi) 10g and *jiŭ zhì dà huáng* (Radix et Rhizoma Rhei, preserved in liquor, decocted later) 6g.

Phlegm

In Chinese medical theory, the spleen is considered as the source of phlegm engenderment. When splenic movement and transformation becomes impaired, this can lead to an accumulation of internal dampness. When dampness persists over a period of time, phlegm will be engendered; other pathologies may follow such as exuberant phlegm-fire or qi constraint with phlegm bind.

Zhang Zi-he was the first physician to establish the theory of "phlegm clouding the orifices of the heart". In the *Confucians' Duties to Their Parents* (*Rú Mén Shì Qīn*) he states, "Heart blood gradually becomes desiccated, and the spleen humor fails to move; with phlegm confounding the heart, withdrawal and mania results." He suggested that stubborn phlegm should be attacked with ejection and purgation methods, and this was a substantial influence on subsequent generations. Purgation of phlegm is still commonly used in contemporary clinics, and this method usually results in immediate relief of many psychiatric conditions.

Use *méng shí* (Chlorite-schist, decocted first) 60g, *chén pí* (Pericarpium Citri Reticulatae) 10g, *bàn xià* (Rhizoma Pinelliae) 10g, *tiān zhú huáng* (Concretio Silicea Bambusae) 15g, *yù jīn* (Radix Curcumae) 30g, *jiǔ zhì dà huáng* (Radix et Rhizoma Rhei, preserved in liquor, decocted later) 15g, *fú líng* (Poria) 30g, and *dǎn nán xīng* (Arisaema cum Bile) 12g.

Historically, *Sān Shèng Sǎn* (Three Sages Powder) and *Guā Dì Sǎn* (Melon Stalk Powder) have been used to promote ejection of phlegm. These formulas are rarely used in contemporary practices because patients tend to reject the idea of vomiting as a treatment method. Clinically, *Qīng Xīn Gǔn Tán Wán* (Heart-Clearing Phlegm-Rolling Pill) is commonly used.

According to the *Prolonging Life and Preserving the Origin* (*Shòu Shì Bǎo Yuán*), this formula consists of *dà huáng* (Radix et Rhizoma Rhei, steamed with liquor) 4 *liang*, *huáng qín* (Radix Scutellariae) 4 *liang*, *qīng méng shí* (Lapis Chloriti) 5 *qian*, *chén xiāng* (Lignum Aquilariae Resinatum) 2.5 *qian*, *yá zào* (Fructus Gleditsiae Abnormalis) 5 *qian*, *xī jiǎo* (Cornu Rhinocerotis) 2 *qian*, *shè xiāng* (Moschus) 5 *fen*, *zhū shā* (Cinnabaris, used as coating) 5 *qian*.

Grind all ingredients to a fine powder and make into pills with water. Each dose is forty to fifty pills, taken with boiled water.

Another commonly used formula is *Ān Shén Gǔn Tán Wán* (Spirit-Calming Phlegm-Rolling Pill). According to the *Supplemental Compilation of Patterns and Treatment* (*Zhèng Zhì Huì Bǔ*), this formula consists of *méng shí* (Chlorite-schist) 1 *liang*, *fēng huà xiāo* (Natrii Sulfas Exsiccatus) 1 *liang*, *zhū shā* (Cinnabaris) 1 *liang*, *chén xiāng* (Lignum Aquilariae Resinatum) 5 *qian*, and *zhēn zhū* (Margarita) 5 *qian*.

Grind the ingredients into powder, mix-fry the resulting powder with *tiān má* (Rhizoma Gastrodiae) paste, and make into pills the size of *qiàn shí* (Semen Euryales) seeds. Take 3 pills each time with ginger juice or bamboo sap.

Fire

Fire-related psychiatric conditions are commonly seen, especially in

Chapter 11
Applications of Chinese Medicine in Psychiatry

the initial stages of mental disorders.

Commonly used medicinals include the following:

For heart heat, use *huáng lián* (Rhizoma Coptidis) 15g, *zhú yè* (Folium Phyllostachydis Henonis) 6g, *zhī zǐ* (Fructus Gardeniae) 15g, and *huáng qín* (Radix Scutellariae) 15g.

For liver fire, use *shēng shí gāo* (Gypsum Fibrosum Cruda) (decocted first) 80g, *shēng shí jué míng* (Concha Haliotidis, raw, decocted first) 60g, *cí shí* (Magnetitum, decocted first) 60g, *dài zhě shí* (Haematitum) 30g and *niú xī* (Radix Achyranthis Bidentatae) 30g.

For exuberant stomach fire, use *shēng shí gāo* (Gypsum Fibrosum Cruda, decocted first) 200–500g and *xuán shēn* (Radix Scrophulariae) 30g.

For exuberant heat in the intestines, use *jiǔ zhì dà huáng* (Radix et Rhizoma Rhei, preserved in liquor, decocted later) 15g.

Medicinals that clear fire-heat should not be taken for extended periods.

Applications and Modifications of Jú Shēn Tāng (Chrysanthemum and Salvia Decoction)

Jú Shēn Tāng (Chrysanthemum and Salvia Decoction) is an empirical formula composed by the author after years of clinical experience in the treatment of psychiatric conditions. It has proven to be very effective for improving the function of the brain-spirit system. When treating brain-related conditions, simply regulating the viscera and bowels is not always sufficient for managing the condition; clearing the brain-spirit with this formula can increase the effectiveness of the other treatments.

For example: in chronic schizophrenia, if there is a pattern of spleen-kidney yang deficiency with failure to nourish to brain, then the simple application of spleen and kidney supplementing therapy for 1–2 months will frequently result in eventual side effects including heat signs of the mouth, tongue, lips and throat, as well as a loss of mental clarity. There are many more examples like this, where the treatment of bowel and viscera patterns fail to resolve the concurrent mental-emotional disorder.

In clinical settings, *Jú Shēn Tāng* can be modified with another modular formula to address the organ patterns. This approach can result in improved outcomes for both deficiency and excess presentations.

For instance, schizophrenic symptoms may change rapidly during the end of an episode. The principle manifestations may include dry stools for several days, irascibility and an unstable mood, impulses to rage, yell or hit people, non-verbal auditory hallucinations, and tinnitus. Such conditions should be treated promptly, before the patient has lost control.

Urgently apply *Jú Shēn Tāng* with added *dà huáng* (Radix et Rhizoma Rhei), *shēng shí gāo* (Gypsum Fibrosum Cruda) and *shēng shí jué míng* (Concha Haliotidis raw), and the condition will resolve in a few days.

The application principles for *Jú Shēn Tāng* are as follows:

Ingredients: *Jú huā* (Flos Chrysanthemi) 15–20g, *chuān xiōng* (Rhizoma Chuanxiong) 10g, and *dān shēn* (Radix et Rhizoma Salviae Miltiorrhizae) 30g.

Functions: Clears the brain and calms the spirit.

Indications: Psychiatric conditions manifesting with dizziness, distending sensations of the head, tinnitus, hallucinations, paranoia, unstable moods, and irascibility.

Analysis:

Jú huā (Flos Chrysanthemi) is neutral and calming in nature and acts to benefit both metal and water in order to calm liver-wood. When wood is calmed, wind will then be extinguished. Blurred vision, dizziness, a distending sensation of the head, and headaches are all associated with effulgent liver-wood fire. This reflects the theory that "all wind, shaking and dizzy vision is ascribed to the liver". Psychiatric symptoms related to the head are mostly associated with fire evil and phlegm. When wood is calmed and wind is extinguished, then the fire will naturally bear downwards.

Chuān xiōng (Rhizoma Chuanxiong) is acrid in flavor and warming, uplifting, and floating in nature. As a qi medicine that works within the blood aspect, it ascends through the *shaoyang* gallbladder channel to open constraint. According to Zhu Dan-xi, "When qi is uplifted, constraint will naturally downbear."

Chuān xiōng (Rhizoma Chuanxiong) also acts to moisten liver dryness, supplement liver deficiency, and move blood stasis within the head and the sea of blood. Therefore, in cases of liver constraint transforming into fire and disturbing brain-spirit, *chuān xiōng* (Rhizoma Chuanxiong) is the

Chapter 11
Applications of Chinese Medicine in Psychiatry

primary choice.

Dān shēn (Radix et Rhizoma Salviae Miltiorrhizae) is neutral and downbearing in nature. It acts to dispel stasis and engender the new in the blood aspect. It is said that "as one single ingredient, *dān shēn* (Radix et Rhizoma Salviae Miltiorrhizae) functions identically to *Sì Wù Tāng* (Four Substances Decoction)". It strongly acts to nourish blood, settle the mind, and free the blood vessels.

Modifications:
- For prominent subjective symptoms of the head such as distending pains in the head or eyes, one can use up to 20g of *jú huā* (Flos Chrysanthemi).
- For liver constraint that has transformed into fire, increase the dosage of *chuān xiōng* (Rhizoma Chuanxiong) to 20g.
- For a persistent condition with inhibited blood vessels and disquieting of the brain-spirit, use *dān shēn* (Radix et Rhizoma Salviae Miltiorrhizae) 30g.

Applications of added medicinals:

1) Liver constraint: *chái hú* (Radix Bupleuri) 6g, *bái sháo* (Radix Paeoniae Alba) 30g, and *dāng guī* (Radix Angelicae Sinensis) 15g.

2) Ascendant liver yang: *shēng shí jué míng* (Concha Haliotidis, raw) 60g, *shēng lóng chǐ* (Dens Draconis, raw) 60g, and *cí shí* (Magnetitum) 60g.

3) Intense internal liver fire: *lóng dǎn cǎo* (Radix et Rhizoma Gentianae) 15g and *niú xī* (Radix Achyranthis Bidentatae) 30g.

4) Intense exuberant stomach fire: *shēng shí gāo* (Gypsum Fibrosum Cruda) 60–300g.

5) Insufficient stomach yin: *shí hú* (Caulis Dendrobii) 30g, *mài mén dōng* (Ophiopogonis) 30g, and *tiān huā fěn* (Radix Trichosanthis) 30g.

6) Liver-kidney yin deficiency: *bái sháo* (Radix Paeoniae Alba) 30g, *dāng guī* (Radix Angelicae Sinensis) 30g, *nǚ zhēn zǐ* (Fructus Ligustri Lucidi) 30g and *gǒu qǐ zǐ* (Fructus Lycii) 15g.

7) Yin-yang dual deficiency of the kidney: *tù sī zǐ* (Semen Cuscutae) 80g.

8) Blood stasis: *táo rén* (Semen Persicae) 10–30g, *hóng huā* (Flos Carthami) 10g, *niú xī* (Radix Achyranthis Bidentatae) 30g and *chì sháo* (Radix Paeoniae Rubra) 30g.

9) Effulgent ministerial fire: *zhī mǔ* (Rhizoma Anemarrhenae) 10g and *huáng bǎi* (Cortex Phellodendri Chinensis) 10g.

10) Exuberant phlegm: *méng shí* (Chlorite-schist) 60g, *fǎ bàn xià* (Rhizoma Pinelliae Praeparatum) 10g, *dǎn nán xīng* (Arisaema cum Bile) 10g, *tiān zhú huáng* (Concretio Silicea Bambusae) 15g, and *yù jīn* (Radix Curcumae) 30g. Proper amounts of *Qīng Xīn Gǔn Tán Wán* (Heart-Clearing Phlegm-Rolling Pill) can be added as well.

11) Non-verbal auditory hallucinations: with yin deficiency, add *shēng dì* (Radix Rehmanniae) 20g, *xuán shēn* (Radix Scrophulariae) 30g, and *dì gǔ pí* (Cortex Lycii) 30g; with qi deficiency, add *shēng huáng qí* (Radix Astragali raw) 20–60g and *tài zǐ shēn* (Radix Pseudostellariae) 30g; with kidney deficiency, add *nǚ zhēn zǐ* (Fructus Ligustri Lucidi) 30g and *gǒu qǐ zǐ* (Fructus Lycii) 15g.

12) Compulsive behavior: *táo rén* (Semen Persicae) 30g, *hóng huā* (Flos Carthami) 10g, and *jī xuè téng* (Caulis Spatholobi) 40g.

13) Excessive sexual desire: *huáng bǎi* (Cortex Phellodendri Chinensis) 10g and *zhī mǔ* (Rhizoma Anemarrhenae) 10g.

14) Irascibility: *shēng shí jué míng* (Concha Haliotidis raw) 60g, *cí shí* (Magnetitum) 60g, *gōu téng* (Ramulus Uncariae Cum Uncis) 30g and *zhī zǐ* (Fructus Gardeniae) 15g.

15) Frequent laughter: *huáng lián* (Rhizoma Coptidis) 15g and *mài mén dōng* (Ophiopogonis) 20g.

16) Frequent weeping: *tài zǐ shēn* (Radix Pseudostellariae) 20g, *bǎi hé* (Bulbus Lilii) 80g and *shā shēn* (Radix Adenophorae) 30g.

17) Susceptibility to fright: *gǒu qǐ zǐ* (Fructus Lycii) 10g, *zhū shā* (Cinnabaris) 0.5g, and *hǔ pò miàn* (Succinum, powdered) 2–6g.

18) Excessive talking: *huáng lián* (Rhizoma Coptidis) 10g, *zhú yè* (Folium Phyllostachydis Henonis) 6g, and *jiǔ zhì dà huáng* (Radix et Rhizoma Rhei, preserved in liquor, added later) 10g.

19) Heart vexation: *huáng lián* (Rhizoma Coptidis) 10g and *zhī zǐ* (Fructus Gardeniae) 10g; with a yellow thick slimy tongue coating, add *pèi lán* (Herba Eupatorii) 10g.

20) Suspicion: with blood stasis, add *táo rén* (Semen Persicae) 20g, *hóng huā* (Flos Carthami) 10g, *chì sháo* (Radix Paeoniae Rubra) 30g and *niú xī* (Radix Achyranthis Bidentatae) 30g; with exuberant phlegm, add *tiān zhú huáng* (Concretio Silicea Bambusae) 15g and *yù jīn* (Radix

Chapter 11
Applications of Chinese Medicine in Psychiatry

Curcumae) 30g.

21) Fear: *shēng huáng qí* (Radix Astragali raw) 30g, *tù sī zǐ* (Semen Cuscutae) 30g and *nǚ zhēn zǐ* (Fructus Ligustri Lucidi) 40g.

22) Slowed thinking: *shí chāng pú* (Rhizoma Acori Tatarinowii) 10g and *hóng huā* (Flos Carthami) 10g.

23) Insomnia and profuse dreaming: *chǎo zǎo rén* (Semen Ziziphi Spinosae, stir-fried) 30 - 80g, *hé huān pí* (Cortex Albiziae) 30g, *yuǎn zhì* (Radix Polygalae) 10g and *hǔ pò miàn* (Succinum, powdered) 2–6g.

24) Declining memory: *gǒu qǐ zǐ* (Fructus Lycii) 15g, *tù sī zǐ* (Semen Cuscutae) 80g and *zhì biē jiǎ* (Carapax Trionycis, processed) 20g.

25) Eye-rolling: *shēng shí gāo* (Gypsum Fibrosum Cruda) 120g.

26) Unclear vision: *shí hú* (Caulis Dendrobii) 30g.

27) Rigidity of the neck and nape: *gé gēn* (Radix Puerariae Lobatae) 25–50g.

28) Shaking limbs: *dāng guī* (Radix Angelicae Sinensis) 30–80g, *jī xuè téng* (Caulis Spatholobi) 40g, *shēng shí gāo* (Gypsum Fibrosum Cruda) 120g, and *xuán shēn* (Radix Scrophulariae) 30g.

29) Heat in the heart of the palms and soles: *qīng hāo* (Herba Artemisiae Annuae) 15g and *dì gǔ pí* (Cortex Lycii) 30g.

30) Dry mouth and tongue: with a red mirror-like tongue with no coating, add *shí hú* (Caulis Dendrobii) 30g, *tiān huā fěn* (Radix Trichosanthis) 30g and *shā shēn* (Radix Adenophorae) 30g; with a red tongue with a slimy coating, add *shēng shí gāo* (Gypsum Fibrosum Cruda) 180g and *huáng lián* (Rhizoma Coptidis) 10g.

31) Fatigue: *shēng huáng qí* (Radix Astragali raw) 30g, *tài zǐ shēn* (Radix Pseudostellariae) 30g and *chì sháo* (Radix Paeoniae Rubra) 30g.

32) Lack of strength: for drug-induced conditions, add *shēng shí gāo* (Gypsum Fibrosum Cruda) 80g and *jī xuè téng* (Caulis Spatholobi) 40g; with spleen deficiency, add *bái zhú* (Rhizoma Atractylodis Macrocephalae) 15g and *dǎng shēn* (Radix Codonopsis) 15g.

33) Shortness of breath: *shēng huáng qí* (Radix Astragali raw) 30g, *tài zǐ shēn* (Radix Pseudostellariae) 15g, *bǎi hé* (Bulbus Lilii) 80g and *dà zǎo* (Fructus Jujubae) 10g.

34) Chest oppression: *chái hú* (Radix Bupleuri) 6g, *bái sháo* (Radix Paeoniae Alba) 30g and *yù jīn* (Radix Curcumae) 30g.

35) Lumbar pain: *dù zhòng* (Cortex Eucommiae) 30g and *sāng jì shēng*

(Herba Taxilli) 20g.

36) Seminal emission: *jīn yīng zǐ* (Fructus Rosae Laevigatae) 15g and *qiàn shí* (Semen Euryales) 15g.

37) Impotence: *yín yáng huò* (Herba Epimedii) 15g, *xiān máo* (Rhizoma Curculiginis) 6g, *tù sī zǐ* (Semen Cuscutae) 60g and *shé chuáng zǐ* (Fructus Cnidii) 10g.

38) Scant semen: *fù pén zǐ* (Fructus Rubi) 15g, *shé chuáng zǐ* (Fructus Cnidii) 15g, *tù sī zǐ* (Semen Cuscutae) 60g and *shā yuàn zǐ* (Semen Astragali Complanati) 15g.

39) Nausea and vomiting: *xuán fù huā* (Flos Inulae) 15g and *dài zhě shí* (Haematitum) 30g.

40) Decreased appetite: *jiāo mài yá* (Fructus Hordei Germinatus Ustus), *jiāo shān zhā* (Fructus Crataegi) and *jiāo shén qū* (Massa Medicata Fermentata Ustus) 10g each.

41) Dry stools: *jiǔ zhì dà huáng* (Radix et Rhizoma Rhei, preserved in liquor, decocted later) 15g.

42) Inhibited urination: *zhū líng* (Polyporus) 15g, *huá shí* (Talcum) 15g and *shēng huáng qí* (Radix Astragali raw) 6g.

43) Drug-induced urinary block: *shēng shí gāo* (Gypsum Fibrosum Cruda) 30g, *chē qián zǐ* (Semen Plantaginis) 15g, *zhū líng* (Polyporus) 15g, and *huá shí* (Talcum) 15g.

44) Drug-induced amenorrhea: *táo rén* (Semen Persicae) 20g, *hóng huā* (Flos Carthami) 10g, *chì sháo* (Radix Paeoniae Rubra) 30g and *niú xī* (Radix Achyranthis Bidentatae) 30g.

45) Profuse menstruation: *dì yú tàn* (Radix Sanguisorbae, charred), *dù zhòng tàn* (Cortex Eucommiae, charred), and *cè bǎi tàn* (Cacumen Platycladi, charred) 30g each.

46) Abnormal liver function: within half a year from the onset, add *bǎn lán gēn* (Radix Isatidis) 30g, *hǔ zhàng* (Rhizoma Polygoni Cuspidati) 30g, and *yīn chén* (Herba Artemisiae Scopariae) 30g; with over half a year from the onset, add *jué míng zǐ* (Semen Cassiae) 15g, *bái sháo* (Radix Paeoniae Alba) 30g, *chì sháo* (Radix Paeoniae Rubra) 30g, *dāng guī* (Radix Angelicae Sinensis) 10g, *gǒu qǐ zǐ* (Fructus Lycii) 10g, and *wǔ wèi zǐ* (Fructus Schisandrae Chinensis) 10g.

47) Drug-related skin eruptions: *bái xiān pí* (Cortex Dictamni) 30g, *jīn yín huā* (Flos Lonicerae Japonicae) 30g, *pú gōng yīng* (Herba Taraxaci) 30g,

Chapter 11
Applications of Chinese Medicine in Psychiatry

mŭ dān pí (Cortex Moutan) 10g, *zĭ huā dì dīng* (Herba Violae) 30g and *huáng lián* (Rhizoma Coptidis) 10g.

48) Extensive depletion of qi and blood due to a chronic condition: *xī yáng shēn* (Radix Panacis Quinquefolii) 30g or *Bā Zhēn Tāng* (Eight Gem Decoction).

49) Deficiency signs among elderly people: *ròu cōng róng* (Herba Cistanches) 30g, *shān zhū yú* (Fructus Corni) 30g, *bā jĭ tiān* (Radix Morindae Officinalis) 15g, and *hé shŏu wū* (Radix Polygoni Multiflori) 30g.

50) Hair loss: *hé shŏu wū* (Radix Polygoni Multiflori) 30g, *hēi zhī má* (Semen Sesami Nigrum), and *shēng dì* (Radix Rehmanniae) 30g.

To successfully treat depression, one should apply modifications *Jú Shēn Tāng* according to the presenting patterns or symptoms. The dosages listed above are merely for reference, and they should always be adjusted carefully according to the condition. These formulas should not be self-prescribed; they should be administered only by a physician or Chinese medical practitioner, and the patient's progress must also be carefully monitored.

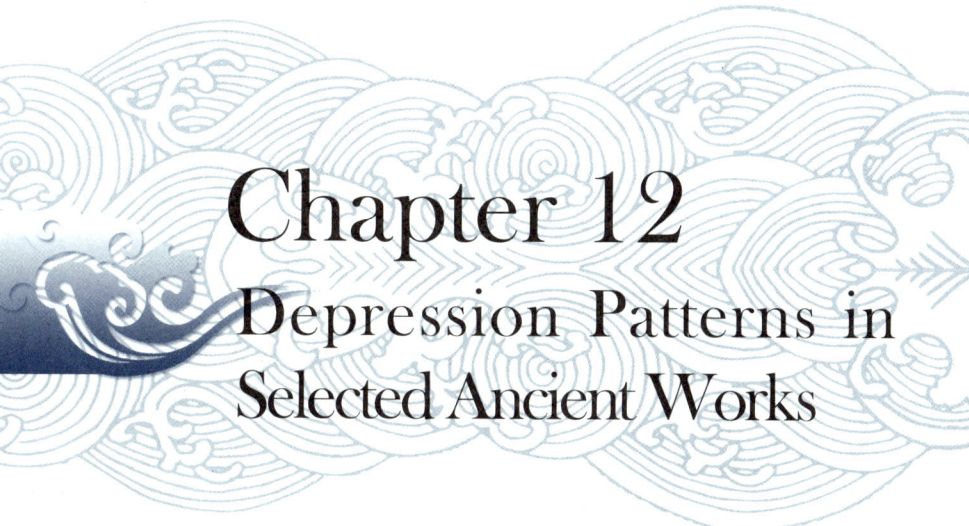

Chapter 12
Depression Patterns in Selected Ancient Works

The *Basic Questions* (Sù Wèn)

《素问》:"精气并于心则喜,并于肺则悲,并于肝则忧,并于脾则畏,并于肾则恐。"

"When essence qi accumulates in the heart then there is joy, when it accumulates in the lung then there is sorrow, when it accumulates in the liver then there is anxiety, when it accumulates in the spleen then there is fear, and when it accumulates in the kidney then there is fright."

"气血上逆,令人能善怒。"

"Counterflow ascent of qi and blood makes people irascible."

"血气内却,令人善恐。"

"Blood and qi declining internally makes people susceptible to fright."

"神有余则笑不休,神不足则悲。"

"If there is a surplus of spirit, there is incessant laughter; if there is insufficiency of the spirit, there is sorrow."

"余知百病生于气也,怒则气上,喜则气缓,悲则气消,恐则气下,寒则气收,炅则气泄,惊则气乱,劳则气耗,思则气结。"

"I know that the hundred diseases are engendered from qi. If there is anger, qi rises; joy, qi slackens; sorrow, qi disperses; fear, qi descends; cold, qi contracts; intense heat, there is discharge of qi; when there is fright, there is disruption of qi; when there is taxation, there is wearing of qi; when there is pensiveness, the qi binds."

The *Spiritual Pivot* (Líng Shū)

《灵枢》:"生之来谓之精,两精相搏谓之神,随神往来者谓之魂,并精而出入者谓之魄,所以任物者谓之心,心有所忆谓之意,意之所存谓之志,因志而存变谓之思,因思而远慕谓之虑,因虑而处物谓之智。"

"That which forms life is called essence; two kinds of essence contending with one another is called spirit; that which comes and goes with the spirit is called the ethereal soul; that which exits and enters along with the essence is called the corporeal soul. That which dominates these things is called the heart; when the heart has a recollection, it is called the intention; the storage of intention is called mind; based on the mind, the observation of changes is called thought; the foresight based on thought is called consideration; and handling things based on consideration is called wisdom."

Chapter 12
Depression Patterns in Selected Ancient Works

"是故怵惕思虑者则伤神，神伤则恐惧流淫而不止。因悲哀动中者，竭绝而失生；喜乐者，神惮散而不藏；愁忧者，气闭塞而不行；盛怒者，迷惑而不治；恐惧者，神荡惮而不收。"

"Therefore apprehensiveness, thought and preoccupation damage the spirit; and when the spirit is damaged, there is fear and incessant flowing and leaking. Sorrow that affects the middle results in exhaustion, expiration [of the vessels and collaterals] and eventually loss of life. Joy results in an unrestrained spirit that cannot be stored. Sorrow results in blockage and stoppage of qi. Exuberant anger results in untreatable confusion. Fear results in an instability of the spirit that cannot be constrained."

"心怵惕思虑则伤神，神伤则恐惧自失，破（䐃）脱肉……。脾愁忧而不解则伤意，意伤则悗乱，四肢不举。肝悲哀动中则伤魂，魂伤则狂忘不精，不精则不正当，人阴缩而挛筋，两胁骨不举……。肺喜乐无极则伤魄，魄伤则狂，狂者意不存人，皮革焦……。肾盛怒而不止则伤志，志伤则喜忘其前言，腰脊不可以俯仰屈伸……。恐惧而不解则伤精，精伤则骨酸痿厥，精时自下。是故五脏主藏精者也，不可伤，伤则失守而阴虚；阴虚则无气，无气则死矣。"

"If there is apprehensiveness, thought, and preoccupation of the heart, there will be damage to the spirit; if there is a damaged spirit, there is involuntary fear resulting in a loss of bulk and the shedding of flesh.

If there is unresolved anxiety of the spleen, there is damage to the intention; if the intention is damaged, there is oppression and derangement which results in an inability to lift the limbs.

If there is sorrow of the liver affecting the center, there will be damage to the ethereal soul; a damaged ethereal soul causes mania and a loss of essence that result in retracted genitals, hypertonicity of the sinews, and pain of the bones in the rib-sides.

When there is incessant joy of the lung, there will be damage to the corporeal soul; if there is damage to the corporeal soul, there is mania with inability to observe, and the skin looks as if it has been scorched.

If there is incessant exuberant anger in the kidney, there will be damage to the mind; if there is a damaged mind, there will be forgetfulness of what one has said and an inability to bend backward and forward in the lumbus and spine.

If there is unresolved fear, there will be damage to the essence. Damaged essence causes aching bones, wilting, reversal, and spontaneous descent of essence.

Since the five viscera govern the storage of essence, they must remain undamaged. Otherwise, they will fail to keep their composure and cause a deficiency of yin. If yin is deficient, the body will be without qi, and without qi there is death."

"是故用针者，察观病人之态，以知精神魂魄之存亡得失之意，五者以伤，针不可以治之也。"

"Therefore, the one who uses needles should observe the status of the patient in order to determine the presence, absence, and gain or loss of the essence, spirit, ethereal soul and corporeal soul. When those five are damaged, it will be impossible to treat with needles."

"肝藏血，血舍魂，肝气虚则恐，实则怒。脾藏营，营舍意，脾气虚则四肢不用，五脏不安，实则腹胀经溲不利。心藏脉，脉舍神，心气虚则悲，实则笑不休。肺藏气，气舍魄，肺气虚，则鼻塞不利少气，实则喘喝胸盈仰息。肾藏精，精舍志，肾气虚则厥，实则胀。

五脏不安，必审五脏之病形，以知其气之虚实，谨而调之也。"

"The liver stores blood and blood is the abode of the ethereal soul. If liver qi is deficient, there will be fear, while with excess there will be anger.

The spleen stores *ying*, and *ying* is the abode of intention. If there is spleen qi deficiency, there will be a loss of use of the limbs and disquiet in the five viscera; with excess, there will be abdominal distention and inhibited menstruation, urination, and defecation.

The heart stores the vessels, and the vessels are the abode of the spirit. If heart qi is deficient, there will be sorrow; with excess, there will be incessant laughing.

The lung stores qi and qi is the abode of the corporeal soul. If there is lung qi deficiency, there will be inhibition and congestion of the nose as well as a shortage of qi, while with excess, there will be rapid breathing with hoarse sounds, fullness of the chest, and panting with one's face turned upward.

The kidney stores essence, and essence is the abode of the mind. If there is kidney qi deficiency, there will be reversal, while with excess, there

Chapter 12
Depression Patterns in Selected Ancient Works

will be swelling.

When the five viscera are not peaceful, one must examine the pathological status of the five viscera to understand the excess or deficiency of qi and cautiously regulate it."

Unified Treatise on Diseases, Patterns and Remedies according to the Three Causes (Sān Yīn Jí Yī Bìng Zhèng Fāng Lùn)

《三因极一病证方论》:"夫五脏六腑,阴阳升降,非气不生。神静则宁,情动则乱,故有喜怒忧思悲恐惊,七者不同,各随其本脏所生所伤而为病。故喜伤心,其气散;怒伤肝,其气激;忧伤肺,其气聚;思伤脾,其气结;悲伤心胞,其气急;恐伤肾,其气怯;惊伤胆,其气乱。虽七诊自殊,无逾于气。黄帝曰:余知百病生于气也。但古论有寒热忧恚,而无思悲恐惊,似不伦类,予恐未然。六腑无说,惟胆有者,盖是奇恒净腑,非转输例,故能蓄惊而为病。"

"The yin and yang, ascending and descending movements of the five viscera and six bowels cannot be created without qi. If the spirit is tranquil, there is peace, while stirred emotions result in turmoil. There are seven distinguishable emotions: joy, anger, anxiety, pensiveness, sorrow, fear and fright. Each emotion can cause diseases according to what their associated viscera are engendered from or damaged by.

So joy damages the heart and causes its qi to disperse; anger damages the liver and causes its qi to surge; anxiety damages the lung and causes its qi to gather; thought damages the spleen and causes its qi to bind; sorrow damages the pericardium and causes its qi to rush; fear damages the kidney and causes qi timidity; fright damages the gallbladder and causes qi disruption. Although the seven diagnoses are different, the cause is no more than qi.

The Yellow Emperor stated: 'I know that the hundred diseases are engendered from qi.' However, this classical statement only includes cold, heat, anxiety and anger; thought, sorrow, fear and fright are omitted. This does not seem to fit the classification, and I am afraid this is not correct. There are no theories regarding the emotional nature of the six bowels except for the gallbladder; this is because the gallbladder is an extraordinary organ that does more than transforming and transporting, therefore fright can amass and cause diseases."

Unified Treatise on Diseases, Patterns and Remedies according to the Three Causes (Sān Yīn Jí Yī Bìng Zhèng Fāng Lùn)

《三因极一病证方论》:"夫喜伤心者,自汗,不可疾行,不可久立,故《经》曰:喜则气散。怒伤肝者,上气,不可忍,时来荡心,短气不得息,欲绝,故《经》曰:怒则气击。忧伤肺气,心系急,上焦闭,荣卫不通,夜卧不安,故《经》曰:忧则气聚。思伤脾者,气留而不行,积聚在中脘,不得饮食,腹胀满,四肢怠惰,故《经》曰,思则气结。悲伤心胞者,善忘,不识人,置物在处,还取不得,筋挛,四肢浮肿,故《经》曰:悲则气急。恐伤肾者,上焦气闭不行,下焦回还不散,犹豫不决,呕逆恶心,故《经》曰:恐则精却。惊伤胆者,神无所归,虑无所定,说物不竟而迫,故《经》曰:惊则气乱。"

"Joy damaging the heart manifests with spontaneous sweating and an inability to walk quickly or stand for long periods; therefore *The Inner Classic* (Nèi Jīng) says: 'Joy causes qi to disperse.'

Anger damaging the liver manifests with an intolerable ascent of qi that constantly affects the heart, and a shortness of qi that makes one unable to breathe and to feel like he is dying; thus *The Inner Classic* says: 'Anger causes qi to attack.'

Anxiety damaging the lung qi manifests with tension of the heart tie, blockage of the upper burner, inhibition of the *ying* and *wei*, and unquiet sleep. Therefore *The Inner Classic* states, 'Anxiety causes qi to gather.'

Thought damaging the spleen manifests with qi retention and stoppage, gatherings and accumulations in the middle stomach duct, inability to eat or drink, abdominal distention and fullness, and fatigue in the extremities. Therefore *The Inner Classic* says: 'Thought causes qi to bind.'

When sorrow damages the pericardium it manifests with forgetfulness, an inability to recognize people or remember where one has put things, hypertonicity of the sinews, and puffy swelling of the limbs. Therefore *The Inner Classic* states, 'Sorrow causes qi to move urgently.'

Fear damaging the kidney manifests with qi blockage in the upper burner and non-dissipation in the lower burner, hesitation, indecision, retching counterflow and nausea. Therefore *The Inner Classic* states, 'Fear causes essence to decline.'

With fright damaging the gallbladder, the spirit has no place to return and the thoughts cannot be settled; when one tries to say something, he

Chapter 12
Depression Patterns in Selected Ancient Works

will feel distressed before he can finish. Therefore *The Inner Classic* states, 'Fright causes qi disruption.'"

Teachings of [Zhu] Dan-xi (*Dān Xī Xīn Fǎ*)

《丹溪心法》:"气血冲和,万病不生,一有怫郁,诸病生焉。故人身诸病,多生于郁。苍术、抚芎,总解诸郁,随证加入诸药。凡郁皆在中焦,以苍术、抚芎开提其气以升之。假如食在气上,提其气则食自降矣。"

"If qi and blood flow in harmony, none of the ten thousand diseases will be engendered; as soon as there is depression, all diseases can potentially be engendered. Thus those various diseases that occur in the human body are commonly engendered from depression. *Cāng zhú* (Rhizoma Atractylodis) and *chuān xiōng* (Rhizoma Chuanxiong) resolve all depressions and may be added to various formulas according to the pattern. All depressions are located in the middle burner. Use *cāng zhú* and *chuān xiōng* to open and uplift qi in order to upbear the depression. If food is stagnated above the qi, upbearing qi will cause the food to downbear spontaneously."

'"戴云:郁者,结聚而不得发越也。当升者不得升,当降者不得降,当变化者不得变化也。传化失常,六郁之病见矣。气郁者,胸胁痛,脉沉涩;湿郁者,周身走痛,或关节痛,遇寒则发,脉沉细;痰郁者,动则喘,寸口脉沉滑;热郁者,瞀闷,小便赤,脉沉数;血郁者四肢无力,能食便红,脉沉;食郁者,嗳酸,腹饱不能食,人迎脉平和,气口脉繁盛者是也。"

"Physician Dai comments: Depression is related to bindings and gatherings that are unable to be brought up and out. Movements of ascending, descent and transformation cannot be carried out. When there is abnormal transport and transformation, the conditions of the six depressions will arise.

Qi depression manifests with pain in the chest and rib-sides and sunken, rough pulses. Damp depression manifests with scurrying pain all over the body or pain in the joints that can be brought on by exposure to cold, and the pulses are sunken and fine. Phlegm depression manifests with panting on exertion and sunken slippery pulses at the inch openings. Heat depression manifests with dizziness, oppression, red urine and sunken rapid pulses. Blood depression manifests with weak limbs, an ability to eat, red stools, and sunken pulses. Food depression manifests with sour belching, a full abdomen with an inability to eat, calm harmonious pulses at *ren ying*, and exuberant pulses at the inch openings."

The Orthodox Tradition of Medicine (Yī Xué Zhèng Chuán)

《医学正传》:"……我丹溪先生触类而长之，而又着为六郁之证，所谓气血冲和，百病不生，一有怫郁，诸病生焉，此发前人之所未发者也。夫所谓六郁者，气、湿、热、痰、血、食六者是也。或七情之抑遏，或寒热之交侵，故为九气怫郁之候。或雨湿之侵凌，或酒浆之积聚，故为留饮湿郁之疾。又如热郁而成痰，痰郁而成癖，血郁而成，食郁而成痞满，此必然之理也。又气郁而湿滞，湿滞而成热，热郁而成痰，痰滞而血不行，血滞而食不消化，此六者皆相因而为病者也。是以治法皆当以顺气为先，消积次之，故药中多用香附、抚芎之类，至理存焉，学人宜知此意。"

"When he encountered this category of conditions, Zhu Dan-xi expanded upon this to invent the patterns of six depressions. It is said that if qi and blood flow are harmonious, none of the ten thousand diseases will be engendered; as soon as there is depression, all diseases can be engendered. This idea was an innovation not seen before. Six depressions refer to qi, dampness, heat, phlegm, blood, and food depression.

Constraint of the seven emotions or invasion of cold and heat can lead to depression of the nine qi. Invasion of rain dampness or the gathering of alcoholic liquids can lead to diseases of rheum retention and damp depression. In addition, depressed heat results in phlegm, depressed phlegm results in aggregation of blood, depressed blood leads to conglomeration of food, and depressed food leads to glomus and fullness; these are the definite rules. Also, depressed qi leads to damp stagnation, depressed heat leads to phlegm, stagnated phlegm leads to blood stoppage, and stagnated blood leads to food indigestion; these six conditions cause one another, therefore the treatment methods should all primarily focus on normalizing qi, and look to disperse the accumulation.

So, among medicinals, *xiāng fù* (Rhizoma Cyperi), *chuān xiōng* (Rhizoma Chuanxiong) and similar things are commonly used. This represents the ultimate truth. Those who study should understand this intention."

Chapter 12
Depression Patterns in Selected Ancient Works

The Gateway to Medicine (Yī Xué Rù Mén)

《医学入门》:"脱营愚者眠食废。

先顺后逆,虽不中邪,病从内生,令人饮食无味,神倦肌瘦,名曰脱营。"

"The fools with *ying* desertion give up sleep and food.

With adversity of life circumstances following prosperity, although there is no strike of external evils, the disease develops from the interior and causes an inability to taste food, fatigue and emaciation. This is called *ying* desertion. "

"有志养阴神自充。

平人上纳下化,水谷滋沛身中,阴气自生。如失名利之士,有志恢图,过于劳倦,形气衰少,谷气不盛,上焦不行,下脘不通而胃热,热熏胸中则内热。……若不早治,复恣酒色,痨瘵之由也。"

"If there is mind to nourish yin, the spirit will be fulfilled naturally.

Normal people receive in the upper body and transform in the lower, thus water and grain nourishes the body and yin qi is naturally engendered. If a man who has lost fame and profit has the notion to stage a comeback, he may suffer from excessive taxation which leads to debilitation of physique and qi, as well as a non-exuberance of grain qi. There will be stoppage in the upper burner and blockage in the lower stomach duct with stomach heat. Heat fumes in the chest and causes internal heat. If treatment is not applied early and there is additional indulgence in alcohol or sexual activities, consumption will result."

Universal Salvation Formulary (Pǔ Jì Fāng)

《普济方》:"惊悸与忪悸不同,惊悸有所大惊,或闻虚响,或见异相,登高陟险,梦寐不祥,惊忤心神,气与涎郁,遂使惊悸,名曰心惊胆寒,在心胆经,属木,内外因,其脉心动。"

"Fright palpitations are different from fearful palpitations. In fright palpitations, there is a great fright, either hearing imaginary sounds or seeing strange images, climbing high mountains, and dreaming of things that seem like bad luck and disturb the heart; qi is constrained by drool, and fright palpitation results. This is called heart fright and gallbladder cold. It is located in the heart and gallbladder channels, ascribed to wood, and is due to neutral causes. The associated pulse is stirring at the heart position."

"怔忡则因汲汲富贵，戚戚贫贱，久思所爱，遽失所重，触事不意，气郁涎聚，遂致怔忡，在心脾经，意思所主，属内所因。"

"Fearful palpitations are related to an eagerness for riches, longstanding poverty, endless pining for that which one loves, a sudden loss of what one treasures, or personal frustration. Qi is constrained and drool gathers, and fearful palpitation results. This is located in the heart and spleen channels, governed by intention and thought, and is due to internal causes."

"或冒风暑湿塞闭诸经，令人忽忽若有所失，恐恐如人将捕，中脘怔忡，此乃外邪，非因心病，况五饮停蓄，闭于中脘，最使人怔忡，治属饮家。除饮悸与外内因所治："

"Due to contraction of wind, summerheat, or dampness, the channels may become congested and blocked. This can cause people to become absent-minded as if emotionally insecure, and afraid as if they are about to be arrested. This fearful palpitation of the middle stomach duct is caused by external evil, not heart conditions. Besides, when the five rheum are retained and block the middle stomach duct, fearful palpitation easily results. Treatment should follow that of a rheum pattern. To eliminate rheum, palpitations, and the external and internal causes, the treatment is as follows:"

"人之所主者心，心之所养者血，心血一虚，神气不守，此惊悸之所肇端也。惊与悸其可无辨，惊者恐怖之谓，悸者怔忪之谓，心虚而郁痰，则耳闻大声，目击异物，遇险临危，触事丧志，心为之忤，使人有惕惕之状，是则为惊，心虚而停水则胸中渗漉，虚气流动，水既上乘，心火恶之，心不自安，使人有怏怏之状，是则为悸。惊者，与之豁痰定惊之剂。悸者，与之逐水消饮之剂，所为扶虚，不过调养心血，和平心气而已。若一切以刚燥用工，或者心火自炎，又有热生风之证。"

"The heart governs the body, and blood nourishes the heart. Once heart blood is deficient, spirit qi will fail to maintain its composure. This is the beginning of fright palpitation. Fright and palpitation should be distinguished. Fright refers to fear and palpitation refers to fearful throbbing. Heart deficiency with constrained phlegm leads to hearing loud sounds, seeing macabre things, encountering danger and deadly peril, or encountering events that make one despondent and cause the

Chapter 12
Depression Patterns in Selected Ancient Works

heart to rebel, also making the person feel apprehensive; this results in fright. On the other hand, heart deficiency with water collecting causes percolating and gurgling in the chest; the deficient qi flows and water rises to overwhelm the upper burner. Heart fire is averse to this, thus the heart cannot calm itself and the person may appear disgruntled; this results in palpitations.

For fright, apply formulas that flush phlegm and settle fright. For palpitations, apply formulas that expel water and disperse phlegm. To support deficiency, the methods are simply to regulate and nourish heart blood while harmonizing and calming the qi of the heart. Take caution, for if the whole treatment is harsh and drying, the result is either heart fire spontaneously flaring up, or a pattern of heat engendering wind."

"心为帝王，神之所舍，诸藏之主，不受外邪。若人动止非宜，寒暄失节，脏腑内损，气血外伤，风邪乘虚入于心经则令人心不定，性识失常，乍喜乍怒，或歌或笑，精神离散，悲乐不恒，故名风邪也。"

"The heart is the emperor and the abode of the spirit. It governs all of the viscera, and does not contract external evil. If a person's way of living is inappropriate or one fails to adjust to the seasons, the viscera and bowels will become damaged interiorly and qi and blood will be harmed at the exterior; wind evil will exploit the deficiency and enter the heart channel. This causes disquietude of the heart manifesting with an abnormal personality and mind, abrupt joy and anger, singing, laughing, separation of essence and spirit, and brief spells of sorrow and happiness. This is therefore called wind evil."

Jing-yue's Complete Works (Jǐng Yuè Quán Shū)

《景岳全书》："凡五气之郁，则诸病皆有，此因病而郁也；至若情志之郁，则总由乎心，此因郁而病也。第自古言郁者，但知解郁顺气，通作实邪论治，不无失矣。兹予辨其三证，庶可无误，盖一曰怒郁，二曰思郁，三曰忧郁。"

"Depression of the five qi can be seen in various diseases; that is to say when disease leads to depression. Depressed emotions are always related to the heart; that is to say when depression leads to disease. With regard to depression since the ancient times, treatment has remained limited to resolving depression and normalizing qi based on the idea that

the pattern is due to excess evils, and this view is not without faults. Here is a differentiation of three patterns, and hopefully they will be borne out in practice. The first is anger-related depression, the second is thought-related depression, and the third is anxiety-related depression."

"如怒郁者，方其大怒气逆之时，则实邪在肝，多见气满腹胀，所当平也。及其怒后而逆气已去，惟中气受伤矣，既无胀满疼痛等证，而或为倦怠，或为少食，此以木邪克土，损在脾矣，是可不知培养而仍在消伐，则所伐者其谁乎？此怒郁之有先后，亦有虚实，所当辨治者如此。"

"For anger-related depression, at a time of great anger with qi counterflow, the excess evil is located in the liver. Common manifestations include qi fullness and abdominal distention. This should be calmed. After the anger has passed, the counterflow qi is eliminated but the middle burner qi remains damaged. There are no symptoms of distention, fullness, or pain, but fatigue or a reduced appetite may occur. This is due to wood evil restraining earth and damaging the spleen. If the physician does not know to bank and nourish the spleen, but rather continues to disperse and attack the liver, then what is being attacked? This exemplifies the sequence of deficiency and excess of anger-related depression that should be differentiated and treated accordingly. "

"又若思郁者，则惟旷女嫠妇，及灯窗困厄，积疑任怨者皆有之。思则气结，结于心而伤于脾也。……然以情病者，非情不解，其在女子，必得愿遂而后可释，或以怒胜思，亦可暂解；其在男子，使非有能屈能伸，达观上智者，终不易却也。若病已既成，损伤必甚，而再行消伐，其不明也亦甚矣。"

"Thought depression can be seen in unmarried girls, widows, men who fail to obtain a career, or in those with accumulated suspicion or deep resentments. Thought causes qi to bind; the bind is located in the heart and this will cause damage to the spleen.

Diseases caused by emotional factors can only be resolved by emotion. For a woman, only if she gets what she wishes for can there be relief; in other cases, when there is anger that overcomes her pensiveness, the condition can also be resolved temporarily. For a man, unless he has a flexible personality, an open mind, and superior wisdom, the condition will be hard to dispel. If the disease has formed, the damage will be

Chapter 12
Depression Patterns in Selected Ancient Works

severe; to disperse and attack on top of that is extremely unwise."

"又若忧郁病者，则全属大虚，本无邪实，此多以衣食之累，利害之牵，及悲忧惊恐而致郁者，总皆受郁之类。盖悲则气消，忧则气沉，必伤脾肺；惊则气乱，恐则气下，必伤肝肾，此其戚戚悠悠，精气但有消索，神志不振，心脾日以耗伤。"

"All anxiety depression is ascribed to great deficiency; there is no evil excess. This kind of depression is commonly caused by the burden of providing for one's daily needs and concerns regarding one's personal interests, as well as sorrow, anxiety, fright and fear. In general, all of this is the contraction of depression.

Sorrow causes qi to disperse and anxiety causes qi to sink; these will damage the spleen and lung. Fright will cause disruption of qi and fear causes qi to descend; these will damage the liver and kidney. With sorrow and sadness, essence and qi can only be dispersed and exhausted; the spirit and mind will be devitalized, and the heart and spleen will be progressively worn and damaged."

"一、怒郁之治：若暴怒伤肝，逆气未解，而为胀满或疼痛者，宜解肝煎、神香散，或六郁汤，或越鞠丸。若怒气伤肝，因而动火，以致烦热，胁痛胀满或动血者，宜化肝煎。若怒郁不解或生痰者，宜温胆汤。若怒后逆气既散，肝脾受伤，而致倦怠食少者，宜五味异功散，或五君子煎，或大营煎、归脾汤之类调养之。"

"1) Treatment for anger-related depression: If sudden violent anger damages the liver and the counterflow qi remains unresolved, distention, fullness and pain will result; *Jiě Gān Jiān* (Liver-Releasing Brew), *Shén Xiāng Sǎn* (Spirit Aroma Powder), *Liù Yù Tāng* (Six-Depression Decoction) and *Yuè Jū Wán* (Depression-Resolving Pill) are recommended.

If anger damages the liver and stirs fire resulting in vexation and heat with rib-side pain, distention, fullness, or stirring of blood, *Huà Gān Jiān* (Liver-Resolving Brew) is recommended.

If anger depression remains unresolved or engenders phlegm, *Wēn Dǎn Tāng* (Gallbladder-Warming Decoction) is recommended.

If after the anger, counterflow qi has dissipated, but damage to the liver and spleen results in fatigue and reduced eating, *Wǔ Wèi Yì Gōng Sǎn* (Five-Ingredients Special Achievement Powder), *Wǔ Jūn Zǐ Jiān* (Five

Gentlemen Brew) or formulas like *Dà Yíng Jiān* (Major Ying Brew) and *Guī Pí Tāng* (Spleen-Restoring Decoction) are recommended for regulation and nourishment."

"一、思郁之治：若初有郁结滞逆不开者，宜和胃煎加减主之，或二陈汤，或沉香降气散，或启脾丸皆可择用。凡妇人思郁不解，致伤冲任之源，而血气日亏，渐至经脉不调，或短少渐闭者，宜逍遥饮，或大营煎。若思忆不遂，以致遗精带浊，病在心肺不摄者，宜秘元煎。若思虑过度，以致遗精滑泄及经脉错乱，病在肝肾不固者，宜固阴煎。若思郁动火，以致崩淋失血，赤带内热，经脉错乱者，宜保阴煎。若思郁动火，阴虚肺热，烦渴，咳嗽见血，或骨蒸夜热者，宜四阴煎，或一阴煎酌宜用之。若生儒寒厄，思结枯肠，及任劳任怨，心脾受伤，以致怔忡健忘，倦怠食少，渐至消瘦，或为膈噎呕吐者，宜寿脾煎，或七福饮；若心膈气有不顺或微见疼痛者，宜归脾汤，或加砂仁、白豆蔻、丁香之类以微顺之。"

"2) Treatment for thought-related depression: when depression, binding and stagnation reversal first appear, modified *Hé Wèi Jiān* (Stomach-Harmonizing Brew) is recommended; *Èr Chén Tāng* (Two Matured Substances Decoction), *Chén Xiāng Jiàng Qì Sǎn* (Aquilaria Qi-Downbearing Powder), or *Qǐ Pí Wán* (Spleen-Arousing Pill) can also be selected.

For women with unresolved thought depression that causes damage to the source of the penetrating and conception vessels leading to gradual depletion of blood and qi which results in irregular menstruation, inhibited scanty menses, or even menstrual block, *Xiāo Yáo Yǐn* (Free Wanderer Beverage) or *Dà Yíng Jiān* (Major Ying Brew) is recommended.

When there is dissatisfaction and pensiveness resulting in seminal emission with turbidity, the disease is associated with heart and lung failing to properly contain, and *Mì Yuán Jiān* (Origin-Securing Brew) is recommended.

With excessive thought and preoccupation resulting in seminal emission, efflux diarrhea, or irregular menstruation, the disease is associated with insecurity of the liver and kidney, *Gù Yīn Jiān* (Yin-Securing Brew) is recommended.

With thought and preoccupation stirring fire resulting in flooding, strangury, blood loss, a red vaginal discharge with internal heat, and irregular menstruation, *Bǎo Yīn Jiān* (Yin-Preserving Brew) is

Chapter 12
Depression Patterns in Selected Ancient Works

recommended.

With thought and preoccupation stirring fire and lung yin deficiency heat manifesting with vexation, thirst, coughing with blood, or steaming bones with night fever, *Sì Yīn Jiān* (Four Yin Brew) is recommended; *Yì Yīn Jiān* (One Yin Brew) is also recommended with proper modifications.

If a Confucian scholar encounters disaster and obstruction in his career with thought binding, hopelessness, taxation, and resentment, the heart and spleen will become damaged and result in fearful throbbing, forgetfulness, fatigue, reduced eating, gradual emaciation, or dysphagia-occlusion and vomiting. *Shòu Pí Jiān* (Spleen-Longevity Brew) or *Qī Fú Yǐn* (Seven Fortune Beverage) is recommended.

With abnormal qi or slight pain in the heart and diaphragm area, *Guī Pí Tāng* (Spleen-Restoring Decoction) is recommended. Medicinals such as *shā rén* (Fructus Amomi), *bái kòu rén* (Fructus Amomi Rotundus) and *dīng xiāng* (Flos Caryophylli) can be added for mild normalization."

"一、忧郁内伤之治：若初郁不开，未至内伤，而胸膈痞闷者，宜二陈汤、平胃散，或和胃煎，或调气平胃散，或神香散、或六君子汤之类以调之。若忧郁伤脾而吞酸呕恶者，宜温胃饮，或神香散。若忧郁伤脾肺而困倦、怔忡、倦怠、食少者，宜归脾汤，或寿脾煎。若忧思伤心脾，以致气血日消，饮食日减，肌肉日削者，宜五福饮、七福饮，甚者大补元煎。"

"3) Treatment for anxiety-related depression with internal damage: with initial depression that has not yet caused internal damage, where only glomus and oppression of the chest and diaphragm is present, *Èr Chén Tāng* (Two Matured Substances Decoction) and *Píng Wèi Sǎn* (Stomach-Calming Powder) are recommended; formulas such as *Hé Wèi Jiān* (Stomach-Harmonizing Brew), *Tiáo Qì Píng Wèi Sǎn* (Qi-Regulating Stomach-Calming Powder), *Shén Xiāng Sǎn* (Spirit Aroma Powder), or *Liù Jūn Zǐ Tāng* (Six Gentlemen Decoction) can also be selected for regulation.

With anxiety-related depression that has damaged the spleen manifesting with acid reflux, nausea and vomiting, select *Wēn Wèi Yǐn* or *Shén Xiāng Sǎn* (Spirit Aroma Powder).

With anxiety depression damaging the spleen and lung manifesting with fatigue, fearful throbbing, and reduced appetite, select *Guī Pí Tāng* (Spleen-Restoring Decoction) or *Shòu Pí Jiān* (Spleen-Longevity Brew).

With anxiety and pensiveness damaging the heart and spleen

resulting in gradual dispersion of qi and blood, reduced food intake and emaciation, select *Wǔ Fú Yǐn* (Five Fortune Beverage), *Qī Fú Yǐn* (Seven Fortune Beverage) or even *Dà Bǔ Yuán Jiān* (Major Origin-Supplementing Brew)."

Jing-yue's Complete Works (*Jǐng Yuè Quán Shū*)

《景岳全书》："附按：丹溪治一室女因事忤意，郁结在脾，半年不食，但日食熟菱枣数枚，遇喜，食馒头弹子大，深恶粥饭。朱意脾气实，非枳实不能散，以温胆汤去竹茹与之，数十帖而愈。"

"Associated commentary:

Zhu Dan-xi treated a virgin with depression binding in the spleen due to personal frustration. For half a year she did not eat anything but a few jujubes each day. When she was happy, she would eat a marble-sized piece of steamed bread. She deeply loathed porridge and rice.

Zhu thought that the excess of spleen qi could only be dissipated with *zhǐ shí*. He prescribed *Wēn Dǎn Tāng* (Gallbladder-Warming Decoction) with *zhú rú* (Caulis Bambusae in Taenia) removed. She was cured after a few dozen doses."

"一女许婚后，夫经商二年不归，因不食，困卧如痴，无他病，多向里床坐。此思想气结也，药难独治，得喜可解；不然令其怒，使其木气升发，而脾气自开，木能制土故也。因自往激之，大怒而哭，良久，令解之，与药一帖，即求食矣。予曰：病虽愈，必得喜方已。乃以夫回，既而果然，病遂不举。"

"A woman was married to a man who left on business just after their wedding and had been gone for more than two years. She refused to eat and would lay about, seemingly drowsy as if feeble-minded. No other signs or symptoms were noted except that she liked to sit next to the wall on the bed. This is qi binding due to pensiveness.

Medicinals would not be effective for this condition, but joy can resolve it. Otherwise, make the person angry so that wood-qi can uplift and diffuse, then the spleen qi will open spontaneously. This is because wood can restrain earth.

The physician went and provoked the woman himself and made her cry out in great anger. After a long time, he told her to stop and prescribed her one dose of medicinals; she immediately asked for food. The physician

Chapter 12
Depression Patterns in Selected Ancient Works

said, 'Although the disease appears to be resolved, joy must be gained to complete the treatment.' The husband was sent for, and then the disease was cured without relapse."

Compilation and Supplementation of Patterns and Treatments (Zhèng Zhì Huì Bǔ)

《证治汇补》:"郁宜调中。治郁之法,多以调中为要者,无他,盖脾胃居中,心肺在上,肾肝处下,四脏所受之邪,过于中者,中气常先受之。况乎饮食不节,寒暑不调,停痰积饮,而脾胃亦先受伤,所以中焦致郁恒多也,治宜开发运动,鼓舞中州,则三阴三阳之郁,不攻自解矣。"

"To treat depression, regulating the middle is recommended. Among the approaches of treating depression, the key is commonly to regulate the middle. This is simply because the spleen and stomach reside in the middle with heart and lung in the upper and kidney and liver in the lower. All the evil that these four viscera contract passes through the middle, and middle qi usually receives it first.

In addition, dietary irregularities, failure to adjust according to seasons, phlegm retention, and rheum accumulation also primarily affect the spleen and stomach. Therefore, depression frequently arises from the middle burner.

Treatment should open, diffuse and move. Once the middle burner earth is invigorated, depression of the three yin and three yang can be resolved without attacking."

"【附失精脱营】

饮食居处,暴乐暴苦,始乐后苦,皆伤精气。病从内生,其先富后贫而病,曰失精。先贵后贱而病,曰脱营。外症身渐瘦,无精神。(钱氏)又有郁结在脾,不思饮食,午后发热,酉戌时退,或烦闷渴呕,或坐卧如痴,喜向暗处,妇人经少,男子溺涩,皆郁病也,更有失名利之士,有志恢图,过于劳倦,形气衰少,谷气不盛,上焦不行,下脘不通,胃气热,热气熏胸中,因而内热,亦郁病也,宜归脾汤随症调之。"

"[Attachment: essence loss and *ying* desertion]

Regarding diet and lifestyle, sudden prosperity and adversity, or prosperity followed by adversity; these can all damage essence and qi. Disease engendered from the interior due to richness followed by poverty is called essence loss. Disease due to nobleness followed by lowness is called *ying* desertion. Physical symptoms include gradual emaciation and low spirits.

Physician Qian also discussed depression binding in the spleen manifesting with no thought for food or drink with heat effusion that occurs after noon and abates between 5pm and 9pm, or vexation with oppression, thirst and retching, or sitting and laying about as if feeble-minded, a preference for dark places, scant menses in women, and difficult urination in men. All these indicate depression disease.

In addition, if there are men who have lost their fame and profit and have the idea of staging a comeback, they may suffer from excessive taxation which leads to debilitation of their physique and qi, as well as non-exuberance of grain qi. There will be stoppage in the upper burner and blockage in the lower stomach duct with stomach heat. Heat fumes in the chest causes internal heat. This is also depression disease. It is recommended to use *Guī Pí Tāng* (Spleen-Restoring Decoction) and to regulate the condition according to the symptoms."

Zhang's Clear View of Medicine (*Zhāng Shì Yī Tōng*)

《张氏医通》:"郁证多缘于志虑不伸,而气先受病,故越鞠、四七始立也。郁之既久,火邪耗血,岂苍术、香附辈能久服乎,是逍遥、归脾继而设也。然郁证多患于妇人,《内经》所谓二阳之病发心脾,及思想无穷,所愿不得,皆能致病,为证不一,或发热头痛者有之,喘嗽气乏者有之,经闭不调者有之,狂癫失志者有之,火炎失血者有之,……治法总不离乎逍遥、归脾、佐金、降气、乌沉七气等方,但当参究新久虚实选用,加减出入可也。"

"Depression patterns are commonly caused by constrained minds and thoughts, and qi is the first affected by disease. Therefore *Yuè Jū Wán* (Depression-Resolving Pill) and *Sì Qī Tāng* (Four Seven Decoction) were created. If depression lasts over a period of time and fire evil wears on blood, how could medicinals like *cāng zhú* (Rhizoma Atractylodis) and *xiāng fù* (Rhizoma Cyperi) be taken for a long time? Therefore *Xiāo Yáo Săn* (Free Wanderer Powder) and *Guī Pí Tāng* (Spleen-Restoring Decoction) were later comprised. However, depression patterns are more commonly seen among women.

The *Inner Classic* stated that diseases of the two yang originate from the heart and spleen; in addition, endless pining or not getting what one

Chapter 12
Depression Patterns in Selected Ancient Works

wishes for can also lead to diseases. The manifestation varies. There may be heat effusion with headache, panting and coughing with lack of qi, menstrual block and irregularities, mania and withdrawal with loss of mind, or fire flaring with bleeding.

Treatment methods always involve formulas like *Xiāo Yáo Sǎn* (Free Wanderer Powder), *Guī Pí Tāng* (Spleen-Restoring Decoction), *Zuǒ Jīn Wán* (Left Metal Pill), *Chén Xiāng Jiàng Qì Sǎn* (Aquilaria Qi-Downbearing Powder), *Wū Chén Tāng* (Lindera and Aquilaria Decoction) and *Qī Qì Tāng* (Seven Qi Decoction). However, one should carefully examine whether the condition is recent or chronic or deficient or excess before selecting a formula, and then apply the proper modifications."

Incisive Light on the Source of Miscellaneous Diseases (*Zá Bìng Yuán Liú Xī Zhú*)

《杂病源流犀烛》："诸郁，脏气病也。其原本由思虑过深，更兼脏气弱，故六郁之病生焉。六郁者，气血湿热食痰也。诸郁之脉皆沉。六郁所挟，则兼芤涩数紧滑缓，或沉结促代，最宜细诊。"

"All depressions are diseases related to visceral qi. The root cause is excessively deep thought combined with weak visceral qi. That is how the diseases of six depressions are engendered. Six depressions refer to qi, blood, dampness, heat, food, and phlegm depression. The pulse image for all depressions is sunken; however, with the six depressions, scallion-stalk, rough, rapid, tight, slippery, and moderate pulses or sunken, bound, skipping and intermittent pulses may also be seen. This should be examined carefully."

"此外又有忧愁思虑之郁，先富后贫曰失精，先贵后贱曰脱荣，此郁开之极难，然究不外木达火发之义。赵献可则又谓东方生生之气在木，治木，诸郁自散，加味逍遥散最妙，柴胡、薄荷能升能清，逆无不达，兼以陈皮、川芎、白芍损肝之过，丹皮、山栀泻肝之实。木盛土衰，甘、术扶之。木伤血病者，当归养之。木实火燥，茯神宁之。

总之，凡治诸郁，均忌酸敛滞腻，宜开发志意，调气散结，和中健脾，如是止耳，否则非其治也。"

"In addition, there is also depression due to anxiety and pensiveness. Wealth followed by poverty is called essence loss; nobleness followed by lowness is called *ying* desertion. These types of depression are very hard to open. However, the principle is no more than freeing wood and diffusing fire. Physician Zhao Xian-ke also said that the qi of the east which engenders life is within wood, therefore, by treating wood all depressions will dissipate spontaneously.

Jiā Wèi Xiāo Yáo Sǎn (Supplemented Free Wanderer Powder) is most effective. *Chái hú* (Radix Bupleuri) and *bò he* (Herba Menthae) are capable of uplifting and clearing; they free all kinds of reversal. *Chén pí* (Pericarpium Citri Reticulatae), *chuān xiōng* (Rhizoma Chuanxiong) and *bái sháo* (Radix Paeoniae Alba) all reduce superabundance of the liver. *Mǔ dān pí* (Cortex Moutan) and *zhī zǐ* (Fructus Gardeniae) drains excess of the liver.

With wood exuberance and earth debilitation, support with *gān cǎo* (Radix et Rhizoma Glycyrrhizae) and *bái zhú* (Rhizoma Atractylodis Macrocephalae). With blood conditions due to wood damage, nourish with *dāng guī* (Radix Angelicae Sinensis). With wood excess and fire dryness, calm with *fú shén* (Sclerotium Poriae Pararadicis).

In a word, when treating all depressions, sour, astringing, stagnating and cloying medicinals are prohibited. It is appropriate to open the mind, regulate qi, dissipate binding, harmonize the middle, and fortify the spleen. Only by doing so can the disease be resolved. There is no other method."

Systematized Patterns with Clear-Cut Treatments (Lèi Zhèng Zhì Cái)

《类证治裁》："经言怵思虑则伤神，忧愁不解则伤意，悲哀动中则伤魂，喜乐无极则伤魄，盛怒不止则伤志，恐惧不解则伤精。此论气血之损。又言尝贵后贱，虽不中邪，病从内生，名曰脱营。尝富后贫，名曰失精，以及病发心脾，不得隐曲，思想无穷，所愿不得，皆情志之郁也。"

"*The Inner Classic* states that apprehensiveness, thought and preoccupation cause damage to the spirit; unresolved anxiety causes damage to the intention; sorrow affecting the middle causes damage to the ethereal soul; incessant joy causes damage to the corporeal soul; incessant exuberant anger causes damage to the mind; and unresolved fear causes damage to the essence.

This section discusses damage to qi and blood and, in addition, it states that in nobleness followed by lowliness, even though there is no strike of evil, there may be a disease engendered from the interior called

Chapter 12
Depression Patterns in Selected Ancient Works

ying desertion. Wealth followed by poverty is called essence loss.

There are also diseases arising from the heart and spleen; an inability to perform sexual activities, endless thinking, and an inability to fulfill one's desires are all related to emotional depression."

"七情内起之郁，始而伤气，继必及血，终乃成劳，主治宜苦辛凉润宣通。苦能泄热，辛能理气，凉润能濡燥，宣通能解结，用剂必气味相投，乃可取效。以郁为燥邪，必肺气失宣，不能升降。中气日结，不能运纳，至血液日涸，肌消骨蒸，经闭失调，乳岩项疬，而郁劳之症成，不止血嗽气膈，狂癫失志而已。"

"Depression can arise from the interior due to the seven emotions damaging qi in the initial stage, subsequently affecting the blood and eventually resulting in taxation. Bitter, acrid, cooling, moistening, diffusing, and freeing medicinals are indicated for this condition. Bitterness can discharge heat, acridity can rectify qi, cooling and moistening can moisten dryness, and the diffusing and freeing can resolve binding depression. Only when medicinals with suitable flavors are selected can there be an effective treatment.

Since depression is related to dryness evil, there will be a failure of lung qi to diffuse with an inability to ascend and descend. The middle qi binds over time and becomes unable to transport and absorb. This causes gradual desiccation of the blood, wasting of the flesh, steaming bones, menstrual block or menstrual irregularities, mammary rocks, scrofula of the nape of the neck, and the condition of depression taxation results. There will also be coughing of blood, qi occlusion, mania, withdrawal, and loss of one's mind."

"今分条列治，如思郁伤脾，气结，宜郁金、贝母、当归、柏子仁、桔梗、木香汁。思郁伤神，精滑。神伤必不摄肾，故遗精淋浊，固阴煎。思郁伤肝，潮热，逍遥散。思郁伤心脾，失血。归脾汤去白术，加白芍。"

"The following is a list of appropriate medicinals for the various treatment methods.

For thought depression damaging the spleen with qi binding: *yù jīn* (Radix Curcumae), *bèi mǔ* (Bulbus Fritillaria), *dāng guī* (Radix Angelicae Sinensis), *bǎi zǐ rén* (Semen Platycladi), *jié gěng* (Platycodonis) and the juice of *mù xiāng* (Radix Aucklandiae) are recommended.

For thought depression damaging the spirit with seminal efflux, the seminal emission and strangury-turbidity are caused by the damaged spirit failing to constrain the kidney. Use *Gù Yīn Jiān* (Yin-Securing Brew).

For thought depression damaging the liver with tidal fever, use *Xiāo Yáo Sǎn* (Free Wanderer Powder).

For thought depression damaging the heart and spleen with blood loss, use *Guī Pí Tāng* (Spleen-Restoring Decoction) with removed *bái zhú* (Rhizoma Atractylodis Macrocephalae) and added *bái sháo* (Radix Paeoniae Alba)."

"忧郁伤肺，气阻，杏仁、瓜蒌皮、郁金、枳壳、枇杷叶、竹沥、姜汁、半夏。忧郁伤中食少，七福饮去熟地，加砂仁。悲忧脏躁欲泣，甘麦大枣汤。"

For anxiety-related depression damaging the lung with qi obstruction, use *xìng rén* (Semen Armeniacae Amarum), *guā lóu pí* (Pericarpium Trichosanthis), *yù jīn* (Radix Curcumae), *zhǐ qiào* (Fructus Aurantii), *pí pá yè* (Folium Eriobotryae), *zhú lì* (Succus Bambusae), *jiāng zhī* (Succus Rhizomatis Zingiberis) and *bàn xià* (Rhizoma Pinelliae).

For anxiety depression damaging the middle with reduced appetite, use *Qī Fú Yǐn* (Seven Fortune Beverage) with removed *shú dì huáng* (Radix Rehmanniae Praeparata) and added *shā rén* (Fructus Amomi).

For sorrow, anxiety, and visceral agitation with a desire to weep, use *Gān Mài Dà Zǎo Tāng* (Licorice, Wheat and Jujube Decoction).

"惊郁胆怯欲迷，人参、枣仁、茯神、龙骨、石菖蒲、南枣、小麦。惊郁神乱欲狂，清心温胆汤。"

"For fright depression with gallbladder timidity on verge of stupor, use *rén shēn* (Radix et Rhizoma Ginseng), *suān zǎo rén* (Semen Ziziphi Spinosae), *fú shén* (Sclerotium Poriae Pararadicis), *lóng gǔ* (Os Draconis), *shí chāng pú* (Rhizoma Acori Tatarinowii), *dà zǎo* (Fructus Jujubae) and *xiǎo mài* (Fructus Tritici).

For fright depression with a deranged spirit on verge of mania, *Qīng Xīn Wēn Dǎn Tāng* (Heart-Clearing Gallbladder-Warming Decoction) is indicated."

"怒郁肝伤气逆，解肝煎。怒郁火升动血，化肝煎。"

Chapter 12
Depression Patterns in Selected Ancient Works

"For anger depression with liver damage and qi reversal, *Jiě Gān Jiān* (Liver-Releasing Brew) is indicated. For anger depression with fire ascending that stirs blood, *Huà Gān Jiān* (Liver-Resolving Brew) is indicated."

"恐郁阳消精怯，八味丸加减，或鹿角胶酒化服。"
"For fear depression with yang dispersion and essence declining, use modified *Bā Wèi Wán* (Eight-Ingredients Pill), or take dissolved *lù jiǎo jiāo* (Colla Cornus Cervi) with wine."

"诸郁久，风阳内生，眩悸咽痛，宜阿胶、生地、石斛、茯神、牡蛎、白芍、麦冬、甘草。"
"For any enduring depression that results in internally engendered wind yang with dizziness, palpitations and sore throat, *ē jiāo* (Colla Corii Asini), *shēng dì* (Radix Rehmanniae), *shí hú* (Caulis Dendrobii), *fú shén* (Sclerotium Poriae Pararadicis), *mǔ lì* (Concha Ostreae), *bái sháo* (Radix Paeoniae Alba), *mài mén dōng* (Ophiopogonis) and *gān cǎo* (Radix et Rhizoma Glycyrrhizae) are recommended."

"气郁脉沉而涩，七气汤。血郁脉涩而芤，四物化郁汤。气郁生涎心悸，温胆汤。血郁络伤胁痛，金铃子散加桃仁、归须、郁金、降真香。"
"For qi depression with sunken rough pulses, use *Qī Qì Tāng* (Seven Qi Decoction).

For blood depression with rough, scallion-stalk pulses, use *Sì Wù Huà Yù Tāng* (Four Substances Depression-Resolving Decoction).

For qi depression with drool and palpitations, use *Wēn Dǎn Tāng* (Gallbladder-Warming Decoction).

For blood depression with damage to the collaterals and rib-side pain, use *Jīn Líng Zǐ Sǎn* (Toosendan Powder) with added *táo rén* (Semen Persicae), *guī xū* (Radicis Angelicae Sinensis Tenuis), *yù jīn* (Radix Curcumae) and *jiàng xiāng* (Lignum Dalbergiae Odoriferae)."

"肺脾郁，营损肌瘦，养营汤去桂心，减熟地黄。心脾郁，怔忡崩漏，归脾汤。肝胆郁，血燥结核，加味逍遥散。若嘈杂吞酸，逍遥佐金汤。脾胃郁，气噎哕呃，金匮麦门冬汤加竹茹、丁香。三焦郁，口干不食，栀子仁姜汁浸炒黑研细，以人参、麦冬、乌梅煎汤服。"

"For depression of the lung and spleen with damaged *ying* and emaciation, use *Yǎng Yíng Tāng* (Ying-Nourishing Decoction) with removed *guì xīn* (Cortex Cinnamomi Rasus) and a reduced dosage of *shú dì huáng* (Radix Rehmanniae Praeparata).

For depression of the heart and spleen with fearful throbbing, and flooding and spotting, use *Guī Pí Tāng* (Spleen-Restoring Decoction).

For depression of the liver and gallbladder with blood dryness binding into nodes, use *Jiā Wèi Xiāo Yáo Sǎn* (Supplemented Free Wanderer Powder); with clamoring stomach and acid swallowing, use *Xiāo Yáo Zuǒ Jīn Tāng* (Free Wanderer Left Metal Decoction).

For depression of the spleen and stomach with qi occlusion and hiccoughing, use *Jīn Guì Mài Mén Dōng Tāng* (Golden Cabinet's Ophiopogon Decoction) with added *zhú rú* (Caulis Bambusae in Taenia) and *dīng xiāng* (Flos Caryophylli).

For triple burner depression with a dry mouth and an inability to eat, soak the *zhī zǐ* (Fructus Gardeniae) in ginger juice, stir-fry until black, grind finely, and decoct with *rén shēn* (Radix et Rhizoma Ginseng), *mài mén dōng* (Ophiopogonis) and *wū méi* (Fructus Mume)."

"若夫六气之火郁,散之。火郁汤。寒郁成热,泻之。羚羊角、山栀、生白芍、丹皮、川黄连、川石斛。湿郁除之。除湿汤、平胃散。痰郁涤之。润下丸,或二陈汤加海石、瓜蒌、贝母、竹沥。食郁消之。保和丸。"

"For fire depression of the six qi, dissipate with *Huǒ Yù Tāng* (Fire-Depression Decoction).

For cold depression resulting in heat, drain with *líng yáng jiǎo* (Cornu Saigae Tataricae), *zhī zǐ* (Fructus Gardeniae), *shēng bái sháo* (Radix Paeoniae Alba, raw), *mǔ dān pí* (Cortex Moutan), *chuān huáng lián* (Rhizoma Coptidis Sichuanense), and *chuān shí hú* (Caulis Dendrobii Sichuanense).

For damp depression, eliminate with *Chú Shī Tāng* (Dampness-Eliminating Decoction) and *Píng Wèi Sǎn* (Stomach-Calming Powder).

For phlegm depression, flush with *Rùn Xià Wán* (Lower-Moistening Pill), or *Èr Chén Tāng* (Two Matured Substances Decoction) with added *hǎi fú shí* (Pumex), *guā lóu* (Fructus Trichosanthis), *bèi mǔ* (Bulbus Fritillaria) and *zhú lì* (Succus Bambusae).

For food depression, disperse with *Bǎo Hé Wán* (Harmony-Preserving Pill)."

Chapter 12
Depression Patterns in Selected Ancient Works

"通治诸郁,用越鞠丸、六郁汤加减。阴阳壅滞,气不升降。沉香降气散。妇人咽中如有炙脔,咯不出,咽不下,半夏厚朴汤。凡怀抱不舒,遭遇不遂,以及怨旷积想在心,莫能排解,种种郁悒,各推其原以治之。然以情病者,当以理遣以命安。若不能怡情放怀,至积郁成劳,草本无能为挽矣,岂可借合欢捐忿,萱草忘忧也哉!"

"For general treatment of all depressions, use modified *Yuè Jū Wán* (Depression-Resolving Pill) and *Liù Yù Tāng* (Six-Depression Decoction).

With yin-yang congestion and qi failing to ascend and descend, use *Chén Xiāng Jiàng Qì Sǎn* (Aquilaria Qi-Downbearing Powder).

For women who have the sensation of a piece of grilled meat in the throat that cannot be spat out or swallowed, use *Bàn Xià Hòu Pò Tāng* (Pinellia and Officinal Magnolia Bark Decoction).

Any constraint of emotions, personal frustration, and resentment, or thoughts that accumulate in the heart which are impossible to resolve can result in depression; treat these according to their respective root causes. However, diseases related to emotions should be eliminated by reason. If one cannot relax the emotions, and the depression accumulates and turns into taxation, medicinals will not be able to remedy this. How can one use *hé huān* (Albiziae) to eliminate anger and *xuān cǎo* (Flos Hemerocallis) to forget anxiety?"

"丹溪立越鞠丸,以治六郁,用香附理气,川芎调血,苍术去湿,山栀泄火,神曲疗食,有痰加贝母。开郁利气为主。"

"Zhu Dan-xi created *Yuè Jū Wán* (Depression-Resolving Pill) for the treatment of the six depressions, using *xiāng fù* (Rhizoma Cyperi) to rectify qi, *chuān xiōng* (Rhizoma Chuanxiong) to regulate blood, *cāng zhú* (Rhizoma Atractylodis) to dispel dampness, *zhī zǐ* (Fructus Gardeniae) to discharge fire, and *shén qū* (Massa Medicata Fermentata) to treat food stagnation. With phlegm, add *bèi mǔ* (Bulbus Fritillaria). The main purpose is to open depression and disinhibit qi."

Selection of Fu-Xi's Treatise on Medicine (*Fú Xī Yī Lùn Xuǎn*)

《鲟溪医论选》:"若郁在情志者,即当以情志解散,此无形之药,病者所自具也。"

"If depression involves the emotions, then these should be resolved and dissipated with emotions. This is a medicine with no physical form that the patient has within himself."

A Clinical Guide with Case Histories (Lín Zhèng Zhǐ Nán Yī Àn)

《临证指南医案》："心藏神，神耗如愦，诸窍失司，非偏寒偏热药治，必得开爽，冀有向安，服药以草木功能，恐不能令其欢悦。"

"The heart stores the spirit; wearing down of the spirit results in fretting and failure to govern the orifices. This cannot be treated with relatively cold or hot medicinals; the person must become gratified in order to get well. The taking of decoctions is to treat the condition, but the medicinal function will probably not make the person happy."

A Clinical Guide with Case Histories (Lín Zhèng Zhǐ Nán Yī Àn)

《临证指南医案》："惊则伤胆，恐则伤肾。大凡可畏之事，猝然而至谓之惊，若从容而至，可以宛转思维者，谓之恐，是惊急而恐缓也。"

"Fright causes damage to the gallbladder, and fear causes damage to the kidney. In general, fright refers to sudden encounters with terrifying things; if those things come gradually so that people can think thoroughly about them, this is referred to as fear. So fright is acute, and fear is insidious."

Wings of the Golden Cabinet (Jīn Guì Yì)

《金匮翼》："肝郁胁痛者，悲哀恼怒，郁伤肝气。"

"Liver constraint with rib-side pain is due to constrained sorrow and anger damaging liver qi."

Essential Cases of Renowned Qing Dynasty Physicians (Qīng Dài Míng Yī Yī Àn Jīng Huá)

《清代名医医案精华》："肝为心母，操用神机，肝木与心火相煽动、肝阳浮。越不僭，彻夜不寐，心悸怔忡，有不能支持之候。"

"The liver is the mother of the heart and facilitates the spirit's dynamic. When liver wood and heart fire fan one another, liver yang floats and goes astray; this results in sleeplessness at night, heart palpitations, and fearful throbbing that is almost unbearable."

Records of Chinese Medicine with Reference to Western Medicine (Yī

Chapter 12
Depression Patterns in Selected Ancient Works

Xué Zhōng Zhōng Cān Xī Lù):

《医学衷中参西录》:"思则心气上通于囟,脑髓实则思易得,过思则心火烁脑"。

"With thinking, the heart qi connects upward with the fontanel. When the brain-marrow is full, thinking will be easy; over-thinking will cause heart-fire to scorch the brain."

Appendix 1
Classifications of Depressive Disorder

A depressive disorder is a mood disorder or affective disorder with mental depression as the main symptom. Although a variety of factors may be involved, the condition is always characterized by a subjectively depressed mood, usually accompanied by emotions of sadness, sorrow, or frustration. Depressed moods arise in all people within their reactions to stress and frustration, the grief of losing a loved one, or temporary feelings of pessimism and despair; these are all common emotions in daily life. A depressed mood is not only an individual experience because such conditions can also involve somatic disease, social factors, and other external factors. Depression often results from marital problems, family crises, poverty, unemployment, aging, and disability.

However, not all reactions to depressing experiences can be regarded as a depressive disorder, and a depressed mood is not equal to a depressive disorder. A depressive disorder is a syndrome consisting also of potentially abnormal biological symptoms and physical signs. In accordance with the basic features of the syndrome, only when the level of depression reaches a certain severity and remains persistent for a certain period of time can it be diagnosed as a depressive disorder.

Current Classification Systems

Although naming a diagnosis is greatly dependent on the particular classification of a disease, there is no classification system that is universally accepted at this time. The *International Classification of Disease* (ICD), (United States) *Diagnostic and Statistical Manual of Mental Disorders* (DSM), and the *Chinese Classification of Mental Disorders* (CCMD) are now the most commonly used classification systems of mental diseases.

The classification of mental and behavioral disorders within the

International Classification of Disease, Tenth Edition (ICD-10, 1992) is the current standard shared by the 170+ member countries of the WHO. The *Diagnostic and Statistical Manual of Mental Disorders, Fourth Edition* (DSM-IV) was established and published in 1994 by the American Psychiatric Association, and most of the content conforms with the ICD-10.

In the ICD-10, depressive disorders are classified under the category of mood disorders, and are subdivided into the following types:

1) Depressive episodes of bipolar affective disorder;
2) Depressive episode;
3) Recurrent depressive disorder;
4) Persistent affective (mood) disorder, including cyclothymia, dysthymia, other persistent mood (affective) disorders, persistent affective (mood) disorders (unspecified);
5) Other affective (mood) disorders.

Depressive episodes are specified as either mild, moderate, or severe, depending on the number and severity of symptoms. The severe depressive episode is further divided into severe depressive episode with psychotic symptoms and severe depressive episode without psychotic symptoms. Mild and moderate depressive episodes are also specified as those with somatic symptoms and those without.

In the DSM-IV, depressive disorder is classified under the category of mood disorders, and these are specified as major depressive disorder (including severe depressive disorder single episode, severe depressive disorder repeated episodes, dysthymic disorder, and unspecified depressive disorder) and bipolar disorder (including bipolar affective disorder unspecified, affective disorder due to somatopathy, materialgenic/substancegenic affective disorder, and unspecified affective disorder).

The ICD-10 and DSM-IV both specify depressive disorder as a persistent syndrome with different severities, conditions lasting for different lengths of time, and those conditions which may or may not be accompanied by psychotic symptoms and somatic symptoms.

The following is a brief ICD-10 description of the "depressive episode" and "dysthymia".

Appendix 1
Classifications of Depressive Disorder

1. Depressive Episodes

To diagnose typical depressive episodes, two out of the following three should be present: 1) lowering of mood, 2) reduction of energy, 3) decrease in activity. A depressive episode may be specified as mild, moderate or severe, depending upon the number, modality, subjective symptoms, and severity of the symptoms.

(1) Mild Depressive Episode

Must fulfill the diagnostic standard of typical cases, but with two of the typical symptoms present and with an additional two symptoms present (i.e. at least 4 symptoms in total). The patient is usually distressed by the symptoms but will be able to continue with most of their social activities and work responsibility.

(2) Moderate Depressive Episode

Must fulfill the diagnostic standard of typical cases, but with two of the typical symptoms present and with an additional four symptoms present (i.e. at least 6 symptoms in total). The patient will typically be able to continue with occupational activities, but will often have greater difficulty with social and household activities.

(3) Severe Depressive Episode

Must fulfill the diagnostic standard of typical cases with all of the 3 symptoms present, but with 5 additional symptoms (at least 8 symptoms in total) and some of the symptoms should be significant. The patient usually suffers great distress, and may also have difficulty in describing the symptoms due to abnormal psychomotor inhibition or excitement. It is almost impossible for the patient to continue with any normal social, occupational, or household activities. A suicide attempt is a significant act defining some extreme cases.

2. Dysthymia

As a unit of diagnostic classification, dysthymia first appeared in the DSM-III to replace the term "depressive neurosis". This syndrome is more moderate than the "major/severe depression" but it may last for several years. Hallucinations and delusions are usually not present in dysthymia, and the patient may sometimes be considered as simply having a depressive personality. Dysthymia may lead to difficulty in social and occupational activities, but the severity is insufficient to be diagnosed as major/severe depression.

Other Categories

1. Persistent Mood (Affective) Disorders: Cyclothymia and dysthymia are under this category in the ICD-10, but listed as individual categories in the DSM-IV.

2. Cyclothymia: The onset is usually at an early age, chronic, and with a lifetime prevalence rate of 0.4%-3.5%. There are no gender differences, and frequently found in the relatives of patients with unipolar or bipolar affective disorders; some patients eventually develop bipolar affective disorder. The mood instability of cyclothymia is usually not related to daily life events, although some patients will have psychoactive substance abuse issues.

3. Melancholia: Melancholia in the DSM-IV is equivalent to the somatic syndrome as described in the ICD-10 and is characterized by the following:
 1) Reduced interest and pleasurable feelings in activities that used to be enjoyed;
 2) Emotional unresponsive to pleasurable circumstances and events;
 3) Waking in the morning several hours before the usual time;
 4) Mood depression worse in the morning;
 5) Marked psychomotor retardation and agitation;
 6) Loss of appetite and weight loss.

A "feeling of guilt" is also mentioned in the DSM-IV, and "loss of libido" is listed in the ICD-10. Some believe that this category is more common in the elderly.

4. Agitated Depression and Retarded Depression: These two categories fall under the traditional classification of depressive disorder, and both terms are still in use in clinical practice for patients with

Appendix 1
Classifications of Depressive Disorder

significant agitation or retardation. It was recently believed that lethargy is an indicator for electroconvulsive therapy, and also that depressive disorder with lethargic symptoms may develop into bipolar disorder.

5. Recurrent Depressive Disorder and Single Episode Depressive Disorder: It is generally believed that the risk of recurrence is higher in patients with previous episodes. However, there are also special groups with a very low risk of recurrence. Some studies suggest two subtypes: single episode depressive disorder and recurrent depressive disorder, with corresponding specifications in both DSM-IV and ICD-10.

6. Dysthymia with Major Depression (Double Depression): The term "double depression" was used to describe an episode of major depression superimposed on an underlying dysthymia (Keller and Shapiro, 1983). An individual suffering from double depression often shows a high incidence of other types of depressive disorder within the family. There are also reports suggesting that the incidence in females is higher than in males.

7. Recurrent Brief Depressive Disorder (RBD): Not all depressive episodes last for 2 weeks or longer, and some may appear for only a few days. Therefore, mild to moderate or even severe depressive episodes will vary in number and severity, but because they do not meet the duration requirement, they cannot be diagnosed as a major depressive episode. However, when brief depressive episodes do recur they will cause significant impact on the patient.

8. Rapid Cycling Bipolar Disorder: Rapid cycling may occur spontaneously (usually longer than the course of chronic bipolar affective disorder) or may be sped up by antidepressants; accompanying thyroid axis conditions may also cause rapid cycling. Some suggest use of alternative mood stabilizers such as anticonvulsant agents carbamazepine or sodium valproate.

Special Types of Depressive Disorders

In addition to the categories listed above, other subtypes of depressive disorder are described in a variety of professional articles.

1. Postpartum Depression:

① Post-partum blues, common and occurring in 1/3 of new mothers in the early postnatal period, this is temporary and usually requires no treatment.

② In the first postnatal year, up to 10% of the new mothers experience mild to moderate postpartum depression. Treatment is the same as the other typical mild to moderate depressions.

③ Postpartum psychosis usually appears as mixed atypical depression and mania, which is also highly relevant to subsequent bipolar disorder and chronic depressions.

2. Seasonal Depressive Disorder:

The key characteristic of seasonal depressive disorder is regular recurrent episodes, usually appearing at a certain time of year (regular onset in autumn or winter with relief in the springtime).

3. Mixed Anxiety-Depression Syndrome:

Some patients have symptoms of both anxiety and depression, but the severity for each group of symptoms does not meet the diagnostic criteria of either anxiety or depression. This category should be differentiated from depressive disorder with anxiety symptoms or anxiety disorder with depression symptoms. In mixed anxiety-depression syndromes, autonomic nervous symptoms will display occasionally (tremor, palpitation, dry mouth, nausea, etc).

4. Primary and Secondary Depressive Disorder:

Primary depressive disorders are depressive disorders not caused by an underlying psychiatric disorder or somatic disease. Secondary depression appears as a result of other underlying psychiatric disorders or somatic diseases (such as post-psychosis depression, pancreatic cancer-induced depression, etc.) or may be caused by substances abuse and chemical dependency.

5. Masked Depression:

Masked depression is when depressive disorder patients report only their somatic symptoms rather than their emotional status. Masked

Appendix 1
Classifications of Depressive Disorder

depression is not a diagnostic criterion, however, because whenever a case is diagnosed as depression, it is no longer masked. Masked depression can show symptoms from all categories of depressive disorders.

6. Menopausal Depressive Disorder:

The onset is usually in late middle age (or post-menopause) and characterized by agitation, hypochondria, and an obsessive-compulsive personality. The term is no longer in use internationally since the validity never met the requirement of the diagnostic criteria. However, there are indeed many patients who experience single episodes of depressive disorder during menopause.

7. Depressive Episode with Stress Symptom:

Also referred to as "depressive stupor". DSM-IV diagnostic criteria: fulfills the criteria of a depressive episode with at least two of the following five characteristics present:

1) Inability to move, appearing as catalepsy or stupor.

2) Significant increase in movement with no purpose and free from external influence.

3) Extreme negativism (marked resistance to all instructions with no purpose, or freezing in certain postures while refusing to move) or silence.

4) Special voluntary mannerisms (remaining in inappropriate or strange postures), stereotyped movements, affectation, or grimacing.

5) Imitative speech or movement.

8. Atypical Depressive Disorder: Atypical depressive disorder is common among young patients and is usually accompanied by temporary increases in appetite and sleep. These symptoms are very rare in most other depressive disorder cases. Patients are usually temporarily emotionally responsive to benign events, but tend to have rapid falls in mood. Sleep and appetite disorders are always present, but patients tend to have excessive sleep and excessive eating rather than insomnia or loss of appetite. Such patients always depend on the recognition of others in interpersonal relationships, and they will feel deeply hurt by any refusal that may significantly impair their social and occupational activities, especially with failure in matters of love.

9. Subclinical Depression: Those conditions that do not meet the diagnostic criteria of the above categories, nor with the frequency, severity or duration of symptoms to meet those requirements. Patients under this category have a high risk of depressive episodes in the future.

Causes of Depressive Disorder

There is not yet a conclusive theory for the exact cause of depressive disorder. Although there are a variety of theories, most studies focus on biological, genetic, and social-psychological factors. Somatic diseases, addictive substances, drug reactions, and environmental toxins may also be contributing factors.

1. Genetic Factors

The onset of depressive disorder is closely associated with genetic factors. Family studies have shown that the incidence of depression is much higher within the same family than in the general population. Incidence among parents, brothers, sisters and children is 12%–24%, and 2.5% among cousins. Twins studies showed an incidence among dizygotic twins of 12%–38%, and 69%–95% among monozygotic twins. Foster care studies showed that the incidence among birth parents of the patient is 31% and only 12% for adoptive parents, suggesting that genetic factors play an important role as the cause. Other studies have shown that 40%–70% of depressive disorder patients have a genetic predisposition, that is, nearly or more than half will have a family history of depression.

Although extensive studies exist on the molecular genetics of bipolar affective disorder, the gene related to the onset of the disease has not yet been identified. Genome scans have excluded the linkage of genetic markers on 2, 3, 4, 7, 9, 10, 11, 22 and X chromosomes. Other evidences showed a locus for bipolar disorder on the long arm of chromosomes 13 and 22.

2. Psychological and Social Factors

Although not all psychological and mental disorders are caused by psychological and social factors, mental stimulations do often induce or trigger depressive disorder episodes.

Appendix 1
Classifications of Depressive Disorder

(1) LIFE EVENTS AND PERSISTENT STRESS

Psychological trauma caused by life changing events and mental stressors frequently result in depression. Studies have shown that 70% of all depressive disorder patients had suffered from negative life events, with 42% showing depressive symptoms within one month after the death of a spouse. At one year after the death of a spouse, 15% were diagnosed with depressive disorder.

These figures show that life events do in fact play an important role in depressive disorder episodes, but the onset of depressive disorder when facing life events also depends on the genetic quality and personality of the individual.

(2) CHILDHOOD EXPERIENCES

Separation from parents and childhood bereavement lower the self-esteem of an individual, and this may develop into depressive disorder in adulthood. In some reports, the risk of depressive disorder was increased in adulthood if the individual experienced bereavement before age 11, but more data is needed to verify this finding. Strict parental control, overprotective behavior, child abuse, and lack of care are all possible factors in the onset of mild depressive episodes. The risk of depressive disorder and other mental disorders also increase significantly with childhood sexual abuse.

(3) PERSONALITY/PERSONAL CHARACTERISTICS

Individuals with significant anxiety, obsessive-compulsion, or impulsive behaviors are more vulnerable to depression. Such personalities may appear as excessively doubtful, cautious, and timid, or overly concerned with detail and always striving for perfection. There may be persistent tension and anxiety, an extremely strong sense of morality, or an excessive adherence to social customs.

(4) INTERPERSONAL RELATIONSHIPS

A lack of intimacy also increases the risk of depressive episodes, but strong social support helps to reduce the impact of negative life events and lower the risk of depressive episodes. Compared to those who have good relationships with friends and relatives, the risk of depressive disorder is three times higher for people facing negative life events.

(5) MARITAL STATUS

The incidence of depressive disorders is lower in happily married people, with the risk being two times higher for those separated. Divorce increases the risk of depressive disorder by five times in both males and females.

3. Biological Factors

Biological factors are critical in the onset of depressive disorder. Researchers in biological psychiatry now employ sophisticated assessment techniques such as radioreceptor assay (RRA), radioimmunoassay, high performance liquid chromatography (HPLC), brain evoked potentials, CT and MRI. Existing data suggests that depressive disorder patients may have abnormalities involving receptors, neurotransmitters, signal transduction, and neuroendocrine levels.

(1) NEUROLOGICAL AND BIOCHEMICAL CHANGES

1) Serotonin (5-HT) Hypothesis: Deficits in serotonergic activity are associated with many of the symptoms of major depression such as depressive mood, loss of appetite, insomnia, circadian rhythm disorders, endocrine dysfunction, sexual dysfunction, anxiety, reduced activity, and an inability to deal effectively with stress. Some tricyclic antidepressants and selective 5-hydroxytryptophan reuptake inhibitors are effective, but selective 5-HT depletion agents (p-alanine) can reverse the effects of tricyclic antidepressants and monoamine oxidase inhibitors (MAOIs) and even cause depression. Reserpine can deplete 5-HT to cause depression, whereas MAOIs inhibit 5-HT degradation and thus show antidepressant effects.

2) Norepinephrine (NE) Hypothesis: Clinical studies show that 3-Methoxy-4-hydroxyphenylglycol, a metabolite of NE, is significant lower in the urine of bipolar depression patients, and MHPG content is increased. The rate-limiting enzyme in the biosynthesis of NE and the TH inhibitor, α-Methylbutyric acid Tyrosine hydroxylase (TH) can control mania but also cause mild depression or worsen depressive symptoms

Appendix 1
Classifications of Depressive Disorder

in recovering patients treated by desipramine. Tricyclic antidepressants inhibit NE recovery and thus can be used to treat depression, whereas reserpine can deplete synaptic NE and cause depression.

3) Dopamine (DA) Hypothesis: Neurochemical pharmacology studies show that brain DA function is lowered in depression and increased in mania. The hypothesis is mainly based on the theory that the dopamine precursor L-DOPA can improve symptoms in some unipolar depression patients, but also cause mania. Dopamine agonists such as pribedil and bromocriptine have antidepressant effects and may also change bipolar depression into mania. Antidepressants such as bupropion mainly inhibit the reuptake of dopamine. The main degradation product of dopamine is homovanillic acid (HVA), and urinary HVA levels are lower in depressive episodes.

4) GABA Hypothesis: GABA is a major inhibitory neurotransmitter of the central nervous system. Clinical studies find that many anticonvulsive drugs such as carbamazepine and sodium valproate can reduce mania and also cause depression. The pharmacological effect is related to the control of brain GABA levels. Studies have found that plasma and cerebrospinal fluid GABA levels are lower in bipolar affective disorder patients.

(2) Neuroendocrine Disorders

Many studies have found that mood disorder patients show functional disorders of the hypothalamic-pituitary-adrenal axis (HPA), hypothalamic-pituitary-thyroid axis (HPT) and the hypothalamic-pituitary growth hormone axis. In plasma cortisol level and 17 - hydroxy corticosteroid level tests, depression patients show excessive cortisol secretion, also suggesting a hypothalamic-pituitary-adrenal axis disorder. There are also changes in the circadian rhythm of cortisol secretion, with a lack of nighttime spontaneous inhibition of cortisol secretion. There are also studies finding that corticotropin-releasing hormone (CRH) is increased in the cerebrospinal fluid of severely depressed patients, suggesting a hypothalamic-pituitary-adrenal axis disorder based on excessive secretion of CRH.

(3) Changes in EEG:

EEG sleep studies find changes in the sleep patterns of depression patients: reduced total sleep time, increased frequency of awakening, and shortening of rapid eye movement (REM). More severe depression also shows shortened REM latency, and this can be used to predict the treatment response.

About 30% of mood disorder patients have electroencephalogram (EEG) abnormalities, with low frequency or high amplitude slow-waves usually appearing in depressive episodes. The average integrated amplitude of the left and right cerebral hemispheres of depression patients have been found to be in negative correlation to the severity of depression. EEG's often show lateralization phenomenon abnormalities (about 70%).

(4) NEUROIMAGING

1) Structural Imaging: CT studies show a 12.5%–42% incidence of ventricular dilatation, with no significant difference in the CT abnormal rates of unipolar and bipolar disorder patients.

2) Functional Imaging: Regional cerebral blood flow (rCBF) of the left frontal area is lower in depression patients, with decreased levels in positive correlation with the severity of depression. Some studies find that rCBF is lower in the left anterior cingulate, also more severe in depression patients with cognitive impairment.

American Criteria

In the third version of *Diagnostic and Statistical Manual of Mental Disorder* (DSM-III) developed by American Psychiatric Association (APA), the different types of depressive disorder are classified under the same category including "dysthymia", which used to be classified as neurosis. The concept of "major depression" is also mentioned while its classification was extended. The term "neurasthenia" has been abandoned since the DSM-III with most neurasthenia conditions being classified as depressive disorder.

The DSM-III-R has clearly defined the symptoms, syndromes, episodes and disorders of depressive disorder. Both the diagnostic criteria and definition of depressive syndrome were clearly indicated. The DSM-IV currently in use has retained parts of the DSM-III-R, also including depressive disorders caused by somatic diseases, psychoactive substances, and also other unspecified depressive disorders.

Appendix 2
Recent studies

Depressive Disorder and CM Syndrome Classifications

Depressive disorder manifests as a persistent state of low mood with somatic discomforts, insomnia, and a variety of other symptoms[1], and falls under the Chinese medicine category of "depression/*yu* disease"[2]. Other syndromes include plum-pit qi (globus hystericus), visceral agitation (hysteria), lily disease, running piglet, also with symptoms of insomnia, hypersomnia, increased dreams, crying, anger, sadness, anxiety, fright, or depressive psychosis (depression accompanied by psychotic symptoms). According to Wang Yan-heng's monograph on the topic, such signs and symptoms are most often associated with *shaoyang* and *shaoyin* syndromes[1]. Depressive disorder may also accompany somatic diseases such as cerebrovascular disease, diabetes, and geriatric diseases.

1. Pathomechanisms

Chen Wen-kai and others[3] suggest that the main syndromes of depression disease include deficiency of both heart and spleen, dampness obstructing the middle, binding constraint of liver qi, disquieting of the heart-spirit, deficiency of both heart and spleen, qi stagnation obstructing the collaterals, qi constraint of both heart and liver, turbid phlegm obstruction, pathogenic heat disturbing the spirit, and deficiency of both spleen and kidney.

The pathomechanism mainly involves binding constraint of spirit-qi, with excess syndromes more commonly present than those of deficiency. Excess syndromes include qi constraint, phlegm dampness, fire, heat and collateral obstruction. Deficiency syndromes include qi and yin deficiency and blood deficiency. Yang deficiency cases are rare.

After investigation, Hu Sui-yu[4] identified the most common

syndromes:
1) Liver constraint with qi stagnation;
2) Liver constraint with spleen deficiency;
3) Liver constraint with phlegm obstruction;
4) Deficiency of both heart and spleen.

However, Tong Jian-ming and others[5, 6] found that most depression cases fall under the category of deficiency syndromes, especially qi deficiency. Zhang Jian[7] summarizes the experiences of Li Fu-ren who suggests that geriatric depression mainly involves the heart, liver, and spleen, and the pathomechanism mainly involves impaired circulation of qi and blood.

2. Syndrome Differentiation and Chinese Medicinal Treatment

Studies have shown certain relationships between subtypes of unipolar depressive disorder and specific CM syndromes. For example, mild and early-stage depression mainly involves syndromes of liver constraint with qi stagnation. Developing stages of the disease and more complicated cases with or without psychotic symptoms involve liver constraint with phlegm obstruction, and recurrent cases are generally characterized by deficiency of both heart and spleen.

In the opinion of Wang Yan-heng[1], mild depression is predominantly associated with the syndromes of liver constraint with qi stagnation, liver constraint with phlegm binding, qi stagnation with static blood, and flaming heat of the heart and liver. Moderate depression is mainly associated with deficiency of both heart and spleen, liver constraint with spleen deficiency, yin deficiency of both liver and kidney, deficiency of both spleen and kidney, and deficiency of both lung and kidney, and severe depression often presents with phlegm-fire syndromes and kidney yang deficiency. Studies of this type can serve as a guideline in clinical practice.

There is not yet one single recognized standard of diagnosis and treatment for depression, but clinical treatment is usually based on syndromes of liver constraint with qi stagnation, pathogenic fire transformed from qi constraint, blood stasis, internal brewing of phlegm-turbidity, deficiency of both heart and spleen, and yin deficiency of both liver and kidney.

Statistically, among the Chinese medicinal formulae for treating depression, over 80% of practitioners report the use of *Chái Hú Shū Gān Sǎn* (Bupleurum Liver-Soothing Powder), *Dān Zhī Xiāo Yáo Sǎn* (Moutan and Gardenia Free Wanderer Powder), *Xuè Fǔ Zhú Yū Tāng* (Blood Stasis Expelling Decoction), *Huáng Lián Wēn Dǎn Tāng* (Coptis Gallbladder-Warming Decoction), *Guī Pí Tāng* (Spleen-Restoring Decoction), *Liù Wèi Dì Huáng Tāng* (Six Ingredients Rehmannia Decoction).

Wang Yan-heng[8] classifies the disease into 5 types:
1) Liver constraint with phlegm bind disturbing the brain-spirit;
2) Liver constraint with qi stagnation obstructing the brain-spirit;
3) Qi stagnation with static blood failing to nourish the brain-spirit;
4) Yin deficiency of both liver and kidney failing to nourish the brain;
5) Liver constraint with spleen deficiency failing to nourish the brain.

Li[9] also classified the disease into 5 types:
1) Binding constraint of liver qi;
2) Internal brewing of phlegm-turbidity;
3) Static blood obstruction;
4) Deficiency of both heart and spleen;
5) Yin deficiency of both heart and spleen.

Yang[10] classified depression into 8 types based on the following liver syndromes:
1) Liver constraint with qi stagnation;
2) Pathogenic fire transformed from liver constraint;
3) Liver constraint with phlegm obstruction;
4) Liver constraint with static blood;
5) Liver constraint with spleen deficiency;
6) Liver constraint with kidney deficiency;
7) Liver constraint with blood deficiency;
8) Liver constraint with qi deficiency.

Han[11] and others classified the disease into the following 6 types:

① Qi constraint with phlegm bind clouding the heart orifice;
② Liver fire combined with phlegm going upward to disturb the heart-spirit;
③ Deficiency of both qi and blood failing to nourish the heart-spirit;
④ Deficiency of both heart and spleen failing to nourish the spirit and mind;
⑤ Non-interaction of heart and kidney, yin deficiency with hyperactive fire;
⑥ Qi deficiency of both heart and gallbladder, disquieting of the spirit.

3. Formula Modifications

Zheng[12] and others successfully treated a group of tumor patients with depression using modifications of *Chái Hú Shū Gān Sǎn* (Bupleurum Liver-Soothing Powder) to improve depressive symptoms.

Lü[13] and others treated 30 depressive patients with *Jiě Yù Tāng* (Depression-Relieving Decoction) (includes *chái hú* (Radix Bupleuri), *xiāng fù* (Rhizoma Cyperi), *yù jīn* (Radix Curcumae) etc.); a control group was treated with Amitriptyline only. The treatment group displayed no obvious side effects, and patient compliance was also higher.

Li Fu-ren[7] studied the effects of modified *Èr Chén Tāng* (Two Matured Substances Decoction) in the treatment of geriatric depression. Quan[14] used modifications of *Bǎi Hé Dì Huáng Tāng* (Lily and Rehmannia Decoction) to treat 30 depressive patients with an overall effective rate of 86.7%.

Wei and others [15] used modifications of *Bǎi Hé Tāng* (Lily Decoction) (including *bǎi hé* (Bulbus Lilii), *shēng dì huáng* (Radix Rehmanniae Recens), *zhī mǔ* (Rhizoma Anemarrhenae), *mài dōng* (Radix Ophiopogonis, *wǔ wèi zǐ* (Fructus Schisandrae Chinensis) in 85 patients with depression, and the overall effective rate was 85.88%.

Others have used *Jiě Yù Tāng* (Depression-Relieving Decoction) (*chái hú* (Radix Bupleuri) etc.) to treat post-schizophrenia depression. The effect was found similar to Amitriptyline but with no obvious side effects[13]. Chen Xiao-shan[16] and others treated geriatric depression based on syndromes of the heart, heart and lung, spleen, spleen and kidney.

Li Jie and others[17] suggest that in clinical practice there are always a variety of syndromes displayed at the same time, and that these syndromes tend to combine and interact. In their opinion, treatment should thus remain flexible and not merely focus on a single syndrome or the use of a single formula.

4. Integrative Treatment

From the data collected, it has been established that superior effects are achieved through integrative treatment that combines Chinese medicinals with Western antidepressant drugs. Chang[18] and others used this approach to treat 44 depression patients. The patients were randomly divided into two groups and both groups were given imipramine. Patients in the treatment group were also given Chinese medicinals according to the presenting syndromes. Results showed an effective rate for the treatment group of 95.65% with side effects significantly reduced, and an effective rate for the control group of 80.95%.

Bai[19] and others treated 54 patients with modifications of *Chái Hú Shū Gān Sǎn* (Bupleurum Liver-Soothing Powder), *Gān Mài Dà Zǎo Tāng* (Licorice, Wheat and Jujube Decoction), *Chái Hú Dá Yuán Yǐn* (Bupleurum Membrane-Source-Opening Decoction), *Èr Yīn Jiān* (Two-Yin Decoction), *Shùn Qì Dǎo Zhì Tāng* (Qi-Balancing and Stagnation-Moving Decoction) combined with Western antipsychotic drugs. The results indicated a short-term cure rate of 94%, suggesting that Chinese medicinals and Western medicines combined are highly effective for mental illnesses, showing rapid effects and a shortened course of disease.

Zhou[20] treated 38 depression patients with Imipramine and *Xiāo Yáo Sǎn* (Free Wanderer Powder) with modifications applied according to the presenting syndrome. The overall effective rate was 100%.

Hou Qin-luan[21] combined *Gēng Nián Ān Tāng* (Climacteric Syndrome Relieving Decoction) with Fluoxetine Hydrochloride to treat menopausal depression and treatment was found to be fairly effective.

5. Acupuncture

Ye[22] selected HT 7 (*shén mén*), SP 6 (*sān yīn jiāo*) and ST 36 (*zú sān lǐ*) as the main acupoints used in the treatment of 36 depression patients, getting an overall effective rate of 83%.

Fu[23] needled RN 12 (*zhōng wǎn*), RN 3 (*zhōng jí*), LI 4 (*hé gǔ*), ST 36 (*zú sān lǐ*) and SP 6 (*sān yīn jiāo*). Compared to their status before acupuncture, all patients tended to show improvement.

Dong[24] applied electro-acupuncture to DU 20 (*bǎi huì*) and *yìn táng* (印堂) in 101 depression cases, with an overall effective rate of 81.2%.

Bai Qiao-ling and others [25] used DU 20 (*bǎi huì*), *yìn táng* (印堂), PC 6 (*nèi guān*), SP 6 (*sān yīn jiāo*), LV 3 (*tài chōng*), and ST 40 (*fēng lóng*) as the basic acupoint selection, also adding HT 7 (*shén mén*) for patients with insomnia; *tài yáng* (太阳), GB 20 (*fēng chí*), and LI 4 (*hé gǔ*) for dizziness and headache; HT 7 (*shén mén*) and RN 17 (*dàn zhōng*) for chest tightness and palpitation; ST 36 (*zú sān lǐ*) for poor appetite; and *sì shén cōng* (四神聪) and ST 36 (*zú sān lǐ*) for patients with slowed thinking and hypomnesis.

Liu Zhi-shun and others[26] treated post-stroke depression with the main acupoints of DU 20 (*bǎi huì*), DU 16 (*fēng fǔ*), GB 20 (*fēng chí*) and upper *yìn táng* (印堂); also adding LV 3 (*tài chōng*) and ST 40 (*fēng lóng*) for patients with wind-phlegm disturbing upward; KI 3 (*tài xī*) and BL 18 (*gān shù*) yin deficiency of both liver and kidney; and RN 12 (*zhōng wǎn*) and SP 10 (*xuè hǎi*) for deficiency of qi and blood. Therapy was given once daily with rest on Saturday and Sunday for one month. In 30 cases, the effective rate was 80%.

Jin Guang-liang and others[27] showed that electro-acupuncture at DU 20 (*bǎi huì*) and *Yìn Táng* (印堂) can significantly reduce the time that test rats could be subjected to an electric shock. Regarding the mechanism of electro-acupuncture, Han Cui[28, 29] concluded that since cytokines have a certain impact in the pathogenesis of depression, the inhibitory effect of electro-acupuncture on cytokines is part of the mechanism; electro-acupuncture at DU 20 (*bǎi huì*) and SP 6 (*sān yīn jiāo*) can also increase both activity and sugar water intake in chronically stress rats.

Results show that electro-acupuncture at DU 20 (*bǎi huì*) and *yìn táng* (印堂) can act as an antidepressant by lowering cortical 5-HT metabolism, providing 5-HT nerve activity, coordinating the balance between NE and 5-HT, protecting BDNF positive neurons in the hippocampus, and adjusting HPA axis function.

In order to analyze the improvement of a depressive state, Yu Jin and others[30] observed the immobility time of mice in forced swimming tests after treatment with a combined therapy of acupuncture and antidepressants. They found that electro-acupuncture used in conjunction with small doses of antidepressants can further enhance the antidepressant effect.

6. Psychotherapy

Chinese medical psychotherapy includes verbal guidance therapy, emotion diversion therapy, restriction therapy using other kinds of emotion, and therapy to satisfy the emotion and desires of the patient. Jiang and others treated stroke patients with depression [31] using Chinese medical psychotherapy together with conventional therapy, using only conventional therapy on the control group. The treatment group displayed significant improvement in both depressive and somatic symptoms.

7. Antidepressant Effects of Single Chinese Medicinals

Wang Bin and others[32] found that saikosaponin can enhance the antidepressant effect of Fluoxetine. Li Ming-ya and others[33] found that decocted *shí chāng pú* (Rhizoma Acori Tatarinowii) has a significant antidepressant effect on the behavioral despair animal model of depression. Molodavkin and others[34] showed that *huáng qí* (Radix Astragali) extract has antidepressant and anxiolytic activity effects.

Cui Cheng-bin and others[35] isolated 5 active ingredients from the Chinese medicinal *bā jǐ tiān* (Radix Morindae Officinalis). It was found after screening different models of depression that *bā jǐ tiān* (Radix Morindae Officinalis) extract can significantly improve the physical signs and brain levels of monoamine in reserpinization of mice, and also significant antidepressant effects. Zhang Zhong-qi and others[36, 37] studied the effect of morinda officinalis oligosaccharides on rats in forced swimming tests and on the acquired helpless rat model of depression. The results indicated that *bā jǐ tiān* (Radix Morindae Officinalis) has an antidepressant effect, and that the dose-response relationship is in a characteristic "U" curve of behavioral pharmacology.

Weng Shen-hong and others[38] showed that *cì wǔ jiā* (Radix et Rhizoma seu Caulis Acanthopanacis Senticosi) capsules show an antidepressant effect in mild to moderate cases of depression. Other studies[39] found hypericum perforatum extract to improve depressive symptoms in test rats. Qin Xiao-song and others [40] found that *yín xìng yè* (Folium Ginkgo) extract used together with the synthetic antidepressants venlafaxine hydrochloride also had a significant antidepressant effect.

Indian scholars found that oral administration of ginkgo acid conjugate can significantly affect the concentration of 5-HT, NE, DA and their metabolites in various parts of the rat brain [41]. The conjugate is confirmed to have antidepressant activity on animal models of anxiety. It may be that part of the active ingredient for the antidepressant effect is contained in *yín xìng yè* (Folium Ginkgo). Chen Yao and others [42] found that the total glucosides of Centella asiatica can adjust the HPA and HPTA axis in depressed rats.

8. Antidepressant Effects of Compound Chinese Medicinal Formulas

Chen Wei-yin and others [43] observed the effect of both Fluoxetine and the compound Chinese medicinal formula *Yù Lè Shū* (Depression Relieving and Emotion Lightening Formula, 郁乐疏) (composed of *chái hú* (Radix Bupleuri), *yù jīn* (Radix Curcumae) etc.) on post stroke depressive symptoms and neurological rehabilitation, concluding that both Fluoxetine and *Yù Lè Shū* are effective for treating post-stroke depression and promoting neurological rehabilitation.

Cao Su [44] used Amitriptyline as a control to study the antidepressant effect, side effects, and safety of the modern formula *Kàng Yì Yù Zhèng Jiāo Náng* (Anti-Depression Capsules, 抗抑郁症胶囊) in treating geriatric depression. Results showed that the group using *Kàng Yì Yù Zhèng Jiāo Náng* had fewer side effects than the Amitriptyline group.

Zhao Zhi-sheng [45] composed his own Chinese medicinal formula, *Yì Lǜ Kāng Jiāo Náng* (Depression and Anxiety Relieving Capsules, 抑虑康胶囊). A study indicated that *Yì Lǜ Kāng Jiāo Náng* can improve symptoms of both depression and anxiety and regulate the emotions with an overall efficacy superior to a control group using Western drugs.

Toshiaki Kita and others [46] confirmed that *Jiā Wèi Xiāo Yáo Sǎn* (Modified Free Wanderer Powder) is effective for somatic and psychologically uncertain depression. Wu Li[47] found that *Wēn Dǎn Tāng* (Gallbladder-Warming Decoction) also has antidepressant effects possibly due to its ability to regulate brain and plasma levels of somatostatin. Xue Zheng[48] found that the qi and blood supplementing formula *Pí Shèn Liǎng Zhù Wán* (Spleen and Kidney Supplementing Pill) is very effective for depression when applied according to syndrome differentiation.

Yang Shi-you, Zhang You-zhi, Yang Jin and others[49-52] studied and verified that compound formulas of Chinese medicinals have definite antidepressant effects and can be used in combination with clinical screening to treat depression. Yang Jin and others[50] concluded that *Chāng Huān Yī Hào* (Acorus and Albizia No. 1, 菖欢1号) mainly act on catechol neurotransmitters, and its therapeutic effect may be performed by increasing NE concentrations in the hypothalamus and hippocampus, by increasing DA concentrations in the striatum and cerebral cortex, and also by lowering their metabolic rates.

9. Summary

To summarize, the effects on depression are most significant when combining Chinese medicine together with Western drugs and psychotherapy. However, many problems still exist:

1) The diagnostic criteria for depression are not standardized. The disease is mainly characterized by subjective symptoms with few laboratory indicators and clinical signs. This causes some difficulty in clinical diagnosis.

2) The syndrome differentiation and criteria for determining therapeutic effects are not standardized. In order to improve clinical efficacy, syndrome differentiation and efficacy evaluation criteria should be established by using modern diagnostic measures and also by combining macro-differentiation and micro-differentiation.

3) Decoctions are the main dosage form as used in clinical practice, the disease is always chronic, and patients need long-term medication. Newer dosage forms should be developed with modern pharmaceutical techniques for the convenience of patients.

Appendix 3
Classical Sources

Chapter 2
Source of Hundreds of Diseases Names in TCM
(Zhōng Yī Bǎi Bìng Míng Yuán Kǎo) 中医百病名源考

The Inner Classic (Nèi Jīng) 内经

The Basic Questions – Great Treatise on the Regular Principles of the Six Origins
(Sù Wèn – Liù Yuán Zhèng Jì Dà Lùn) 素问·六元正纪大论

The Basic Questions – Treatise on Pain
(Sù Wèn – Jǔ Tòng Lùn) 素问·举痛论

The Spiritual Pivot – Spirit
(Líng Shū – Běn Shén) 灵枢·本神

The Basic Questions – Treatise on Sickness
(Sù Wèn – Běn Bìng Lùn) 素问·本病论

The Basic Questions – Qi and Manifestations of Healthy Persons
(Sù Wèn – Píng Rén Qì Xiàng Lùn) 素问·平人气象论

The Basic Questions – Essentials of Needling
(Sù Wèn – Cì Yào Lùn) 素问·刺要论

The Grand Chinese Medical Dictionary
(Zhōng Guó Yī Xué Dà Cí Diǎn) 中国医学大辞典

Appendix 3
Classical Sources

Treatise on Cold Damage
(*Shāng Hán Lùn*) 伤寒论

Essentials of the Golden Cabinet
(*Jīn Guì Yào Lüè*) 金匮要略

The Pulse Classic
(*Mài Jīng*) 脉经

Treatise on the Origins and Manifestations of Various Diseases
(*Zhū Bìng Yuán Hòu Lùn*) 诸病源候论

Important Formulas Worth a Thousand Gold Pieces for Emergency
(*Bèi Jí Qiān Jīn Yào Fāng*) 备急千金要方

Arcane Essentials from the Imperial Library
(*Wài Tái Mì Yào*) 外台秘要

Comprehensive Recording of Divine Assistance
(*Shèng Jì Zǒng Lù*) 圣济总录

Discourse on Tracing Back to the Medical Classics
(*Yī Jīng Sù Huí Jí*) 医经溯洄集

Teachings of [Zhu] Dan-xi
(*Dān Xī Xīn Fǎ*) 丹溪心法

The Orthodox Tradition of Medicine
(*Yī Xué Zhèng Zhuàn*) 医学正传

The Complete Compendium of Ancient and Modern Medical Works
(*Gǔ Jīn Yī Tǒng Dà Quán*) 古今医统大全

The Complete Works of [Zhang] Jing-yue
(*Jǐng Yuè Quán Shū*) 景岳全书

The Yellow Emperors Inner Classic
(*Huáng Dì Nèi Jīng*) 黄帝内经

Key Link of Medicine
(*Yī Guàn*) 医贯

Black Pearl from Red Waters
(*Chì Shuǐ Xuán Zhū*) 赤水玄珠

Shen's Books on Respecting Life
(*Shěn Shì Zūn Shēng Shū*) 沈氏尊生书

Case Records as a Guide to Clinical Practice
(*Lín Zhèng Zhǐ Nán Yī Àn*) 临证指南医案

Categorized Patterns with Clear-cut Treatments
(*Lèi Zhèng Zhì Cái*) 类证治裁

Non-retention Collection
(*Bù Jū Jí*) 不居集

Standards for Diagnosis and Treatment
(*Zhèng Zhì Zhǔn Shéng*) 证治准绳

Chapter 3

The Basic Questions – Treatise Explaining the Five Qi
(*Sù Wèn – Xuān Míng Wǔ Qì Piān*) 素问·宣明五气篇

Secret Records of the Brocade Sack
(*Jǐn Náng Mì Lù*) 锦囊秘录

The Spiritual Pivot – the Engendering and Interaction of Ying and Wei
(*Líng Shū – Yíng Wèi Shēng Huì*) 灵枢·营卫生会

The Basic Questions – Great Treatise on the Correspondences and Manifestation of Yin and Yang

Appendix 3
Classical Sources

(*Sù Wèn – Yīn Yáng Yìng Xiàng Dà Lùn*) 素问 · 阴阳应象大论

The Basic Questions – Treatise on Pain
(*Sù Wèn – Jǔ Tòng Lùn*) 素问 · 举痛论

The Spiritual Pivot – Spirit
(*Líng Shū – Běn Shén*) 灵枢 · 本神

Revised Popular Guide to 'Treatise on Cold Damage'
(*Chóng Dìng Tōng Sú Shāng Hán Lùn*) 重订通俗伤寒论

The Classified Classic
(*Lèi Jīng*) 类经

Precepts for Physicians
(*Yī Mén Fǎ Lǜ*) 医门法律

The Classified Classic – Volume Fifteen
(*Lèi Jīng – Juàn Shí Wǔ*) 类经 · 卷十五

Essentials of the Medical Classics
(*Yī Jīng Jīng Yì*) 医经精义

Treatise on Diseases, Patterns, and Formulas Related to the Unification of the Three Etiologies – Patterns and Treatment of the Seven Qi
(*Sān Yīn Jí Yī Bìng Zhèng Fāng Lùn – Qī Qì Zhèng Zhì*) 三因极一病证方论 · 七气证治

Wondrous Lantern for Peering into the Origin and Development of Miscellaneous Diseases
(*Zá Bìng Yuán Liú Xī Zhú*) 杂病源流犀烛

Treatise on Blood Syndromes
(*Xuě Zhèng Lùn*) 血证论

The Basic Questions – Treatise on the Secret Scriptures of the Chamber of

Spiritual Orchids
(Sù Wèn – Líng Lán Mì Diǎn Lùn) 素问·灵兰秘典论

The Basic Questions – Treatise on the Nature of Life in the Distant Past
(Sù Wèn – Shàng Gǔ Tiān Zhēn Lùn) 素问·上古天真论

The Spiritual Pivot – Channels and Vessels
(Líng Shū – Jīng Mài Piān) 灵枢·经脉篇

The Basic Questions – Treatise on the Engenderment of Five Viscera
(Sù Wèn – Wǔ Zàng Shēng Chéng Piān) 素问·五脏生成篇

The Compendium of Materia Medica – Flos Magnoliae
(Běn Cǎo Gāng Mù – Xīn Yí Tiáo) 本草纲目·辛夷条

Correction of Errors in Medical Works
(Yī Lín Gǎi Cuò) 医林改错

Standards for Diagnosis and Treatment – General Introduction
(Zhèng Zhì Zhǔn Shéng – Zǒng Lùn) 证治准绳·总论

Chapter 4
Black Pearl from Red Waters – Categories of Depression
(Chì Shuǐ Xuán Zhū – Yù Mén) 赤水玄珠·郁门

Chapter 6
The Great Compendium of Acupuncture and Moxibustion – Attending Function of the Points of the Governing Vessel
(Zhēn Jiǔ Dà Chéng – Dū Mài Jīng Xué Zhǔ Zhì) 针灸大成·督脉经穴主治

The Great Compendium of Acupuncture and Moxibustion – Indications of Hand Taiyin Channel and Points
(Zhēn Jiǔ Dà Chéng – Shǒu Tài Yīn Jīng Xué Zhǔ Zhì) 针灸大成·手太阴经穴主治

The Spiritual Pivot – Knowledge from the Masters

(Líng Shū – Shī Chuán) 灵枢·师传

Chapter 7
The Basic Questions – Treatise Explaining the Five Qi
(Sù Wèn – Xuān Míng Wǔ Qì Piān) 素问·宣明五气论

Basic Questions – Treatise on Wilting
(Sù Wèn – Wěi Lùn) 素问·痿论

The Spiritual Pivot – Spirit
(Líng Shū – Běn Shén) 灵枢·本神

Explanation of Mysterious Pathogeneses and Etiologies Based on the 'Basic Questions'
(Sù Wèn Xuán Jī Yuán Bìng Shì) 素问玄机原病式

Chapter 9
Formulas from Benevolent Sages Compiled during the Taiping Era
(Tài Píng Shèng Huì Fāng) 太平圣惠方

Chapter 11
Introduction to Medicine
(Yī Xué Rù Mén) 医学入门

Correction of Errors in Medical Works
(Yī Lín Gǎi Cuò) 医林改错

Confucians' Duties to Their Parents
(Rú Mén Shì Qīn) 儒门事亲

Prolonging Life and Preserving the Origin
(Shòu Shì Bǎo Yuán) 寿世保元

Supplemental Compilation of Patterns and Treatment
(Zhèng Zhì Huì Bǔ) 证治汇补

Chapter 12 Depression Patterns in Selected Ancient Works

The *Basic Questions – Treatise Explaining the Five Qi*
(*Sù Wèn – Xuān Míng Wǔ Qì Lùn*) 素问·宣明五气论

The *Basic Questions – Treatise on Needling with and against the Four Seasons*
(*Sù Wèn – Sì Shí Cì Nì Cóng Lùn*) 素问·四时刺逆从论

The *Basic Questions – Treatise on Needling with and against the Four Seasons*
(*Sù Wèn – Sì Shí Cì Nì Cóng Lùn*) 素问·四时刺逆从论

The *Basic Questions – Treatise on Regulating the Channels*
(*Sù Wèn – Tiáo Jīng Lùn*) 素问·调经论

The *Basic Questions – Treatise on Pain*
(*Sù Wèn – Jǔ Tòng Lùn*) 素问·举痛论

The *Spiritual Pivot – The Spirit*
(*Líng Shū – Běn Shén*) 灵枢·本神

Unified Treatise on Diseases, Patterns and Remedies according to the Three Causes, Volume 8, Discussion on the Seven Qi
(*Sān Yīn Jí Yī Bìng Zhèng Fāng Lùn – Juàn Zhī Bā – Qī Qì Xù Lùn*)
三因极一病证方论·卷之八·七气叙论

Unified Treatise on Diseases, Patterns and Remedies according to the Three Causes, Volume 8, Discussion on the Seven Qi
(*Sān Yīn Jí Yī Bìng Zhèng Fāng Lùn – Juàn Zhī Bā – Qī Qì Zhèng Zhì*)
三因极一病证方论·卷之八·七气证治

Teachings of [Zhu] Dan-xi, Volume 3, Six Depressions
(*Dān Xī Xīn Fǎ – Juàn Sān – Liù Yù*) 丹溪心法·卷三·六郁

Appendix 3
Classical Sources

The Orthodox Tradition of Medicine, Depression Pattern
(Yī Xué Zhèng Zhuàn – Yù Zhèng) 医学正传·郁证

The Gateway to Medicine – Depression
(Yī Xué Rù Mén – Yù) 医学入门·郁

Universal Salvation Formulary, Volume 18, Heart Viscus, Fearful Throbbing and Fright Palpitations
(Pǔ Jì Fāng – Juàn Shí Bā – Xīn Zàng Mén – Zhēng Chōng Jīng Jì)
普济方·卷十八·心脏门·怔忡惊悸

Jing-yue's Complete Works, Volume 19, Miscellaneous Diseases, Depression Pattern, Discussion on the Patterns and Treatment of the Three Depressions Associated with Emotion
(Jǐng Yuè Quán Shū – Juàn Zhī Shí Jiǔ – Zá Zhèng Mò – Yù Zhèng – Lùn Qíng Zhì Sān Yù Zhèng Zhì)
景岳全书·卷之十九·杂证谟·郁证·论情志三郁证治

Jing-yue's Complete Works, Volume 19, Miscellaneous Diseases, History of Depression Patterns (Jǐng Yuè Quán Shū – Juàn Zhī Shí Jiǔ – Zá Zhèng Mò – Yù Zhèng Shù Gǔ)
景岳全书·卷之十九·杂证谟·郁证述古

Compilation and Supplementation of Patterns and Treatments, Volume 2, Internal Causes, Depression
(Zhèng Zhì Huì Bǔ – Juàn Zhī Èr – Nèi Yīn Mén – Yù Zhèng)
证治汇补·卷之二·内因门·郁症

Zhang's Clear View of Medicine, Volume 3, Various Qi, Depression
(Zhāng Shì Yī Tōng – Juàn Sān – Zhū Qì Mén – Yù)
张氏医通·卷三·诸气门·郁

Incisive Light on the Source of Miscellaneous Diseases, Volume 18, Internal Damage and External Contraction, Sources of Various Depressions
(Zá Bìng Yuán Liú Xī Zhú – Juàn Shí Bā – Nèi Shāng Wài Gǎn Mén – Zhū

Yù Yuán Liú)
杂病源流犀烛·卷十八·内伤外感门·诸郁源流

Systematized Patterns with Clear-Cut Treatments, Volume 3, Treatise and Treatments of Depression Disease
(Lèi Zhèng Zhì Cái – Juàn Zhī Sān – Yù Zhèng Lùn Zhì)
类证治裁·卷之三·郁症论治

Selection of Fu-Xi's Treatise on Medicine
(Fú Xī Yī Lùn Xuǎn)
俫溪医论选

A Clinical Guide with Case Histories, Depression
(Lín Zhèng Zhǐ Nán Yī Àn – Yù) 临证指南医案·郁

A Clinical Guide with Case Histories, Fright
(Lín Zhèng Zhǐ Nán Yī Àn – Jīng) 临证指南医案·惊

Wings of the Golden Cabinet, An Overall Treatise on Rib-side Pain
(Jīn Guì Yì – Xié Tòng Tǒng Lùn) 金匮翼·胁痛统论

Essential Cases of Renowned Qing Dynasty Physicians, Cases of Ling Xiao-wu
(Qīng Dài Míng Yī Yī Àn Jīng Huá – Líng Xiǎo Wǔ Yī Àn) 清代名医医案精华·凌晓五医案

Records of Chinese Medicine with Reference to Western Medicine
(Yī Xué Zhōng Zhōng Cān Xī Lù) 医学衷中参西录

References

1. Wang Yan-heng. *Differentiation and Treatment of Depressive Disorder by Integration of Traditional Chinese Medicine and Western Medicine* (中西医结合论治抑郁障碍). Beijing: The People's Medical Publishing House; 2006.

2. Wang Yong-yan. *Traditional Chinese Internal Medicine* (中医内科学). Shanghai: Shanghai Scientific and Technical Publishers; 1998. p.274.

3. Chen Wen-kai, Zhou Ling, etc. Research on Traditional Chinese Medicine Syndromes and Clinical Epidemiology of 571 Depression Cases (571例抑郁症中医证候学临床流行病学调查). *Zhejiang Journal of Traditional Chinese Medicine* (浙江中医杂志). 2007, 5: 262-264.

4. Hu Sui-yu, Zhang Hong-geng, Zheng Lin, etc. An Analysis on the Proportion of Different Traditional Chinese Medical Syndromes in 1997 Depression Patients (1977例抑郁症患者中医不同证型构成比分析). *Journal of Chinese Physician* (中国医师杂志). 2003, 5(10): 1312-1314.

5. Tong Jian-ming, Liu Hong, Lan Jia-fa, Li Jian-hua. Depression and Functional Disorder of the Spleen and Stomach (抑郁症与脾胃功能障碍). *Traditional Chinese Medicinal Research* (中医研究). 1993, 2(6): 12-13.

6. Yang Zheng-chun, Tong Jian-ming, etc. Further Discussion on the Traditional Chinese Medical Pathomechanism of Depression (抑郁症的中医病机再探讨). *Journal of Luzhou Medical College* (泸州医学院学报). 2006, 3(29): 220-221.

7. Zhang Jian. Experiences of Li Fu-ren in Treating Elderly Depression (李辅仁治疗老年抑郁症经验). *Journal of Traditional Chinese Medicine* (中医杂志). 2000, 41(4): 208-209.

8. Guo Ya-ming, Liu Cui-feng. Experiences of Wang Yan-heng in Treating Depression (王彦恒治疗抑郁症经验). *Hebei Journal of Traditional Chinese Medicine* (河北中医). 2002, 24(2): 100-101.

9. Li Jie. A Brief Discussion on the Syndrome Differentiation and Treatment of Depression (浅谈抑郁症的辨证施治). *Hubei Journal of Traditional Chinese Medicine* (湖北中医杂志). 2002, 24(2): 28-29.

10. Yang Lin. A Discussion on Liver Constraint and Depression (论肝郁与抑郁症). *Shaanxi Journal of Traditional Chinese Medicine* (陕西中医). 2002, 21(6): 260-261.

11. Han Xu, Fan Sheng-kai, Zhang Jie. Clinical Observation of 50 Depression Cases Treated with Syndrome Differentiation (抑郁症的辨证施治临床观察50例). *Beijing Journal of Traditional Chinese Medicine* (北京中医). 2003, 22(1): 31-32.

12. Zheng Jian-jun, Wu Xin-hua, Li Guang-ming. Treating 63 Patients with Tumor and Depression with *Chái Hú Shū Gān Sǎn* (柴胡疏肝散治疗肿瘤患者抑郁症63例). *Shandong Journal of Traditional Chinese Medicine* (山东中医杂志). 2002, 21(9): 530.

13. Lü Ya-qin, Wang Cai-lu, Du Hong. Treating 30 Post-Schizophrenia Depression

Cases with *Jiě Yù Tāng* (解郁汤治疗精神分裂症后抑郁30例). *Liaoning Journal of Traditional Chinese Medicine* (辽宁中医杂志). 2002, 29(6): 350.

14. Quan Shi-jian. Efficacy Observation in 30 Depression Cases Treated with Modified *Bǎi Hé Dì Huáng Tāng* (百合地黄汤加减治疗抑郁症30例疗效观察). *New Journal of Traditional Chinese Medicine* (新中医). 1999, 31(2): 16-17.

15. Wei Xu-huan, Tang Qing-jun. Treating 85 Depression Cases with Modified Self-composed *Bǎi Hé Tāng* (自拟百合汤加减治疗抑郁症85例). *Jiangsu Journal of Traditional Chinese Medicine* (江苏中医药). 2002, 23(7): 25.

16. Chen Xiao-shan, Zhang Li-hui. Traditional Chinese Medical Syndrome Differentiation and Treatment of Elderly Depression (老年抑郁症的中医辨治). *Chinese Journal of School Doctors* (中国校医). 2005, 1(19): 96.

17. Li Jie. A Brief Discussion on the Syndrome Differentiation and Treatment of Depression (浅谈抑郁症的辨证施治). *Hubei Journal of Traditional Chinese Medicine* (湖北中医杂志). 2002, 4(24): 28.

18. Chang Fa-wei, Ma Yu-hong. Clinical Observation of 23 Depression Cases Treated by Integrated Therapy of Traditional Chinese Medicine and Western Medicine (中西医结合治疗抑郁症23例临床观察). *Forum on Traditional Chinese Medicine* (国医论坛). 2002, 17(3): 36-37.

19. Bai Xiao-ying, Zhang Wei. Treating 54 Mental Disorder Cases with Integrated Therapy of Traditional Chinese Medicine and Western Medicine (中西医结合治疗精神障碍54例). *Shaanxi Journal of Traditional Chinese Medicine* (陕西中医). 2002, 23(2): 118-120.

20. Zhou Zheng-rong. Treating 38 Cases of Reactive Depression with Integrated Therapy of Traditional Chinese Medicine and Western Medicine (中西医结合治疗反应性抑郁症38例). *Journal of Practical Traditional Chinese Medicine* (实用中医药杂志). 2001, 17(10): 30.

21. Hou Qin-luan. Using *Gēng Nián Ān Tāng* with Fluoxetine Hydrochloride to Treat Menopause Depression (更年安汤联合盐酸氟西汀治疗绝经期抑郁症). *Journal of Zhejiang College of Traditional Chinese Medicine* (浙江中医学院学报). 2005, 6(29).

22. Ye Guo-chuan. Treating 36 Depression Cases with Acupuncture Therapy (针灸治疗抑郁症36例). *Shanghai Journal of Acupuncture and Moxibustion* (上海针灸杂志). 2000, (6): 30.

23. Fu Wen-yan. The Application of Acupuncture Therapy in the Elderly (针灸疗法在老年人的应用). *Foreign Medical Sciences (Section of Traditional Chinese Medicine and Medicinals)* (国外医学.中医中药分册). 1999, (4): 46.

24. Dong Zi-ping. Treating 101 Depression Cases with Electro-Acupuncture (电针治疗抑郁症101例). *Chinese Acupuncture & Moxibustion* (中国针灸). 2001, (1): 6

25. Bai Qiao-ling, Ma Xiao-jing, etc. Clinical Observation of 30 Depression Cases Treated with Acupuncture Therapy (针刺治疗抑郁症30例临床疗效观察). *Journal of Chinese Physician* (中国临床医生). 2004, 32 (8): 52-53.

References

26. Liu Zhi-shun. Clinical Observation of 30 Post-Stroke Depression Cases Treated with Regulating the Sea of Marrow Therapy (调理髓海法治疗中风后抑郁症30例临床观察). *Chinese Acupuncture & Moxibustion* (中国针灸). 1997, 9: 543-544

27. Jin Guang-liang. The Effect of Electro-Acupuncture on the Brain Monoamine Neurotransmitters in Rat Models of Depression (电针对慢性应激抑郁模型大鼠脑内单胺类神经递质的影响). *Chinese Journal of Psychiatry* (中华精神科杂志). 1999, 32(4): 220.

28. Han Cui, Wang Lei, etc. The Effect of Electro-Acupuncture on Serum Cytokine in Depression Patients (电针对抑郁症患者血清细胞因子的影响). *Chinese Journal of Behavioral Medical Science* (中国行为医学科学). 2002, 3(11): 277-279.

29. Han Cui, Li Xue-wu. The Effect of Electro-acupuncture on the Hippocampus DNF in Chronic Stress Rat Models of Depression (电针对慢性应激抑郁模型大鼠海马DNF的影响). *Chinese Journal of Basic Medicine in Traditional Chinese Medicine* (中国中医基础医学杂志). 2001, 7(7): 535.

30. Yu Jin, Li Xiao-yan. Using Electro-acupuncture with Antidepressants to Significantly Reduce Immobility Time in Forced Swimming Tests on Mice (电针合用抗抑郁药能明显减少小鼠强迫游泳实验中的静止时间). *Acupuncture Research* (针刺研究). 2002, 27(2): 119-123.

31. Jiang Ling-ling, Xu Qian-fang, Zheng Chao-ying, etc, Treating 30 Cases of Stroke Patients with Depression by the Associated Therapy of Traditional Chinese Medical Psychotherapy (中医心理疗法配合治疗中风病伴抑郁症30例). *Shanghai Journal of Traditional Chinese Medicine* (上海中医药杂志). 2002, 36(8): 17-18.

32. Wang Bin, Liu Tian-pei. Saikosaponin Enhancement in the Antidepressant Effect of Fluoxetine in Forced Swimming Test Models (柴胡皂甙加强氟西汀在强迫游泳模型上的抗抑郁作用). *Chinese Traditional and Herbal Drugs* (中草药). 1997, 28(12): 729-731.

33. Li Ming-ya, Chen Hong-mei. The Antidepressant Effect of Rhizoma Acori Tatarinowii on Behavioral Despair Animal Models of Depression (石菖蒲对行为绝望动物抑郁模型的抗抑郁作用). *Journal of Chinese Medicinal Materials* (中药材). 2001, 24(1): 40-41.

34. Molodavkin GM, Aldarmaa Zh, Voronina TA, et al. Khim_FarmZh, 1998, 32(4), 35

35. Cui Cheng-bin, Yang Ming. Research on the Active Antidepressant Ingredients in the Chinese Medicinal Morinda Officinalis (中药巴戟天中抗抑郁活性成分的研究). *China Journal of Chinese Materia Medica* (中国中药杂志). 1995, 20(1): 36.

36. Zhang Zhong-qi, Huang Shi-jie, Yuan Li, etc. The Effect of Morinda Officinalis Oligosaccharides on Rats in Forced Swimming Tests and Acquired Helpless Models of Depression of Rats (巴戟天寡糖对鼠强迫性游泳和获得性无助抑郁模型的影响). *Chinese Journal of Pharmacology and Toxicity* (中国药理学与毒理学杂志). 2001, 15(4): 262-265.

37. Zhang Zhong-qi, Yuan Li. The Antidepressant Effect of Morinda Officinalis Extract (巴戟天醇提物的抗抑郁作用). *Chinese Pharmacological Journal* (中国药学杂志). 2000, 35(11): 739-1226.

38. Weng Shen-hong, Cheng Zi-li, Wang Gao-hua. Study on the Clinical Control of Treating Depression with Radix et Rhizoma seu Caulis Acanthopanacis Senticosi Capsules (刺五加胶囊治疗抑郁症的临床对照研究). *Hubei Journal of Traditional Chinese Medicine* (湖北中医杂志). 2001, 23(6): 8-9.

39. Si Yin-chu, Sun Jian-ning. The Effect of Hypericum Perforatum Extract on the Behavior, Brain 5HT and NE Expression of Chronic Stress Rat Models of Depression (贯叶连翘提取物对慢性应激抑郁大鼠行为及脑内5HT，NE表达的影响). *Journal of China Medical University* (中国医科大学学报). 2003, 34(1): 70-73.

40. Qin Xiao-song, Jin Kui-he, Ding Bao-kun. The Effect of Ginkgo Biloba Extract with Venlafaxine Hydrochloride on NOS Protein Expression and NO Levels in the Hippocampus of Depression Rats. (银杏叶提取物联合盐酸文拉法辛对抑郁大鼠海马NOS蛋白表达及NO水平的影响). *Chinese Mental Health Journal* (中国心理卫生杂志). 2003, 17(12): 828-831.

41. Satyan KS, Jaiswal AK, Ghosal S, et al. Effect of Ginkgolic Acid Conjugates on Brain Monoamines and Metabolites in Rodents. Biog.Amines, 1997, 13(2): 143.

42. Chen Yao, Qin Lu-ping. The Effect of Total Glucosides of Centella Asiatica on the Neuroendocrine Function of Depression Rats (积雪草总甙对抑郁症大鼠神经内分泌功能的影响). *Academic Journal of Second Military Medical University* (第二军医大学学报). 2002, 23(11): 1224-1226.

43. Chen Wei-yin, Liu Fu-you. Research on the Effect of Compound Chinese Medicinal Formulas and Fluoxetine on Post-Stroke Depression and Neurological Rehabilitation (中药复方与氟西汀对卒中后抑郁神经功能康复影响的研究). *Journal of Chengdu University of Traditional Chinese Medicine* (成都中医药大学学报). 2001, 24(4): 20-23.

44. Cao Su. Clinical Study of Treating Elderly Depression with *Kàng Yì Yù Zhèng Jiāo Náng* (抗抑郁症胶囊治疗老年抑郁症的临床研究). *China Journal of Chinese Medicine* (中国中医药学报). 2001, 16(3): 32-34.

45. Zhao Zhi-sheng. Efficacy Observation of Treating Depressive Syndrome (Anxiety, Depression) with "*Yì Yù Kāng*" ("抑郁康"治疗郁证(焦虑、抑郁)的疗效观察). *Shanghai Journal of Traditional Chinese Medicine* (上海中医药杂志). 1999, 33(2):12

46. Tong Jian-ming, Lin De-yun. Recent Foreign Studies on Treating Dysthymia with Chinese Medicinals (中药治疗心境恶劣的国外研究近况). *Foreign Medical Sciences* (*Section of Traditional Chinese Medicine and Medicinal*) (国外医学. 中医中药分册). 2000, 22(4): 203.

47. Wu Li, Zhang Li-ping, etc. The Effect of Modified *Wēn Dǎn Tāng* on the Behavior and Plasma Somatostatin Levels in Rat Models of Depression (加减温胆汤对

References

抑郁模型大鼠行为学和血浆生长抑素含量的影响). *Chinese Journal of Clinical Rehabilitation* (中国临床康复). 2005, 9(8):114-116.

48. Xue Zheng. An Experimental Study on the Antidepressant Effect of *Pǐ Shèn Liǎng Zhù Wán* (脾肾两助丸抗抑郁作用的实验研究). *Journal of Shanxi College of Traditional Chinese Medicine* (山西中医学院学报). 2003, 4(4): 14-16.

49. Yang Shi-you, Huang Shi-fu. The Effects of *Jiě Bǎi Yōu Kǒu Fú Yè* on the Behavior and Central Neurotransmitters in Rat Models of Depression (解百忧口服液对抑郁模型大鼠行为及中枢神经递质的影响). *Chinese Journal of Basic Medicine in Traditional Chinese Medicine* (中国中医基础医学杂志). 2000, 6(11): 56.

50. Yang Jin, Xie Zhong-li. The Effect of *Chāng Huān Yī Hào* on the Brain Monoamine Neurotransmitters in Rat Models of Depression (菖欢1号对大鼠抑郁症模型脑内单胺类神经递质的影响). *Journal of Nanjing University of Traditional Chinese Medicine* (南京中医药大学学报). 2001, 17(5): 294.

51. Zhang You-zhi, Nie Hui-min. Effects of the Compound Formula Radix Bupleuri and Radix Rehmanniae on the Cerebral Prefrontal Cortex and Hippocampus Monoamine Neurotransmitters of Chronic Stress Rat Models of Depression (柴地合方对慢性应激大鼠大脑前额皮质和海马单胺类神经递质的影响). *Journal of Anhui Traditional Chinese Medical College* (安徽中医学院学报). 2005, 24(1): 34-36.

52. Zhang You-zhi, Nie Hui-min. Behavioral Study of Treating Depression Animal Models with Classical Formulas such as *Chái Hú Jiā Lóng Gǔ Mǔ Lì Tāng* (柴胡加龙骨牡蛎汤等经方治疗抑郁症的动物行为学研究). *Chinese Journal of Basic Medicine in Traditional Chinese Medicine* (中国中医基础医学杂志). 2001, 7(7): 511.

53. Xin Qian, Jin You-yu, Tang Guang, editors. *New Compilation of Pharmacology* (新编药物学). 15th ed. Beijing: The People's Medical Publishing House; 2004.

54. Chen Yan-fang, editor. *The Treatment and Care of CCMD-3 Related Disorders* (CCMD-3相关障碍的治疗与护理). Shandong: Shandong Science & Technology Press; 2001.

55. Gong Shao-lin, editor. *Depression* (抑郁症). Beijing: The People's Medical Publishing House; 2003.

56. Leng Fang-nan, editor. *The Criterion of Pattern Differentiation and Treatment in Traditional Chinese Medicine* (中医证候辨治规范). Beijing: The People's Medical Publishing House; 1989.

57. Shen Yu-cun, editor. *Psychiatry* (精神病学). 4th ed. Beijing: The People's Medical Publishing House; 2001.

58. Fan Xiao-dong, Wang Xiang-dong, Yu-xin, etc, translators. *ICD-10 Classification of Mental and Behavioral Disorders* (ICD-10精神与行为障碍分类：临床描述与诊断要点). Beijing: The People's Medical Publishing House; 1993.

59. Wang Qi, editor. *The Study of Visceral Manifestation of Traditional Chinese Medicine* (中医藏象学). Beijing: The People's Medical Publishing House; 1997.

60. Wang Yan-heng, editor. *The Practical Chinese Medical Psychiatry* (实用中医精神病学). Beijing: The People's Medical Publishing House; 2000.

61. Wang Yong-yan, Shen Shao-gong, editors. *Traditional Chinese Internal Medicine in Modern Day* (今日中医内科). Beijing: The People's Medical Publishing House; 2000.

62. Wang Yong-yan, Zhang Tian, Li Di-chen, etc, editors. *Clinical Traditional Chinese Internal Medicine* (临床中医内科学). Beijing: Beijing Publishing House; 1994.

63. Yan Wen-wei, editor. *Clinical Psychopharmacology* (临床精神药理学). Changsha: Hunan Science and Technology Press; 1998.

64. Yang Bao-feng, editor. *Pharmacology* (药理学). 6th ed. Beijing: The People's Medical Publishing House; 2004.

65. Yang Quan. *Diagnosis and Treatment of Depressive Disorder* (抑郁障碍的诊断与治疗). Chengdu: Sichuan Science and Technology Press; 2003.

66. Zhang Ji-zhi, Ji Zhong-fu, editors. *The Rational Use of Psychotropic Drugs* (精神药物的合理应用). 3rd ed. Beijing: The People's Medical Publishing House; 2003.

67. Cai Zuo-ji, editor. *The Fundamentals and Clinical Practice of Depression* (抑郁症基础与临床). 2nd ed. Beijing: Science Press; 2002.

68. Pharmacopoeia Commission of the Chinese Ministry of Public Health. *Pharmacopoeia of the People's Republic of China* (中华人民共和国药典). Volume 2. 2005 ed. Beijing: Chemical Industry Press; 2005.

69. Chinese Society of Psychiatry. *The Chinese Classification of Mental Disorders* (中国精神障碍分类与诊断标准). 3rd ed. Shandong: Shandong Science & Technology Press; 2001.

70. Zhu Zi-qing, editor. *The Key to Diagnosis and Treatment of Depressive Disorder* (抑郁障碍诊疗关键). Nanjing: Jiangsu Science and Technology Press; 2003.

71. A Brief Discussion of the Relationship between *Xie Yi* and Depressive Disorder with Report of 58 Clinical Cases (解依与抑郁性精神障碍的关系浅探—附58例临床报道). *Shanghai Journal of Traditional Chinese Medicine* (上海中医药杂志). 1994, 2: 14-16.

72. Qian Hui-nan. A Brief Investigation of the Origin of Constraint Syndrome (郁证源流考略). *Chinese Journal of Basic Medicine in Traditional Chinese Medicine* (中国中医基础医学杂志). 1995, 1(3): 55.

73. Zhang An-ling, Qi Ke-jian. A Discussion of Constraint from the Perspective of Lung (从肺论郁). *Journal of Shandong College of Traditional Chinese Medicine* (山东中医学院学报). 1994, 18(5).

74. Qin Bo-wei. *Medical Lectures Notes of Qian-zhai* (谦斋医学讲稿). Shanghai: Shanghai Scientific and Technical Publishers; 1964.

References

75. Zhang Gang. *Investigations of the Naming and Origin of a Hundred Diseases in Traditional Chinese Medicine* (中医百病名源考). Beijing: The People's Medical Publishing House; 1997.

76. Jin Shi-hua. *The Likes and Dislikes of Brain-Shen* (脑神的喜与恶). Copy of manuscript with other information unknown.

Index by Disease Names and Symptoms

A

a bitter taste in the mouth, 61
abdominal distention, 53, 94, 113, 166
abdominal fullness, 175
abdominal pain, 216
aching cold lumbus and knees, 70
aching limp lumbus and back, 173
aching limp lumbus and knees, 177
acid reflux, 61
agitation, 62, 64, 112, 201
amenorrhea, 63, 126, 164, 199, 232
amnesia, 92
anxiety depression, 13
anxiety, 60, 73, 82, 93, 216
auditory hallucinations, 93, 228, 242

B

belching, 61, 103, 112, 222
bipolar disorder, 3
blood stasis, 237, 241
blurred vision, 16, 61, 94
bulimia nervosa, 232
bulimia, 137, 234

C

chest impediment, 177
chest oppression, 110, 175, 243
chest tightness, 53
constipation, 32, 72, 94, 212
cyclothymia, 278

D

decreased libido, 75
delirious speech, 228
depressive disorder, 2, 275
depressive episode, 276
despair, 71
diarrhea, 83, 94
difficulty falling asleep, 67, 107
distending fullness of rib-sides, 53
dizziness, 38, 61, 62, 82, 83, 85, 90, 109, 171, 218, 240
drug-induced symptoms, 4
dry bound stools, 166
dry eyes, 111
dry mouth, 94, 111, 192, 243
dry stools, 62, 214
dysmenorrhea, 83
dysthymia, 276, 277

E

emaciation, 66, 232
enuresis, 94
exuberant phlegm, 73

F

fatigue, 17, 54, 119, 173, 243
Fear, 133
fibromyalgia, 11
fidgetiness, 63
fifth-watch diarrhea, 75

fine sunken pulses, 66, 69
fine wiry pulses, 67, 68
food accumulation, 140
forgetfulness, 62, 81, 120, 123, 124, 127
frequent sighing, 60, 62, 70
frequent urination, 66
fullness and oppression of chest, 32

G

geriatric depressive disorder, 147

H

hair loss, 245
hallucinations, 2, 92, 240
headache, 62, 92, 109, 171, 218
heart vexation, 12, 63
hiccoughing, 222
hiccoughs, 167

I

impotence, 75, 126, 131, 195, 196, 244
incontinence, 71
infertility, 126
insomnia, 55, 73, 81, 89, 105, 109, 124, 197, 243
irascibility, 61, 102, 112, 242
irregular menstruation, 82
irritability, 55
irritation, 85, 93

K

kidney yang deficiency, 70

L

liver constraint and spleen deficiency, 83
loose stools, 66, 125, 216
low appetite, 109
low libido, 67, 68, 195, 196
low spirits, 54, 58, 61, 67, 68, 69, 72, 74, 75, 103, 218
lumbar pain, 120

M

mania, 55
manic episodes, 3
melancholia, 278
migraines, 93

N

nausea, 54, 94, 113, 168, 244
neurasthenia, 216, 236
night sweats, 68, 71

O

obesity, 94, 170
olfaction disorders, 94
overeating, 232

P

palpitations, 26, 27, 66, 81, 86, 178, 180, 181, 200, 211
paranoia, 2, 27
persistent mood (affective) disorders, 278
pessimism, 69, 71, 72, 75, 103
poor appetite, 35, 62
poor memory, 67, 123
poor sleep, 211
postpartum depression, 13
premature ejaculation, 126, 131
profuse dreaming, 66, 92, 109, 111, 124, 243
profuse nightmares, 67
psycholepsy, 216
psychological symptoms, 2

R

red eyes, 61
red face, 64, 72

Index by Disease Names and Symptoms

red tongue, 61
rib-side pain, 82, 93

S
sadness, 70
scant menses, 26
schizophrenia, 98
seminal emission, 68, 94, 126, 195, 244
shortness of breath, 27, 70, 76, 243
sighing, 32
sleeplessness, 60, 63, 66, 81, 107, 112, 216
somatic symptoms, 2
somnolence, 54, 116
sorrow, 129
spontaneous sweating, 109
stomach pain, 83

T
tardive dyskinesia, 188
thirst, 64, 109

timidity, 27, 135
tinnitus, 61, 93, 240

U
unstable mood, 64, 73, 102
urinary retention, 94

V
vertigo, 85
vexation, 62, 64, 102, 178
vexing heat in the five hearts, 68
vexing heat in the hearts of palms and soles, 111
vomiting, 61, 82, 113

W
weeping, 70, 242
weight loss, 232
withdrawal disease, 98

Index by Chinese Medicinals and Formulas

A
Ān Shén Gŭn Tán Wán, 238
Arillus Longan, 211
Arisaema cum Bile, 62

B
bái fú líng, 173
băi hé, 32, 66, 70, 242
Bái Hŭ Tāng, 162
bái jí lí, 61, 68
bái kòu rén, 171
bái sháo, 68, 74, 76, 135, 158, 181, 227, 231
bái zhú, 66, 131, 142, 171, 173
bā jĭ tiān, 70, 75, 152
bàn xià, 113, 114, 171
Bàn Xià Hòu Pò Tāng, 13
Băo Hé Wán, 112, 140
Bā Zhèng Săn, 185
Bā Zhēn Tāng, 76
biē jiă, 71, 76
bò he, 176
bŭ gŭ zhī, 66, 70, 74
Bulbus Allii Macrostemi, 164
Bulbus Lilii, 32, 66, 70, 242
Bŭ Zhōng Yì Qì Tāng, 143, 187

C
cāng zhú, 14, 67, 118, 174
căo dòu kòu, 74
Carapax et Plastrum Testudinis, 70, 71, 76, 104, 151
Carapax Trionycis, 71, 76

Caulis Bambusae in Taenia, 62, 114, 128
Caulis Spatholobi, 163
chái hú, 60, 63, 103, 110, 121, 143, 157, 158, 176, 191, 200, 236
Chái Hú Shū Gān Săn, 60, 179
chăo bái zhú, 74, 110
chăo zăo rén, 68, 70, 74, 108, 110, 111, 132
Chéng Qì Tāng, 162
chén pí, 62, 109, 113, 118, 128, 140, 142
chén xiāng, 186
chē qián zĭ, 185
chì sháo, 153, 158, 174, 179, 231
chuān liàn zĭ, 61
chuān niú xī, 63
chuān xiōng, 14, 63, 67, 69, 72, 174, 240
Chūn Zé Tāng, 187
Cinnabaris, 183
cí shí, 61, 73, 74, 112
Colla Corii Asini, 181
Colla Cornus Cervi, 75
Concha Arcae, 61
Concha Haliotidis, 61
Concha Margaritiferae Usta, 183, 230
Concha Ostreae, 73
Concha Ostreae Cruda, 184
Concretio Silicea Bambusae, 61, 66, 73, 103, 238
Cortex Cinnamomi, 188
Cortex Eucommiae, 69, 75, 120, 152
Cortex Lycii, 69, 71
Cortex Magnoliae Officinalis, 139, 166
Cortex Mori, 186

Cortex Moutan, 121
Cortex Phellodendri Chinensis, 64, 196

D

dà huáng, 61, 62, 64, 102, 114, 128, 166, 168, 236
dài zhě shí, 143, 233
dāng guī, 63, 76, 122, 131, 135, 181, 237
dǎng shēn, 66, 104, 110, 121, 125, 131, 136, 173, 201
dǎn nán xīng, 62
dān shēn, 69, 73, 108, 240
Dàn Zhú Rú Tāng, 13
dà zǎo, 66, 70, 121, 136, 211
Dens Draconis, 73
Diān Kuáng Mèng Xǐng Tāng, 237
dì gǔ pí, 69, 71
dù zhòng, 69, 75, 120, 152

E

ē jiāo, 181
é zhú, 63
Èr Chén Tāng, 175
Èr Zhú Fú Líng Tāng, 175

F

fǎ bàn xià, 62, 128, 139, 140, 142, 145
Flos Carthami, 63, 73, 153, 158, 174, 179, 197, 202, 237
Flos Chrysanthemi, 61, 68, 69, 72, 108, 240
Flos Farfarae, 32
Flos Inulae, 143, 233
Folium Eriobotryae, 145
Folium Mori, 108
Folium Perillae, 139
Folium Phyllostachydis Henonis, 167, 239
fó shǒu, 74, 158
Fructus Alpiniae Oxyphyllae, 66

Fructus Amomi, 61, 74, 172
Fructus Amomi Rotundus, 171
Fructus Aurantii, 63, 236
Fructus Aurantii Immaturus, 114, 166
Fructus Cannabis, 166
Fructus Citri, 74, 158
Fructus Citri Sarcodactylis, 74, 158
Fructus Corni, 67, 69, 71, 75, 119, 120, 126
Fructus Crataegi, 112, 140, 176
Fructus Gardeniae, 63, 64, 67, 102, 171
Fructus Gardeniae Praeparatus (scorched-fried), 174
Fructus Hordei Germinatus, 62, 71, 176
Fructus Jujubae, 66, 70, 121, 136, 211
Fructus Ligustri Lucidi, 66, 68, 69, 71, 108, 127, 195
Fructus Lycii, 68, 69, 74, 75, 76, 105, 120, 152
Fructus Mori, 120
Fructus Psoraleae, 66, 69, 70, 74
Fructus Rosae Laevigatae, 244
Fructus Schisandrae Chinensis, 71, 76, 105, 120, 121
Fructus Toosendan, 61
Fructus Tribuli, 61, 68
Fructus Trichosanthis, 164
Fructus Tritici, 132
Fructus Tritici Levis, 71
fú líng, 62, 63, 66, 67, 104, 110, 118, 121, 126, 128, 131, 142, 158, 180
fú xiǎo mài, 71
fù zǐ, 188

G

gān cǎo, 183
Gān Mài Dà Zǎo Tāng, 13, 211
gé gēn, 69, 163, 194
gǒu qǐ zǐ, 68, 69, 74, 75, 76, 105, 120, 152
gōu téng, 61

Index by Chinese Medicinals and Formulas

guā lóu, 164
guī jiǎ, 70, 71, 76, 104, 151
Guī Pí Tāng, 110, 181
guì zhī, 142, 183
Guì Zhī Gān Cǎo Lóng Gǔ Mǔ Lì Tāng, 183
Gypsum Crudum, 163, 165
Gypsum Fibrosum, 189
Gypsum Fibrosum Cruda, 61, 73, 167, 192, 194, 230

H

Haematitum, 143, 233
Heart-Clearing Phlegm-Rolling Pill, 73
Herba Artemisiae Annuae, 69
Herba Cistanches, 228
Herba Dianthi, 185
Herba Epimedii, 67, 70, 71, 75, 228
Herba Eupatorii, 73, 111, 118, 231
Herba Houttuyniae, 186
Herba Leonuri, 197, 201
Herba Lycopi, 63
Herba Menthae, 176
hé shǒu wū, 108, 127, 196, 245
hóng huā, 63, 73, 153, 158, 174, 179, 197, 202, 237
hòu pò, 139, 166
huái shān yào, 75
huáng bǎi, 64, 196
huáng lián, 64, 73, 102, 111, 168, 178, 231, 239
Huáng Lián Ē Jiāo Tāng, 111
huáng qí, 236
huáng qín, 64, 102, 168, 171, 186
huǒ má rén, 166
Huō Tán Qīng Nǎo Tāng, 72
Radix Polygoni Multiflori, 245

J

jiāo zhī zǐ, 174
jié gěng, 32
jīn yīng zǐ, 244
Jì Shēng Shèn Qì Wán, 188
jiǔ zhì dà huáng, 231
jī xuè téng, 163
jú huā, 61, 68, 69, 72, 108, 240
jú pí, 145
Jú Pí Zhú Rú Tāng, 145
Jú Shēn Tāng, 239

K

kuǎn dōng, 32

L

lái fú zǐ, 62, 73, 113, 128, 140, 166, 231, 236
lián zǐ, 211
Liáng Gé Sǎn, 171
Lignum Aquilariae Resinatum, 186
Líng Guì Zhú Gān Tāng, 141, 177
lóng dǎn cǎo, 61
lóng gǔ, 184
lóng yǎn ròu, 211
lù jiǎo jiāo, 75

M

Magnetitum, 61, 73, 74, 112
Má Zǐ Rén Wán, 166
mài mén dōng, 63, 68, 70, 105, 163, 182
Mài Wèi Dì Huáng Wán, 112
mài yá, 62, 71, 176
Massa Medicata, 140
Massa Medicata Fermentata, 62, 67, 71, 112, 140, 174, 176, 228
méng shí, 128, 238
mǔ dān pí, 121

mǔ lì, 73
mù xiāng, 172

N
niú xī, 62, 73, 158, 231
nǚ zhēn zǐ, 66, 68, 69, 71, 108, 127, 195

O
Os Draconis, 184

P
páo fù zǐ, 119
pèi lán, 73, 118, 231
Pericarpium Citri Reticulatae, 62, 109, 113, 118, 128, 140, 142, 145
Pericarpium Citri Reticulatae Viride, 113, 118
Phlegm-Flushing Brain-Clearing Formula, 72
pí pá yè, 145
Poria, 62, 63, 66, 67, 104, 110, 118, 121, 126, 128, 131, 142, 158, 180
Poria Alba, 173

Q
Qi-Benefiting Lily Bulb Decoction, 70
qīng pí, 113, 118
Qīng Xīn Gǔn Tán Wán, 73, 238, 242
Qù Dāi Xǐng Nǎo Tāng, 104
qú mài, 185
Qù Yù Yì Nǎo Tāng, 68

R
Radix Achyranthis Bidentatae, 62, 73, 158, 231
Radix Aconiti Lateralis (blast-fried), 119
Radix Aconiti Lateralis Praeparata, 173, 188
Radix Adenophorae, 70, 169

Radix Angelicae Sinensis, 63, 76, 122, 131, 135, 181, 237
Radix Asparagi, 182
Radix Astragali, 70, 74, 110, 121, 125, 136, 200, 236
Radix Aucklandiae, 172
Radix Bupleuri, 60, 63, 103, 110, 121, 143, 157, 158, 176, 191, 200, 236
Radix Codonopsis, 66, 104, 110, 121, 125, 131, 136, 173, 201
Radix Curcumae, 60, 62, 63, 67, 103, 110, 111, 141
Radix Cyathulae, 63
Radix et Rhizoma Asteris, 32, 70, 132
Radix et Rhizoma Gentianae, 61
Radix et Rhizoma Ginseng, 180, 187
Radix et Rhizoma Ginseng Cruda, 76
Radix et Rhizoma Glycyrrhizae, 183
Radix et Rhizoma Glycyrrhizae Praeparata cum Melle, 66, 131, 132
Radix et Rhizoma Rhei, 61, 62, 102, 114, 128, 166, 168, 236
Radix et Rhizoma Rhei (preserved in liquor), 64
Radix et Rhizoma Salviae Miltiorrhizae, 69, 73, 108, 240
Radix Morindae Officinalis, 70, 75, 152
Radix Ophiopogonis, 63, 68, 70, 105, 163, 182
Radix Paeoniae Alba, 68, 74, 76, 135, 158, 181, 227, 231
Radix Paeoniae Rubra, 153, 158, 174, 179, 231
Radix Platycodonis, 32
Radix Polygalae, 125
Radix Polygoni Multiflori, 108, 127, 196
Radix Pseudostellariae, 67, 74, 104
Radix Puerariae Lobatae, 69, 163, 194
Radix Rehmanniae, 111, 127, 163, 169,

Index by Chinese Medicinals and Formulas

173, 190
Radix Rehmanniae Praeparata, 75, 119, 126, 127, 134, 152
Radix Scrophulariae, 63, 68, 127, 163
Radix Scutellariae, 64, 102, 168, 171, 186
Ramulus Cinnamomi, 142, 183
Ramulus Uncariae Cum Uncis, 61
rén shēn, 180, 187
Rhizoma Acori Tatarinowii, 118
Rhizoma Alismatis, 122, 126
Rhizoma Anemarrhenae, 196
Rhizoma Atractylodis, 14, 67, 118, 174
Rhizoma Atractylodis Macrocephalae, 66, 131, 142, 171, 173
Rhizoma Atractylodis Macrocephalae (stir-fried), 74, 110
Rhizoma Chuanxiong, 14, 63, 67, 69, 72, 174, 240
Rhizoma Cimicifugae, 143, 187
Rhizoma Coptidis, 64, 73, 102, 111, 168, 178, 231, 239
Rhizoma Corydalis, 74
Rhizoma Curculiginis, 70, 75
Rhizoma Curcumae, 63
Rhizoma Cyperi, 60, 103, 113
Rhizoma Dioscoreae, 75, 119
Rhizoma Gastrodiae, 171
Rhizoma Pinelliae, 113, 114, 171
Rhizoma Pinelliae Praeparatum, 62, 128, 139, 140, 142, 145
Rhizoma Zingiberis Recens, 139
ròu cōng róng, 228
ròu guì, 188

S
sāng bái, 186
sāng shèn, 120
sāng yè, 108
Sān Huáng Zhī Zǐ Tāng, 102

Sān Rén Tāng, 171
Sān Zǐ Yǎng Qīn Tāng, 175
Semen Aesculi, 61
Semen Alpiniae Katsumadai, 74
Semen Armeniacae Amarum, 32, 166, 171
Semen Coicis, 171
Semen Cuscutae, 67, 69, 71, 75, 108, 120, 127, 135, 195, 228, 241
Semen Euryales, 244
Semen Nelumbinis, 211
Semen Persicae, 63, 73, 158, 179, 197, 202, 237
Semen Plantaginis, 185
Semen Pruni, 166
Semen Raphani, 62, 73, 113, 128, 140, 166, 231, 236
Semen Ziziphi Spinosae, 73, 108, 132
Semen Ziziphi Spinosae (stir-fried), 68, 70, 74, 108, 110, 111
shā rén, 61, 74, 172
shā shēn, 70, 169
shān yào, 119
shān zhā, 112, 140, 176
shān zhū yú, 69, 71, 75, 119, 120, 126
shēng dì, 111, 127, 163, 169, 173, 190
shēng huáng qí, 70, 74, 110, 121, 125, 136, 200
shēng jiāng, 139
shēng lóng chǐ, 73
shēng má, 143, 187
Shēng Mài Sǎn, 164
Shēng Mài Yǐn, 5, 220
shēng mǔ lì, 184
shēng shài shēn, 76
shēng shí gāo, 61, 73, 163, 167, 189, 192, 194, 230
Shēn Líng Bái Zhú Sǎn, 175
shén qū, 62, 67, 71, 112, 140, 174, 176, 228
shí chāng pú, 118

shí gāo, 165
shí jué míng, 61
shú dì huáng, 75, 119, 126, 127, 134, 152
Shū Gān Hé Wèi Yǐn, 74
Sì Huáng Zhī Zǐ Tāng, 64
Sì Jūn Zǐ Tāng, 66, 180
Sì Nì Sǎn, 56
Spleen-Restoring Decoction, 110
suān zǎo rén, 73
Suān Zǎo Tāng, 13
suō luó zǐ, 61

T

tài zǐ shēn, 67, 74, 104
Táo Hóng Sì Wù Tāng, 202
táo rén, 63, 73, 158, 179, 197, 202, 237
tiān má, 171
tiān mén dōng, 182
Tiān Wáng Bǔ Xīn Dān, 112, 182, 233
tiān zhú huáng, 61, 66, 73, 103, 238
Torpidity-Eliminating Brain-Awakening Decoction, 104
tù sī zǐ, 67, 69, 71, 75, 108, 120, 127, 135, 195, 228, 241

W

wǎ léng zǐ, 61
Wēn Dǎn Tāng, 62, 176
Wǔ Líng Sǎn, 175
Wū Tù Tāng, 108
wǔ wèi zǐ, 71, 76, 105, 120, 121

X

xiān líng pí, 67, 70, 71, 75, 228
xiān máo, 70, 75
xiāng fù, 60, 103, 113
xiāng yuán, 74, 158
Xiǎo Bàn Xià Tāng, 141
Xiǎo Chái Hú Tāng, 12

xiǎo mài, 132
Xiāo Yáo Sǎn, 16
xiè bái, 164
xìng rén, 32, 166, 171
Xuán Fù Dài Zhě Tāng, 143, 236
xuán fù huā, 143, 233
xuán shēn, 63, 68, 127, 163
Xuè Fǔ Zhú Yū Tāng, 63, 179

Y

yán hú suǒ, 74
yì mǔ cǎo, 197, 201
Yì Qì Bǎi Hé Tāng, 70
Yì Wèi Tāng, 145
yì yǐ rén, 171
yì zhì rén, 66
Yì Zhì Xǐng Shén Tāng, 69
Yòu Guī Wán, 75
yuǎn zhì, 125
Yuè Jú Wán, 14, 67
yù jīn, 60, 62, 63, 67, 103, 110, 141
yù lǐ rén, 166
yú xīng cǎo, 186

Z

zé lán, 63
zé xiè, 122, 126
Zé Xiè Tāng, 175
zhēn zhū mǔ, 183, 230
zhì fù zǐ, 173
zhì gān cǎo, 66, 131, 132
zhī mǔ, 196
zhǐ qiào, 63, 236
zhǐ shí, 114, 166
Zhǐ Zhú Wán, 175
zhī zǐ, 63, 64, 67, 102, 171
Zhū Líng Tāng, 5
zhú rú, 62, 114, 128
zhū shā, 183

Index by Chinese Medicinals and Formulas

Zhū Shā Ān Shén Wán, 112, 182
zhú yè, 167, 239
Zhú Yè Shí Gāo Tāng, 167
Zhú Yè Tāng, 13

zǐ sū yè, 139
zǐ wǎn, 32, 70, 132
Zuǒ Jīn Wán, 168

General Index

A

abdominal distention, 53, 94, 113, 166
abdominal fullness, 175
abdominal pain, 216
a bitter taste in the mouth, 61
aching cold lumbus and knees, 70
aching limp lumbus and back, 173
aching limp lumbus and knees, 69, 177
acid reflux, 61
acupuncture, 80
agitation, 62, 64, 112, 201
amenorrhea, 73, 63, 126, 164, 199, 232
amnesia, 92
Ān Shén Gǔn Tán Wán, 238
anxiety, 60, 73, 82, 93, 216
anxiety depression, 13
Arillus Longan, 211
Arisaema cum Bile, 62
auditory hallucinations, 93, 228, 242

B

bái fú líng, 173
bǎi hé, 32, 66, 70, 242
bǎi huì, 81, 92, 95, 123
Bái Hǔ Tāng, 162
bái jí lí, 61, 68
bái kòu rén, 171
bái sháo, 68, 74, 76, 135, 158, 181, 227, 231
bái zhú, 66, 131, 142, 171, 173
bā jǐ tiān, 70, 75, 152
bàn xià, 113, 114, 171
Bàn Xià Hòu Pò Tāng, 13
Bǎo Hé Wán, 112, 140
Bā Zhèng Sǎn, 185
Bā Zhēn Tāng, 76
bēi dié, 18
belching, 61, 103, 112, 222
biē jiǎ, 71, 76
bipolar disorder, 3
BL 15, 91
BL 17, 89
BL 18, 83, 84, 91
BL 19, 83
BL 20, 84, 91, 93
BL 23, 84, 86
blood deficiency with stasis, 202
blood stasis, 29, 38, 55, 85, 197, 226, 241
blurred vision, 16, 61, 94
brain-spirit, 22, 23, 26
bǔ gǔ zhī, 66, 70, 74
Bulbus Allii Macrostemi, 164
Bulbus Lilii, 32, 66, 70, 242
bulimia, 137, 234
bulimia nervosa, 232
Bǔ Zhōng Yì Qì Tāng, 143, 187

C

cāng zhú, 14, 67, 118, 174
cǎo dòu kòu, 74
Carapax et Plastrum Testudinis, 70, 71, 76, 104, 151
Carapax Trionycis, 71, 76

Caulis Bambusae in Taenia, 62, 114, 128
Caulis Spatholobi, 163
chái hú, 60, 63, 103, 110, 121, 143, 157, 158, 176, 191, 200, 236
Chái Hú Shū Gān Săn, 60, 179
chăo bái zhú, 74, 110
chăo zăo rén, 68, 70, 74, 108, 110, 111, 132
chē qián zĭ, 185
chén pí, 62, 109, 113, 118, 128, 140, 142
chén xiāng, 186
Chéng Qì Tāng, 162
chest impediment, 177
chest oppression, 110, 175, 243
chest tightness, 53
chì sháo, 153, 158, 174, 179, 231
chuān liàn zĭ, 61
chuān niú xī, 63
chuān xiōng, 14, 63, 67, 69, 72, 174, 240
Chūn Zé Tāng, 187
Cinnabaris, 183
cí shí, 61, 73, 74, 112
Colla Corii Asini, 181
Colla Cornus Cervi, 75
Concha Arcae, 61
Concha Haliotidis, 61
Concha Margaritiferae Usta, 183, 230
Concha Ostreae, 73
Concha Ostreae Cruda, 184
Concretio Silicea Bambusae, 61, 66, 73, 103, 238
constipation, 32, 72, 94, 212
constraint pattern, 8, 14
corporeal soul, 30
Cortex Cinnamomi, 188
Cortex Eucommiae, 69, 75, 120, 152
Cortex Lycii, 69, 71
Cortex Magnoliae Officinalis, 139, 166
Cortex Mori, 186

Cortex Moutan, 121
Cortex Phellodendri Chinensis, 64, 196
Cyclothymia, 278

D

dà huáng, 61, 62, 64, 102, 114, 128, 166, 168, 236
dà líng, 86, 91
dài zhĕ shí, 143, 233
damp-heat in the bladder, 184
dampness encumbering spleen-yang, 118
dà zăo, 66, 70, 121, 136, 211
dà zhuī, 89, 91
dăn nán xīng, 62
dān shēn, 69, 73, 108, 240
dăn shù, 83
dàn zhōng, 89, 84
Dàn Zhú Rú Tāng, 13
dāng guī, 63, 76, 122, 131, 135, 181, 237
dăng shēn, 66, 104, 110, 121, 125, 131, 136, 173, 201
decreased libido, 75
deficiency patterns, 55
delirious speech, 228
Dens Draconis, 73
depressed earth, 9
depressed wood, 9
depressive disorder, 2, 275
depressive episode, 276
despair, 71
Diān Kuáng Mèng Xǐng Tāng, 237
diarrhea, 83, 94
difficulty falling asleep, 67, 107
dì gŭ pí, 69, 71
discharge liver fire, 83
disharmony of liver and stomach, 91
distending fullness of rib-sides, 53

General Index

dizziness, 38, 61, 62, 82, 83, 85, 90, 109, 171, 212, 218, 240
drug-induced symptoms, 4
dry bound stools, 166
dry eyes, 111
dry mouth, 94, 111, 192, 243
dry stools, 62, 214
DU 14, 89, 91
DU 16, 80
DU 20, 81, 92, 95, 123
DU 24, 81, 93
DU 26, 92, 93, 123
du channel, 80
dù zhòng, 69, 75, 120, 152
dysmenorrhea, 83
dysthymia, 276, 277

E

ē jiāo, 181
é zhú, 63
electro-acupuncture, 92
emaciation, 66, 232
enuresis, 94
Èr Chén Tāng, 175
Èr Zhú Fú Líng Tāng, 175
etiology, 48
excess patterns, 60
extrapyramidal reactions, 162
exuberant phlegm, 73

F

fǎ bàn xià, 62, 128, 139, 140, 142, 145
fatigue, 17, 54, 119, 173, 243
fear, 133
fēng chí, 123
fēng fǔ, 80
fēng lóng, 84, 91
fibromyalgia, 11
fidgetiness, 63

fifth-watch diarrhea, 75
fine sunken pulses, 66, 69
fine wiry pulses, 67, 68
fire constraint, 10
five phases, 16
five spirits, 22
five transport points, 84
Flos Carthami, 63, 73, 153, 158, 174, 179, 197, 202, 237
Flos Chrysanthemi, 61, 68, 69, 72, 108, 240
Flos Farfarae, 32
Flos Inulae, 143, 233
Folium Eriobotryae, 145
Folium Mori, 108
Folium Perillae, 139
Folium Phyllostachydis Henonis, 167, 239
food accumulation, 140
food stagnation, 140
forgetfulness, 62, 81, 120, 123, 124, 127
fó shǒu, 74, 158
four gates, 82
frequent sighing, 60, 62, 70
frequent urination, 66
fright and fear, 49
Fructus Alpiniae Oxyphyllae, 66
Fructus Amomi, 61, 74, 172
Fructus Amomi Rotundus, 171
Fructus Aurantii, 63, 236
Fructus Aurantii Immaturus, 114, 166
Fructus Cannabis, 166
Fructus Citri, 74, 158
Fructus Citri Sarcodactylis, 74, 158
Fructus Corni, 67, 69, 71, 75, 119, 120, 126
Fructus Crataegi, 112, 140, 176
Fructus Gardeniae, 63, 64, 67, 102, 171
Fructus Gardeniae Praeparatus (scorched-

fried), 174
Fructus Hordei Germinatus, 62, 71, 176
Fructus Jujubae, 66, 70, 121, 136, 211
Fructus Ligustri Lucidi, 66, 68, 69, 71, 108, 127, 195
Fructus Lycii, 68, 69, 74, 75, 76, 105, 120, 152
Fructus Mori, 120
Fructus Psoraleae, 66, 69, 70, 74
Fructus Rosae Laevigatae, 244
Fructus Schisandrae Chinensis, 71, 76, 105, 120, 121
Fructus Toosendan, 61
Fructus Tribuli, 61, 68
Fructus Trichosanthis, 164
Fructus Tritici, 132
Fructus Tritici Levis, 71
fú líng, 62, 63, 66, 67, 104, 110, 118, 121, 126, 128, 131, 142, 158, 180
fullness and oppression of chest, 32
fú xiǎo mài, 71
fù zǐ, 188

G

gān cǎo, 183
Gān Mài Dà Zǎo Tāng, 13, 211
gān shù, 83, 84, 91
GB 20, 123
GB 24, 82
GB 34, 83, 84, 90, 93
GB 39, 90
GB 40, 83, 86
gé gēn, 69, 163, 194
geriatric depressive disorder, 147
gé shù, 89
gōng sūn, 83
gǒu qǐ zǐ, 68, 69, 74, 75, 76, 105, 120, 152
gōu téng, 61
guā lóu, 164

guān yuán, 82, 91
guī jiǎ, 70, 71, 76, 104, 151
Guī Pí Tāng, 110, 181
guì zhī, 142, 183
Guì Zhī Gān Cǎo Lóng Gǔ Mǔ Lì Tāng, 183
Gypsum Crudum, 163, 165
Gypsum Fibrosum, 189
Gypsum Fibrosum Cruda, 61, 73, 167, 192, 194, 230

H

Haematitum, 143, 233
hair loss, 245
hallucinations, 2, 92, 240
headache, 62, 82, 92, 109, 171, 218
Heart-Clearing Phlegm-Rolling Pill, 73
heart-spirit, 24
heart-spleen dual deficiency, 104, 124, 232
heart and liver heat ascending, 64
heart and liver heat disturbing the brain-spirit, 102
heart and lung qi dual deficiency, 131
heart and spleen dual deficiency, 66, 109, 120
heart blood insufficiency, 181
heart fire, 28
heart heat, 239
heart qi insufficiency, 180, 236
heart vexation, 12, 63
heart yin depletion, 182
hé gǔ, 82, 91, 94
Herba Artemisiae Annuae, 69
Herba Cistanches, 228
Herba Dianthi, 185
Herba Epimedii, 67, 70, 71, 75, 228
Herba Eupatorii, 73, 111, 118, 231
Herba Houttuyniae, 186

General Index

Herba Leonuri, 197, 201
Herba Lycopi, 63
Herba Menthae, 176
hé shǒu wū, 108, 127, 196, 245
hiccoughing, 222
hiccoughs, 167
hóng huā, 63, 73, 153, 158, 174, 179, 197, 202, 237
hòu pò, 139, 166
hòu xī, 81
HT 7, 82, 91, 92, 93
huái shān yào, 75
huáng bǎi, 64, 196
huáng lián, 64, 73, 102, 111, 168, 178, 231, 239
Huáng Lián Ē Jiāo Tāng, 111
huáng qí, 236
huáng qín, 64, 102, 168, 171, 186
huǒ má rén, 166
Huō Tán Qīng Nǎo Tāng, 72

I

impotence, 75, 126, 131, 195, 196, 244
incontinence, 71
individual constitution, 50
infertility, 126
insomnia, 55, 28, 73, 81, 89, 93, 105, 109, 124, 197, 243
insufficiency of heart blood, 27
insufficiency of kidney essence, 40
insufficiency of the sea of marrow, 151
insufficiency of the spleen and kidney, 152
insufficiency of yang qi, 54
intangible phlegm, 32
Intelligence-Benefiting Spirit-Awakening Decoction, 69
internal fire, 54
internal heat, 55

irascibility, 61, 102, 112, 242
irregular menstruation, 82
irritability, 55
irritation, 85, 93

J

jiāo zhī zǐ, 174
jié gěng, 32
jīn yīng zǐ, 244
Jì Shēng Shèn Qì Wán, 188
jiǔ zhì dà huáng, 231
jī xuè téng, 163
jú huā, 61, 68, 69, 72, 108, 240
jú pí, 145
Jú Pí Zhú Rú Tāng, 145
Jú Shēn Tāng, 239

K

KI 3, 82, 84, 86, 94
kidney-essence depletion, 119, 126
kidney-essence insufficiency, 134
kidney deficiency, 216
kidney yang debilitation, 188
kidney yang deficiency, 41, 70, 91, 119
Kidney yang depletion, 74
kidney yang insufficiency, 195
kidney yin deficiency, 39
kidney yin insufficiency, 196
kuǎn dōng, 32

L

lái fú zǐ, 62, 73, 113, 128, 140, 166, 231, 236
láo gōng, 82, 91
LI 4, 82, 91, 94
Liáng Gé Sǎn, 171
lián zǐ, 211
Lignum Aquilariae Resinatum, 186
lí gōu, 86

Líng Guì Zhú Gān Tāng, 141, 177
liver-gallbladder damp-heat, 121
liver-gallbladder dual deficiency, 135
liver-kidney yin deficiency, 241
liver-stomach disharmony, 73, 139
liver and kidney deficiency, 11
Liver and kidney yin deficiency, 68, 91, 107
liver and stomach disharmony, 221
liver constraint, 51, 227, 241
liver constraint and blood stasis, 225
liver constraint and qi stagnation, 52, 60, 215
liver constraint and spleen deficiency, 83, 84, 158
liver constraint combining with phlegm, 156
liver constraint transforming into fire, 223
liver constraint with blood stasis, 203
liver constraint with phlegm binding, 61, 91
liver constraint with qi stagnation, 83, 91, 236
liver constraint with spleen deficiency, 37, 67, 91
liver qi constraint, 36, 82, 98, 103, 186
liver qi invading the spleen, 61
liver qi stagnation, 49, 191
liver yang hyperactivity, 61
liver yin insufficiency, 190
lóng dǎn cǎo, 61
lóng gǔ, 184
lóng yǎn ròu, 211
loose stools, 66, 125, 216
low appetite, 109
low libido, 67, 68, 195, 196
low spirits, 54, 58, 61, 67, 68, 69, 72, 74, 75, 103, 218

LU 9, 89, 91
lù jiǎo jiāo, 75
lumbar pain, 120
Lung and kidney dual deficiency, 70, 91
lung heat exuberance, 186
LV 13, 88
LV 14, 82, 83, 91, 93
LV 2, 82, 83
LV 3, 82, 85, 91, 94
LV 5, 86

M

Magnetitum, 61, 73, 74, 112
mài mén dōng, 63, 68, 70, 105, 163, 182
Mài Wèi Dì Huáng Wán, 112
mài yá, 62, 71, 176
mania, 55
manic episodes, 3
Massa Medicata, 140
Massa Medicata Fermentata, 62, 67, 71, 112, 140, 174, 176, 228
Má Zǐ Rén Wán, 166
melancholia, 278
méng shí, 128, 238
metal constraint, 9
migraines, 93
moxibustion, 92
mǔ dān pí, 121
mǔ lì, 73
mù xiāng, 172

N

nausea, 54, 94, 113, 168, 244
nèi guān, 81, 83, 85, 86, 91
neurasthenia, 216, 236
night sweats, 68, 71
niú xī, 62, 73, 158, 231

non-interaction of heart and kidney, 127
nǚ zhēn zǐ, 66, 68, 69, 71, 108, 127, 195

O

obesity, 94, 170
olfaction disorders, 94
Os Draconis, 184
overeating, 232

P

palpitations, 26, 27, 66, 81, 86, 178, 180, 181, 200, 211
páo fù zǐ, 119
paranoia, 2, 27
PC 6, 81, 83, 85, 86, 91
PC 7, 86, 91
PC 8, 82, 91
pèi lán, 73, 118, 231
Pericarpium Citri Reticulatae, 62, 109, 113, 118, 128, 140, 142, 145
Pericarpium Citri Reticulatae Viride, 113, 118
persistent mood (affective) disorders, 278
pessimism, 69, 71, 72, 75, 103
phlegm, 237, 242
phlegm-fire, 72, 91, 106
phlegm-fire disturbing the heart, 113, 178
Phlegm-Flushing Brain-Clearing Formula, 72
phlegm-heat, 109, 216
phlegm accumulation, 55
Phlegm constraint, 54
Phlegm turbidity, 128
pí pá yè, 145
pí shù, 84, 91, 93
plum-pit qi, 13
poor appetite, 35, 62

poor memory, 67, 123
poor sleep, 211
Poria, 62, 63, 66, 67, 104, 110, 118, 121, 126, 128, 131, 142, 158, 180
Poria Alba, 173
postpartum deficiency vexation, 13
postpartum depression, 13
premature ejaculation, 126, 131
profuse dreaming, 66, 92, 109, 111, 124, 243
profuse nightmares, 67
psycholepsy, 216
psychological symptoms, 2

Q

Qi-Benefiting Lily Bulb Decoction, 70
qi and blood depletion, 136
qi and blood dual deficiency, 75
qi and blood insufficiency, 218
qi constraint, 52
qi deficiency, 30
qi deficiency and blood stasis, 153, 200
qī mén, 82, 83, 91, 93
qīng pí, 113, 118
Qīng Xīn Gǔn Tán Wán, 73, 238, 242
qi stagnation and blood stasis, 62, 157, 174, 177, 179, 199, 228
qi stagnation with static blood, 91
qiū xū, 83, 86
Qù Dāi Xǐng Nǎo Tāng, 104
qú mài, 185
Qù Yù Yì Nǎo Tāng, 68

R

Radix Achyranthis Bidentatae, 62, 73, 158, 231
Radix Aconiti Lateralis (blast-fried), 119
Radix Aconiti Lateralis Praeparata, 173,

188
Radix Adenophorae, 70, 169
Radix Angelicae Sinensis, 63, 76, 122, 131, 135, 181, 237
Radix Asparagi, 182
Radix Astragali, 70, 74, 110, 121, 125, 136, 200, 236
Radix Aucklandiae, 172
Radix Bupleuri, 60, 63, 103, 110, 121, 143, 157, 158, 176, 191, 200, 236
Radix Codonopsis, 66, 104, 110, 121, 125, 131, 136, 173, 201
Radix Curcumae, 60, 62, 63, 67, 103, 110, 111, 141
Radix Cyathulae, 63
Radix et Rhizoma Asteris, 32, 70, 132
Radix et Rhizoma Gentianae, 61
Radix et Rhizoma Ginseng, 180, 187
Radix et Rhizoma Ginseng Cruda, 76
Radix et Rhizoma Glycyrrhizae, 183
Radix et Rhizoma Glycyrrhizae Praeparata cum Melle, 66, 131, 132
Radix et Rhizoma Rhei, 61, 62, 102, 114, 128, 166, 168, 236
Radix et Rhizoma Rhei (preserved in liquor), 64
Radix et Rhizoma Salviae Miltiorrhizae, 69, 73, 108, 240
Radix Morindae Officinalis, 70, 75, 152
Radix Ophiopogonis, 63, 68, 70, 105, 163, 182
Radix Paeoniae Alba, 68, 74, 76, 135, 158, 181, 227, 231
Radix Paeoniae Rubra, 153, 158, 174, 179, 231
Radix Platycodonis, 32
Radix Polygalae, 125
Radix Polygoni Multiflori, 108, 127, 196, 245
Radix Pseudostellariae, 67, 74, 104
Radix Puerariae Lobatae, 69, 163, 194
Radix Rehmanniae, 111, 127, 163, 169, 173, 190
Radix Rehmanniae Praeparata, 75, 119, 126, 127, 134, 152
Radix Scrophulariae, 63, 68, 127, 163
Radix Scutellariae, 64, 102, 168, 171, 186
Ramulus Cinnamomi, 142, 183
Ramulus Uncariae Cum Uncis, 61
red eyes, 61
red face, 64, 72
red tongue, 61
regulate qi, 52
rén shēn, 180, 187
Rhizoma Acori Tatarinowii, 118
Rhizoma Alismatis, 122, 126
Rhizoma Anemarrhenae, 196
Rhizoma Atractylodis, 14, 67, 118, 174
Rhizoma Atractylodis Macrocephalae, 66, 131, 142, 171, 173
Rhizoma Atractylodis Macrocephalae (stir-fried), 74, 110
Rhizoma Chuanxiong, 14, 63, 67, 69, 72, 174, 240
Rhizoma Cimicifugae, 143, 187
Rhizoma Coptidis, 64, 73, 102, 111, 168, 178, 231, 239
Rhizoma Corydalis, 74
Rhizoma Curculiginis, 70, 75
Rhizoma Curcumae, 63
Rhizoma Cyperi, 60, 103, 113
Rhizoma Dioscoreae, 75, 119
Rhizoma Gastrodiae, 171
Rhizoma Pinelliae, 113, 114, 171
Rhizoma Pinelliae Praeparatum, 62, 128, 139, 140, 142, 145
Rhizoma Zingiberis Recens, 139

rib-side pain, 82, 93
RN 12, 82, 88, 91, 92, 94
RN 17, 89, 84
RN 3, 94
RN 4, 82, 91
ròu cōng róng, 228
ròu guì, 188

S

sadness, 70
sāng bái, 186
sāng shèn, 120
sāng yè, 108
Sān Huáng Zhī Zǐ Tāng, 102
Sān Rén Tāng, 171
sān yīn jiāo, 82, 84, 91
Sān Zǐ Yǎng Qīn Tāng, 175
scant menses, 26
schizophrenia, 98
Semen Aesculi, 61
Semen Alpiniae Katsumadai, 74
Semen Armeniacae Amarum, 32, 166, 171
Semen Coicis, 171
Semen Cuscutae, 67, 69, 71, 75, 108, 120, 127, 135, 195, 228, 241
Semen Euryales, 244
Semen Nelumbinis, 211
Semen Persicae, 63, 73, 158, 179, 197, 202, 237
Semen Plantaginis, 185
Semen Pruni, 166
Semen Raphani, 62, 73, 113, 128, 140, 166, 231, 236
Semen Ziziphi Spinosae, 73, 108, 132
Semen Ziziphi Spinosae (stir-fried), 68, 70, 74, 108, 110, 111
seminal emission, 68, 94, 126, 195, 244
seven emotions, 15, 48

shān yào, 119
shān zhā, 112, 140, 176
shān zhū yú, 69, 71, 75, 119, 120, 126
shā rén, 61, 74, 172
shā shēn, 70, 169
shén mén, 82, 91, 92, 93
shén qū, 62, 67, 71, 112, 140, 174, 176, 228
shèn shù, 84, 86
shén tíng, 81, 93
shēng dì, 111, 127, 163, 169, 173, 190
shēng huáng qí, 70, 74, 110, 121, 125, 136, 200
shēng jiāng, 139
shēng lóng chǐ, 73
shēng má, 143, 187
Shēng Mài Sǎn, 164
Shēng Mài Yǐn, 5, 220
shēng mǔ lì, 184
shēng shài shēn, 76
shēng shí gāo, 61, 73, 163, 167, 189, 192, 194, 230
Shēn Líng Bái Zhú Sǎn, 175
shí chāng pú, 118
shí gāo, 165
shí jué míng, 61
shortness of breath, 27, 70, 76, 243
shú dì huáng, 75, 119, 126, 127, 134, 152
Shū Gān Hé Wèi Yǐn, 74
shuǐ gōu, 92, 93, 123
SI 3, 81
side-effects, 162
sighing, 32
Sì Huáng Zhī Zǐ Tāng, 64
Sì Jūn Zǐ Tāng, 66, 180
Sì Nì Sǎn, 56
Sì Shén Cōng, 81
sì shén cōng, 92, 93

sleeplessness, 60, 63, 66, 81, 107, 112, 216
slimy white coating, 61
slippery and rapid pulses, 166
slippery rapid pulses, 128
somatic symptoms, 2
somnolence, 54, 116
soothing the liver and regulating qi, 82
sorrow, 129
SP 10, 82
SP 3, 86, 91
SP 4, 83
SP 6, 82, 84, 91
SP 9, 82
spleen-kidney deficiency, 200
Spleen-kidney dual deficiency, 103
spleen-kidney qi deficiency, 175
Spleen-Restoring Decoction, 110
spleen and kidney deficiency, 173, 190
spleen and kidney dual deficiency, 69, 216
spleen and stomach deficiency, 143
spleen deficiency, 172
spleen deficiency with damp exuberance, 201
spontaneous sweating, 109
ST 25, 94
ST 36, 86, 94
ST 40, 84, 91
stomach pain, 83
stomach qi disharmony, 112
Stomach yin insufficiency, 145, 192
suān zǎo rén, 73
Suān Zǎo Tāng, 13
suicidal tendencies, 71
suō luó zǐ, 61

T

tài bái, 84, 86, 91
tài chōng, 82, 85, 91, 94
tài xī, 82, 84, 86, 94
tài yáng, 83, 92, 93
tài yuān, 89, 91
tài zǐ shēn, 67, 74, 104
Táo Hóng Sì Wù Tāng, 202
táo rén, 63, 73, 158, 179, 197, 202, 237
tardive dyskinesia, 188
thirst, 64, 109
tiān má, 171
tiān mén dōng, 182
tiān shū, 94
Tiān Wáng Bǔ Xīn Dān, 112, 182, 233
tiān zhú huáng, 61, 66, 73, 103, 238
timidity, 27, 135
tinnitus, 61, 93, 240
Torpidity-Eliminating Brain-Awakening Decoction, 104
tù sī zǐ, 67, 69, 71, 75, 108, 120, 127, 135, 195, 228, 241

U

unstable mood, 64, 73, 102
urinary block, 184
urinary retention, 94

V

vertigo, 85
vexation, 62, 64, 102, 178
vexing heat in the five hearts, 68
vexing heat in the hearts of palms and soles, 111
viscera-spirits, 23
visceral agitation, 13
vomiting, 61, 82, 113

W

wǎ léng zǐ, 61
water constraint, 9

General Index

weeping, 70, 242
weight loss, 232
Wēn Dǎn Tāng, 62, 176
wiry fine pulses, 73, 190
wiry pulses, 103
wiry rapid pulses, 64
withdrawal disease, 98
Wǔ Líng Sǎn, 175
Wū Tù Tāng, 108
wǔ wèi zǐ, 71, 76, 105, 120, 121

X

xiāng fù, 60, 103, 113
xiāng yuán, 74, 158
xiān líng pí, 67, 70, 71, 75, 228
xiān máo, 70, 75
Xiǎo Bàn Xià Tāng, 141
Xiǎo Chái Hú Tāng, 12
xiǎo mài, 132
Xiāo Yáo Sǎn, 16
xiè bái, 164
xie yi, 10
xíng jiān, 82, 83
xìng rén, 32, 166, 171
xīn shù, 91
Xuán Fù Dài Zhě Tāng, 143, 236
xuán fù huā, 143, 233
xuán shēn, 63, 68, 127, 163
xuán zhōng, 90
Xuè Fǔ Zhú Yū Tāng, 63, 179
xuè hǎi, 82

Y

yáng líng quán, 83, 84, 90, 93
yán hú suǒ, 74
yellow slimy coating, 62, 64, 121
yì mǔ cǎo, 197, 201
yin and yang dual deficiency, 196
yin deficiency of the liver and kidney, 84
yin deficiency with effulgent fire, 111
yīn líng quán, 82
yìn táng, 81, 82, 92
Yì Qì Bǎi Hé Tāng, 70
Yì Wèi Tāng, 145
yì yǐ rén, 171
yì zhì rén, 66
Yì Zhì Xǐng Shén Tāng, 69
Yòu Guī Wán, 75
yuǎn zhì, 125
Yuè Jú Wán, 14, 67
yù jīn, 60, 62, 63, 67, 103, 110, 141
yù lǐ rén, 166
yú xīng cǎo, 186

Z

zé lán, 63
zé xiè, 122, 126
Zé Xiè Tāng, 175
zhāng mén, 88
zhēn zhū mǔ, 183, 230
zhì fù zǐ, 173
zhì gān cǎo, 66, 131, 132
zhī mǔ, 196
zhǐ qiào, 63, 236
zhǐ shí, 114, 166
Zhǐ Zhú Wán, 175
zhī zǐ, 63, 64, 67, 102, 171
zhōng jí, 94
zhōng wǎn, 82, 88, 91, 92, 94
Zhū Líng Tāng, 5
zhú rú, 62, 114, 128
zhū shā, 183
Zhū Shā Ān Shén Wán, 112, 182
zhú yè, 167, 239
Zhú Yè Shí Gāo Tāng, 167
Zhú Yè Tāng, 13
zǐ sū yè, 139

335

zǐ wǎn, 32, 70, 132
zong qi, 27

Zuǒ Jīn Wán, 168
zú sān lǐ, 86, 94

图书在版编目（CIP）数据

中西医结合治疗抑郁障碍=The Treatment of Depressive Disorders with Chinese Medicine-An Integrative Approach：英文/王彦恒等主编.—北京：人民卫生出版社，2010.12
ISBN 978-7-117-12729-5

Ⅰ.①中… Ⅱ.①王… Ⅲ.①抑郁症-中西医结合疗法-英文 Ⅳ.①R749.405

中国版本图书馆CIP数据核字（2010）第138706号

门户网：www.pmph.com	出版物查询、网上书店
卫人网：www.ipmph.com	护士、医师、药师、中医师、卫生资格考试培训

中西医结合治疗抑郁障碍（英文）

主　　编：王彦恒　康玉春
出版发行：人民卫生出版社（中继线 +8610-5978-7399）
地　　址：中国北京市朝阳区潘家园南里19号
　　　　　世界医药图书大厦B座
邮　　编：100021
网　　址：http://www.pmph.com
E - mail：pmph @ pmph.com
发　　行：pmphsales@gmail.com
购书热线：+8610-5978 7399/5978 7338（电话及传真）
开　　本：787×1092　1/16
版　　次：2010年12月第1版　2010年12月第1版第1次印刷
标准书号：ISBN 978-7-117-12729-5/R·12730

版权所有，侵权必究，打击盗版举报电话：+8610-5978-7482
（凡属印装质量问题请与本社销售中心联系退换）